T0319504

POSTCOLONIAL DISORDERS

POSTCOLONIAL DISORDERS

Edited by
Mary-Jo DelVecchio Good,
Sandra Teresa Hyde,
Sarah Pinto, and
Byron J. Good

University of California Press   Berkeley Los Angeles London

University of California Press, one of the most distinguished
university presses in the United States, enriches lives around
the world by advancing scholarship in the humanities, social
sciences, and natural sciences. Its activities are supported by the
UC Press Foundation and by philanthropic contributions from
individuals and institutions. For more information, visit
www.ucpress.edu.

University of California Press
Berkeley and Los Angeles, California

University of California Press, Ltd.
London, England

Library of Congress Cataloging-in-Publication Data

Postcolonial disorders / edited by Mary-Jo DelVecchio
    Good . . . [et al.].
        p.   cm.
    Includes bibliographical references and index.
    ISBN 978-0-520-25223-3 (cloth : alk. paper).—
    ISBN 978-0-520-25224-0 (pbk. : alk. paper)
      1. Medical anthropology.   2. Diseases—Social aspects.
    3. Colonization—Social aspects.   4. Globalization—Social
    aspects.   5. Subjectivity.   I. Good, Mary-Jo DelVecchio.

GN296.P67   2008
306.4'61—dc22   2007029461

Manufactured in the United States of America

17   16   15   14   13   12   11   10   09   08
10   9   8   7   6   5   4   3   2   1

Dedicated to Begoña Aretxaga
(1960–2002)

CONTENTS

ACKNOWLEDGMENTS

Many people have been involved in energizing the ongoing conversations from which this volume originated. The editors thank the National Institute of Mental Health and its support for the seminar that led to this volume. The 2000–01 seminar entitled "Postcolonialism, Psychiatry, and Lived Experience" was part of the Harvard Training Program in Culture and Mental Health Services Research, which has been funded by grant MH 18006 from 1984 until the present and which is directed by Byron Good, Arthur Kleinman, and Mary-Jo DelVecchio Good. For over twenty years, the Friday Morning Seminar on Medical Anthropology and Cultural Psychiatry has been a core activity of the Harvard Program in Medical Anthropology, which resides both in the Department of Social Medicine, Harvard Medical School, and the Department of Anthropology, Harvard University. We thank faculty, fellows, guest lecturers, and students in these programs who have contributed to the conversation represented by the papers in this volume.

We express our appreciation to Stanley Holwitz, Randy Heyman, and Mary Severance, our editors at the University of California Press, for their support for the project, to Tom Csordas and Tanya Lurhmann for their careful reading and suggestions for revisions, and to Julie Van Pelt for her elegant and knowledgeable copyediting. At Harvard, we are grateful to Seth Hannah, Laura Delano, and Martha Fuller, who labored through the many renditions and complexities of final manuscript preparation. We also thank our many friends, colleagues, graduate students, and postdoctoral fellows who read earlier versions of this volume and made helpful suggestions, including Andrew Lakoff, postdoctoral fellow, who recommended the abbreviated current title. We acknowledge the generosity of Entang Wiharso, who has granted us permission to reproduce his painting *Don't Touch Me* for the jacket cover.

Postcolonial Disorders is dedicated to the memory of Begoña Aretxaga, a dear friend, creative spirit, and pioneer in the work represented by this collection. Begoña, an anthropologist of Northern Ireland and of the Basque Country, was a member of the faculty of Harvard University's Department of Anthropology, where she held the John L. Loeb Associate Professorship of the Social Sciences (1992–99). Our friendship with "Bego" flourished intellectually and affectively during her Harvard years, influencing our intellectual endeavors and in particular the theme for our seminar of 2000–01. She thus played an important role in the evolution of this collection. In 1999, Bego joined the anthropology faculty at the University of Texas at Austin, albeit she returned frequently to Harvard. Begoña's publications include *Shattering Silence: Women, Nationalism, and Political Subjectivity in Northern Ireland* (Princeton University Press, 1997); *Los Funerales en al Nacionalismo Radical Vasco* (San Sebastian, 1987); "Maddening States," *Annual Review of Anthropology* 32 (2003): 393–410; *Empire and Terror: Nationalism/Postnationalism in the New Millennium*, Center for Basque Studies Conference Papers Series, edited with Dennis Dworkin, Joseba Gablondo, and Joseba Zulaika (University of Nevada Press, 2005); and *States of Terror: Begoña Aretxaga's Essays*, edited by Joseba Zulaika (Center for Basque Studies, 2005). We are grateful to Joseba for his support.

Kay Warren, graduate advisor and friend, wrote in her memorial note for *Anthropology News* (May 2003), "Bego was famed for the power and humanism of her ethnographies of political movements and state repression, and for sophisticated theoretical engagement with postmodern literatures on subjectivity, power and the state in the face of intensified globalization." Begoña's influence in anthropology, through her essays, books, and posthumous edited collections with her colleagues in Basque studies, continues through the extraordinary enduring presence of her ideas and her passion. Her untimely death as we were preparing this volume represents an enormous personal loss to her many colleagues and students and a great loss to our field. We hope this book contributes to advancing the enterprise to which she was so central.

Mary-Jo DelVecchio Good
Byron J. Good
Sandra Teresa Hyde
Sarah Pinto
Harvard University
September 22, 2006

POSTCOLONIAL DISORDERS: REFLECTIONS ON SUBJECTIVITY IN THE CONTEMPORARY WORLD

Byron J. Good, Mary-Jo DelVecchio Good,
Sandra Teresa Hyde, and Sarah Pinto

This book is a collection of essays reflecting on the nature of subjectivity—on everyday modes of experience, the social and psychological dimensions of individual lives, the psychological qualities of social life, the constitution of the subject, and forms of subjection found in the diverse places where anthropologists work at the beginning of the twenty-first century. The essays are a conscious effort to find new ways to link the social and the psychological, to examine how lives of individuals, families and communities are affected by large-scale political and economic forces associated with globalization, and to theorize subjectivity within this larger context. And the essays explore the role of colonialism in shaping postcolonial states and distinctive forms of subjectivity increasingly characteristic of contemporary societies.

Although these essays address the "nature" of subjectivity, they are ethnographic rather than primarily theoretical or philosophical; they are efforts to understand persons and lives lived under extraordinary conditions all too common in much of the world today. But it is precisely by attempting to make sense of lives that challenge comprehension—lives of Basque youth engaged in acts of revolutionary violence viewed as utterly mad by most of their Basque compatriots; visionary artists and a provincial politician gone psychotic, responding to social breakdown at the end of the Suharto regime in Indonesia; local officials and international specialists engaged in often fantastic humanitarian ventures in the Balkans or attempting to control AIDS in China and the Republic of Congo; women responding to the deaths of their infants in India; and persons with mental illness caught up with psychiatrists and old colonial hospitals in Ireland and Morocco—that the authors in this volume address the most difficult problems of history, methodology, and theory.

Despite great diversity in the ways the essays in this book explore lives such as these, taken together they provide the basis for three broad, interconnected claims. First, these essays suggest that ethnographic studies of subjectivity are both feasible and productive, and that the analytic term "subjectivity" denotes a set of critical issues for anthropologists working in contemporary societies, issues different than those raised by classic studies of "self" or "person and emotion," opening new domains for ethnographic investigation. Second, taken as a whole, these essays support the claim that viewing subjectivity through the lens of the "postcolonial" provides a language and analytic strategies, often derived from the work of historians and literary critics, valuable for investigations of lives, institutions, and regimes of knowledge and power in the societies in which anthropologists work today. Indeed, the book suggests that whether directly addressed or not, the figure of the colonial haunts ethnographic writing today, and that thematizing the postcolonial has the potential to transform ethnographic writing about subjectivity. Third, this volume suggests that contemporary studies of subjectivity must necessarily address "disorders"—the intertwined personal and social disorders associated with rampant globalization, neoliberal economic policies, and postcolonial politics; and whether read as pathologies, modes of suffering, the domain of the imaginary, or as forms of repression, disordered subjectivity provides entrée to exploring dimensions of contemporary social life as lived experience.

We briefly examine these three key terms—subjectivity, postcolonial, and disorders—in turn.

SUBJECTIVITY

The increasing use of the terms "subject" and "subjectivity" in anthropology points to widespread dissatisfaction with previous efforts to understand psychological experience and inner lives in particular cultures, characteristic of an earlier generation of psychological and cultural anthropologists—however important and incomplete that work was. "Subjectivity" immediately signals awareness of a set of historical problems and critical writings related to the genealogy of the subject and to the importance of colonialism and the figure of the colonized "other" for writing about the emergence of the modern (rational) subject. Subjectivity denotes a new attention to hierarchy, violence, and subtle modes of internalized anxieties that link subjection and subjectivity, and an urgent sense of the importance of linking national and global economic and political processes to the most intimate forms of everyday experience. It places the political at the heart of the psychological and the psychological at the heart of the political. Use of the term "subject" by definition makes analysis of the state and forms of citizenship immediately relevant in ways that analysis of the "self" or "person" does not, and "disordered states" is a trope for both the political and the subjective. It is thus little wonder that subjectivity becomes a framing device for exploring lives and motives in relation to the nearly incomprehensible social and political conditions described by the authors in this book.

In much of the literature on subjectivity, "subject" references the *sujet* of French psychoanalytic, poststructuralist, and feminist writing, locating discussions in theoretical territories that evoke strong reactions—positive and negative—within anthropology. Whether responding to Foucault's archaeology of the modern subject (Foucault 1997, 1998, 2000), Lacanian analyses of political subjectivity and gender (e.g., Žižek 1997, 1998, 1999; Copjec 1994; Kristeva 1982; Stavrakakis 1999), or Judith Butler's linking of subjectivity and subjection (1997), the resulting debates have opened new territories for anthropologists, cutting across subdisciplines and linking ethnographic work to feminist writing and gender studies, literary criticism, and diverse forms of cultural studies. This work has begun to create a new language and new forms of analysis for studies focused on subjective experience.

Given this promise, there are several reasons why much contemporary writing on subjectivity seems either overly theorized, lacking grounding in reflections on individual lives, or undertheorized, descriptive of social experience and emotions, but dependent largely on the analysis of cultural categories. First, poststructuralist writing has reinforced a broad anthropological suspicion of studies of individual lives and psychological experience. Critique of the humanist subject and the resort to analyzing "subject position" over actual lives in all their complexity have meant that the apparent promise of this theoretical configuration remains unrealized in much anthropological writing.[1] Second, however strong the conviction that the social and the psychological, the political and personal experience, are essential for understanding subjectivity, models for carrying out such analyses remain elusive. The social and the psychological are often brought together through assertion or the sleight of hand of metaphorical linkages: psychotic individuals linked metaphorically to mad crowds, as in popular discourse;[2] traumatic memory as individual and communal; anxiety, insecurity, paranoia, and dissociation of whole societies as well as individual experience. Deep analyses of individual lives are too seldom found in such studies, while the use of psychological terms for understanding group processes remains undertheorized. One of the central questions of this book is whether current forms of theorizing, particularly those associated with writings on post-colonialism, offer new ways to link the social and the psychological.

Third, anthropological research, the authorial voice of the ethnographer, and the classic genre of ethnographic representations of the "other"—efforts to make sense of the difficult to comprehend, of a culture or tradition foreign to the writer or assumed reader, of the subaltern or persons belonging to stigmatized groups, or of lives lived under duress—are now subject to postcolonial anxiety. For example, Linda Tuhiwai Smith (1999: 1), director of the International Research Institute for Maori and Indigenous Education at the University of Auckland, writes, "From the vantage point of the colonized, a position from which I write, and choose to privilege, the term 'research' is inextricably linked to European imperialism and colonialism. The word itself, 'research', is probably one of the dirtiest words in the indigenous world's vocabulary. When mentioned in many indigenous contexts, it stirs up silence, it conjures up bad memories, it raises a smile that is knowing and distrustful." Anthropologists are well aware of the colonial history of the discipline, and while "writing culture" has become subject to Orientalist critique, representing individual lives of others is often contested as speaking for the other. An important question for this book, therefore, is whether postcolonial theorizing suggests new positions for the ethnographic voice and new ways of writing for those interested in subjectivity under current conditions.

It was the conviction that developing new means of ethnographic analysis of subjectivity is critical for anthropology and the social sciences more generally, and an enormous respect for the difficulties in doing so, that led to this book. We remain convinced that some of the most interesting and creative writing in the social sciences and humanities is focused around studies of subjectivity. Our intuition that addressing issues of colonialism, postcoloniality, and neo-colonialism is necessary to move the field forward led to the specific focus of the essays in this collection.

POSTCOLONIAL

Many of the essays in this volume were first presented in Harvard's Friday Morning Seminar on Medical Anthropology and Cultural Psychiatry.[3] For two years, this seminar met weekly to explore anthropological approaches to the study of "subjectivity"—in relation to illness and suffering, psychological experience and psychopathology, medicine and psychiatry. The first year addressed general theoretical and methodological issues associated with research and writing about culture, subjectivity, and human experience.[4] In the second year, we invited those who presented in the seminar to rethink some aspect of their work on subjectivity by replacing the common anthropological trope "culture" with the category "postcoloniality" or "the postcolonial," entitling the seminar "Postcolonialism, Psychiatry, and Lived Experience." This challenge to reflect on subjectivity through the lens of the postcolonial was intended not as a commitment to the tradition of postcolonial scholarship, but as a provocation. It served as a challenge to members of the seminar to work through issues raised by postcolonial theorists, and as a provocation for presenters to rethink the place of "culture" in theorizing subjectivity in studies of the broad array of disordered experience investigated by medical anthropologists today; to place medical and psychiatric anthropology, studies of political subjectivity, and postcolonial theorizing in conversation; and to insert detailed ethnographic studies into a theoretical corpus that is often largely literary and seldom seems "experience-near."

Examining subjectivity through the lens of the postcolonial was not intended to replace consideration of globalization, neoliberal policies, medicalization, or other pervasive political and economic forces that increasingly shape modes of experience and what it means to be a subject in many parts of the world. It was certainly not meant to suggest a singularity of "the" postcolonial, as though colonialism were uniform or produced uniform subjects, or a sense of temporal or developmental linearity. These issues have long been discussed critically within historical and literary studies of the postcolony.[5] And it was not meant to suggest a single overarching theoretical position, as any reading of the essays in this book will quickly make evident. Our intention instead was to bring explicit attention to the haunting presence of the colonial, a specter often present but in only ghostly forms in current anthropological writings on subjectivity. Our goal is to recognize a set of problems that cannot be avoided and to develop new ways to address them in thinking and writing about subjectivity.

Introduction of the category "postcoloniality" into a seminar that had long focused on mental health services in the United States had particular meaning, provoking a reexamination of thinking on race, ethnicity, and culture, and on their relevance for psychiatry. A formal conceptualization of psychology and psychopathology in relation to the colonial legacy has been most clearly articulated by American Indian psychologists, where the examination of "postcolonial psychology," the effects for mental health of the "American Indian holocaust," "historical" or multigenerational trauma, and "historical unresolved grief," is well underway, and where the implications for healing and health care as well as for empirical research are being explored.[6] Attention to colonialism and the postcolonial movements of peoples, however, runs throughout ethnic studies in this country. For example, the language of postcoloniality makes classic writing on slavery and the "racial self" among African Americans (Gates 1987) or on the border wars and the colonial history of Mexican Americans (Limon 1998) relevant to discussions of "health disparities," culturally appropriate services, difficulties in engaging minority patients in psychotherapy, and rates of involuntary confinement of the mentally ill among minority populations, in ways that analyses of "culture" or "ethnicity" or "cultural competence" often do not.[7] A focus on postcolonialism in the context of a long-running seminar on psychiatric services thus served as a reminder that the issues being discussed were as important for American society and its postcolonial peoples as for many of the former colonial societies in which anthropologists work.

What emerged in the seminar was a rich, diverse, and yet surprisingly coherent set of explorations and conversations, suggesting the great importance for anthropological studies to engage colonial, postcolonial, and neocolonial dimensions of both social pathologies and subjective experience. The presenters dealt with societies with varied relationships to European colonialism: Brazil, Haiti, Morocco, Ireland, Indonesia, Congo, Vietnam, India, Spain, the Balkans, and China. This diversity made obvious the plurality of experiences of colonialism, depending both on the colonizing nation (French, Dutch, British, American) and local civilizations. But the conversations nonetheless suggested the importance of rethinking some classic issues of psychological, cultural, and medical anthropology in relation to the postcolonial literature.

In one of the early presentations in the seminar, which we reproduce as the first chapter of this collection, Begoña Aretxaga, to whom this book is dedicated, made explicit how she would appropriate the category "postcolonial" for her writing about "political madness" in the Basque Country of Spain, and several themes she would trace through her essay. "At the risk of using postcoloniality here as a metaphor of a particular existential state," she wrote for this volume, "let me say nevertheless that something that characterizes the postcolonial state and the transitional state of countries like Spain or those of the former socialist bloc is a marginal status within the global political and economic order." Querying the "lived experience of politics in these altered states," as well as "the changing nature of the state in our postmodern global world," which for Aretxaga was more about fantasies of the state than about institutions, was the task she set for herself in the presentation to the seminar. And it is this task that occupied many of the authors of the texts that make up this volume.

We use "postcolonialism" in this book in the broad way suggested by Aretxaga to indicate an era and a historical legacy of violence and appropriation, carried into the present as traumatic memory, inherited institutional structures, and often unexamined assumptions. Postcolonialism denotes relationships between members of societies that were colonial powers and those that were colonies or "crypto-colonies" (Herzfeld 2002); between powerful political, economic, and state entities and those that are marginalized; between knowledge structures and modes of experience shaped by the often violent relationships of colonialism; as well as a body of theoretical writing. We assume, as has often been pointed out, that the "post" in this terminology is seldom far from the "neo" of new and emergent forms of global hierarchy and domination. To attempt further definitions of postcolonialism, however, or an overview of a field as diverse and unruly as postcolonial studies, would hardly capture the wide-ranging ideas explored in the essays in this volume or the ideas that emerged in the discussions in the seminar.

DISORDERS

The theme of toleration, thought to be the hallmark of civilization in the seventeenth and eighteenth centuries, at least in certain corners of Europe, was believed to carry the promise of ending all kinds of brutality. . . . For those who wanted to believe that superstition was on the way out, that a more rational and humane public and private existence was possible, there were reasons for confidence, and these prevailed well into the nineteenth century, reinforced by what were thought to be the marvels of modern science and technology. Such confidence has not survived our own century of violence, and is not likely to be restored very soon.

(Graubard 1996: vi–vii)

The strategic assemblage of ideas, institutions, and forms of domination that constituted colonialism—in the name of God, science, and capital or under the rubric of civilization, commerce, and Christianity—all functioned to establish and maintain a distinctive "order," a mode of social life and an enactment of "the Real" characteristic of a particular Enlightenment vision of reason, progress, and freedom.[8] As João Biehl's essay in this volume shows clearly, the establishment of this order and of bourgeois colonial governance in settings such as nineteenth-century Brazil required that authorities respond with harsh violence to any rebellion against this order, particularly if based on an affirmation of an autonomous symbolic order. This was as true of other colonial settlers as of indigenous peoples. Indeed, as Biehl's essay suggests, the very origins of the modernist equation of disorder with the mad, the primitive, and the bestial— all characteristics of "the Other"—are found in the efforts to enact and instantiate this particular colonial order. The theorization of madness and violence of individuals, in the formal languages of psychopathology, and the interpretations of political violence of groups, using similar pathologizing terms, share these historical origins in the pragmatics and imagination of colonial rule and colonial order.

The third key term in this book, "disorders," thus provides an opportunity to explore modalities of social life and subjectivities that reflect, ironically, the establishment of political, moral, and epistemic *orders* through state violence that reproduces *disorder*.[9] "Disorder" and "disorders" therefore provide a lens for investigating the contradictions that emerge in postcolonial societies and the social conditions they produce. These include "disorderly states," both those that are autocratic and those that are weak or failed and depend on privatized militias and violence; conflicts between "imagined" national communities and primordial commitments, leading to forms of religious and ethnic violence perceived as new but often reflecting colonial strategies of domination via ethnic conflict; and social pathologies that occur differentially at the centers and margins of state power, mimicking those at the centers and peripheries of colonial governance. These also include the disorders emanating from the "new world order," the contradictions made apparent when the personal mobility and transnational identities of intellectuals are juxtaposed with the vast numbers of violently displaced persons; when mobile capital and emerging middle classes are viewed side by side with extreme poverty and the wide insecurity of increasing numbers of persons; and when social breakdown or natural disasters are responded to with new modes of mobile sovereignty emerging from global institutions of finance, development, and humanitarian relief.[10]

The essays in this volume examine subjectivity in relation to contemporary forms of just such postcolonial disorders and interventions aimed at remedying them. Authors here explore the complex lives of those affected by terrorism and political violence—perpetrators, victims, politicians, and activists—and the pervasive insecurity and trauma associated with the breakdown of state structures. They describe how dislocation and labor migration differentially affect poor women, and how these women's "unruly agency" disrupts their characterization as victims of "trafficking" or as "sex workers." The authors describe the emergence of new categories of "international crises" and "emergencies," from ethnic cleansing in the Balkans to HIV/AIDS in China and Africa; the global, humanitarian assemblages and "mobile sovereignties" organized to respond to these; and the complex positioning of actors—members of NGOs, government officials at national and local levels, human rights psychiatrists—within these assemblages. And they explore how the subjectivity of persons suffering clinical psychopathology inevitably is caught up in complexes of social and personal meanings that reflect colonial discourses on rationality and superstition, current versions of psychiatric science, and institutional histories of the asylum and the clinic. Some of the essays reveal the darker sides of the global flows of capital and labor, which have produced the "flexible citizens" and "hybrid identities" of postcolonial theorizing (e.g., Bhabha 1994; Ong 1999). All of the essays examine the complex relationships between the social and the psychological, linking the "disordered states" of individuals and polities, exploring how and why the language of rationality and madness is so commonly used to make sense of political violence.

It is inevitable that anthropologists working as field researchers and advocates in "unstable places" (Greenhouse, Mertz, and Warren 2002) would attempt to represent the lives and experiences of individuals, families, and communities with whom they work as richly and sympathetically as possible. Reflections on the meaning of subjectivity and on the difficult theoretical and methodological problems that emerge in ethnographic representation of persons living in disordered polities are therefore not surprising. However, the challenge of understanding and representing the complexity of individual lives and of families and communities across cultures cannot be underestimated, and for anthropologists writing about persons attempting to fashion lives under extreme conditions the challenge is much greater.

We might note three broad strands of thinking and writing that have emerged in recent anthropological accounts of this kind. First, poststructuralist writing brought attention to the place of power in shaping any subject and to the place of "subjection" (particularly to Foucauldian disciplinary practices) and "subjugation" (to state domination) in shaping subjectivity.[11] But an immediate hazard of this framing is the representation of individuals as victims and an overdeterminist view of the role of governmentalities in producing unitary subjects and modes of consciousness. In response, "agency" and "resistance" have become key terms for exploring "where and how marginalization, dispossession and exploitation form the grounds of subjectivities in very different postcolonies" (Werbner 2002: 3), and writers find it necessary to stress contingency and creativity or "playful or aestheticised self-fashioning" (Werbner 2002: 2) to portray individual lives, for whom the image "victim" often seems inaccurate, partial at best, and demeaning.[12]

Second, there has been an increasing engagement with psychiatry and the clinical sphere among ethnographers attempting to write about the suffering of persons who experience severe violence, loss, insecurity, and oppressive conditions. The language of "trauma" has become ubiquitous, whether used generically to describe acute suffering, clinically to describe the dynamics of individuals with overt psychopathology, or critically to challenge the medicalization of forms of extreme human experience and avoid close attention to the social and the moral.[13] Clinical terms—depression and melancholia, anxiety, dissociation, and paranoia—are increasingly present, employed in similarly diverse ways.[14] And awareness of the richness of psychotherapeutic literatures and techniques for exploring personal subjectivity is reentering anthropology, now with reference to psychological and psychoanalytic writing quite different from that of the 1940s and 1950s.[15] When used with technical precision, clinical language has the potential to distinguish between normal human responses to loss or violence and those that represent more extreme or pathological "clinical" responses, illuminating the role of individual psychology in coping with social conditions experienced by many. At the same time, diagnostic language has the potential to reproduce medicalizing tendencies or to assert universal categories without warrant. When used generically, clinical terms convey important everyday meanings of lived experience, but may be incomprehensible to those who work clinically with persons suffering from clinical syndromes.

Third, in part as critical response to these two forms of analysis, some have advocated "suffering" or "social suffering" as a more experience-near language of analysis. Arthur Kleinman and his colleagues undertook a series of workshops and conversations, supported in part by the Social Science Research Council, on social suffering and subjectivity, which led to three edited volumes.[16] If a language of power and political agency marks writing originating within the poststructuralist tradition, and the language of psychopathology and psychology marks that engaged with clinical practice, the work on social suffering, read as "the devastating injuries that social force inflicts on human experience" (Kleinman, Das, and Lock 1996), places particular primacy on the existential, the phenomenological, and the moral. Ethnographers and humanists sometimes make use of "suffering"—drawn from the language of religion and morality—as an analytic category, without fully exploring the complexity of using moral categories for ethnographic analysis and without detailing the relevance of the category "suffering" for local religious traditions or individual lives. The question of the validity of essentializing "suffering" as a distinctive mode of experience, a term akin to "victim," is thus raised by this work. Kleinman and his colleagues have attempted to clarify many of these issues and to further a humane, ethnographic voice that brings wide-ranging and theoretically diverse writing into conversation.

The essays in this book may be read as an effort to build on and explore alternatives to these three approaches.

We recognize that there is an obvious hazard to approaching subjectivity among postcolonial societies through a focus on disorder or pathology. If "research" is as suspect among indigenous peoples as Linda Tuhiwai Smith indicates, research on social pathologies is particularly problematic, laden with colonial history and power relations. In the colonial context, the pathologies of native cultures were routinely cited as evidence of the inferiority of the colonized and as a mandate for intervention. In liberal societies, focus on the pathologies of indigenous peoples—or of the poor—is often equally used as mandate for intervention by powerful bureaucracies as well as social-service organizations. Recognizing, labeling, studying, and responding to social pathologies are thus located in complex terrains of postcolonial histories and relationships.

This book is of course not a set of analyses of disorders that purport to provide a mandate for interventions. Indeed, a benefit of linking "disorders" to "subjectivity" is the potential for increasing understanding of the lived experience of persons caught up in complex, threatening, and uncertain conditions of the contemporary world. Such a linking provides a focus on the historical genealogy of normative conceptions associated with order and disorder, rationality and pathology, and brings analytic attention to everyday lives and routine practices instantiated in complex institutions. Indeed, the essays in this book provide a critical examination of conflicting interpretations of postcolonial disorders and the local and global interventions undertaken to respond to them.

POSTCOLONIAL SUBJECTS, POSTCOLONIAL DISORDERS: LOOKING BACKWARD AND FORWARD

The authors of this volume provide strikingly innovative responses to the challenge of exploring subjectivity in relation to individual and social disorders, engaging the legacy of colonialism and its enduring effects in the societies studied and the intellectual traditions through which we investigate the modern subject and subjectivity. The result, we believe, opens new ways for engaging literatures often peripheral to much anthropological writing on subjectivity, for bringing psychological writing into conversation with the historical and political, for exploring how states and their peripheries figure in the imaginary and the everyday experience of social actors, and for suggesting a place for the uncanny as critical to subjective experience and its analysis. Running throughout is a sense of the hidden, the unspoken and the unspeakable, that appears in the fissures and gaps of the everyday and is very much a part of subjectivity in all its complexity. What begins to take form in the pages of this book is the outline of a project to develop new strategies for investigating and theorizing subjects in postcolonial societies and situations. We hope this book will contribute to initiating just such a project.

From the perspective that emerges within these essays, several literatures, pointing both backward and forward, become relevant to the project of investigating postcolonial subjectivities and postcolonial disorders within contemporary ethnographic research. First, much of the classic scholarship on colonial and postcolonial subjectivity becomes relevant to such a project in new ways. A powerful tradition of writing about colonial subjectivity begins with Frantz Fanon, the psychiatrist born in Martinique and educated in France, who found his mission in Algeria during the violent struggle to "decolonize" the nation. Fanon (1963) wrote vividly about violence as the means by which colonial powers and their settlers established and maintained domination of colonized peoples. He drew an absolute contrast, a "Manichean" dichotomy, between two "species" of men—the colonizers and the colonized (1963: 42, 93). As theorist and psychiatrist, his interest was in the consciousness of the colonized, in the traumatizing effects of experiencing and witnessing colonial violence, in the constant humiliation and degradation inflicted in the name of colonial mastery, and in how these produced the "mental disorders" he saw and treated in his clinical practice. Fanon's Manichean views and rejection of the "native" bourgeoisie who were educated in French schools meant that he sometimes—particularly in his earlier writings—gave little attention to the internalization of the colonial ideology, the development of a dual consciousness as part of colonial subjectivity, and the diverse forms of multiple and "hybrid" consciousness that emerged both in the colonial and postcolonial eras. In contrast, Ashis Nandy, Homi Bhabha, and others have made these diverse forms of consciousness central to understanding postcolonial subjectivity. But Fanon's theorization of the consciousness of the colonized *and* the colonizers, his placing of psychopathology within this context, his reflections on "the so-called dependency complex," and his linking of racism and colonialism are of ongoing relevance to anthropological rethinking of subjectivity.[17]

For Ashis Nandy (1983, 1995), the "intimate enemy" of colonialism, the internalization of colonial disregard for local cultures and values and the resulting self-hatred imposed through colonial rule, produced—and continue to produce in the postcolony—a split self in which one element is repressed or denied. For Nandy and others, including Tanya Luhrmann (1996), who explored self-criticism among the postcolonial Parsi elite of India that arose through identification with the colonizers, this schizoid quality of experience and identity is seen as being at once condition and consequence of colonial and postcolonial discourses and forms of oppression. Paul Gilroy draws on W. E. B. DuBois's notion of double consciousness to describe "the core dynamic of racial oppression as well as the fundamental antinomy of diaspora blacks" (Gilroy 1993: 30); Fredric Jameson (1991) describes the split subject as the indexical figure of postmodernity and its requisite ruptures of space and time. The latter is a move Homi Bhabha (1994: 90) evokes in his descriptions of the "not quite/not white" identity of the postcolonial writer/subject and also in his discussion of mimicry (91). What is wonderful about Nandy's writing, of course, is that he does not stop with a caricatured reading of Indian consciousness as ultimately self-hating, but goes on to provide detailed accounts of Indian intellectuals, Western medicine in India, and the emergence of Indian cinema, all describing complex forms of colonial and postcolonial subjectivity. Such forms of subjectivity are often discussed in postcolonial studies in the language of "hybridity"—a term derived from colonial racist ideologies often celebrated, oddly enough, with little sense of irony. Following Bhabha, the ambiguous, mixed identities common in the postcolonies are often elegized as spaces for creative subversion of master discourses. Remaining at the heart of this work, however, is the ongoing tension between modern, rational modes of subjectivity and selves and the "traditional," and the linking of this duality to colonial memories of power and humiliation. The essays in this book suggest ways in which this literature has special importance for anthropological studies of subjectivity.

Critics of postcolonial theory rightly express a sense of irony that a body of inquiry founded on consideration of difference remains mired in a language of singularity: "the postcolonial condition," "the postcolonial subject," "the postcolonial nation." This irony is akin to Bhabha's sense that in the sites of alterity, "the postcolonial perspective . . . resists the attempt at holistic forms of social explanation . . . forc[ing] us to rethink the profound limitations of a consensual and collusive liberal sense of cultural community" (1994: 173, 175). In quite practical ways, it also forces anthropologists to explore diverse "colonialisms" and "postcolonialisms," in much the same way that recent scholarship has urged the pluralizing of modernity ("modernities").[18] The project of developing new ethnographies of subjectivity, postcolonial subjects, and postcolonial disorders thus links directly with a second body of diverse literatures that critique unitary and evolutionary theories of modernity and the modern subject,[19] including criticisms of the absence of the analysis of colonialism in Foucault's critical genealogy of the modern subject;[20] widely accepted arguments about the emergence of contemporary taken-for-granted categories of gender, race, and the "stranger" in colonial societies and colonial theorizing; as well as a body of studies that set out to explore the diversity of modernities and forms of modern experience that emerge within the centers and peripheries of major colonial empires. Charles Taylor's exploration of the "massive errors" of acultural theories of modernity, including the "Enlightenment package error" (2001: 180), which assumes that all societies have to undergo a range of cultural changes experienced in Europe and North America (for example, secularization and the growth of "atomistic forms of self-identification"), points to the sweeping range of issues encountered as anthropologists write about subjectivity in the societies in which they work. Our argument here is that normative assumptions about the modern subject surface at times unexpectedly in this work, challenging anthropological writing and any easy claims about cultural diversity (for example, do we really accept that secularizing forces are not inherent in modernizing processes?), and that addressing these issues adds to the dynamic quality of the project outlined here. It is also our argument that local and regional experiences with diverse European and American colonialisms (and crypto-colonialisms) shape not only "modernities" and "postcolonialities" but the theoretical traditions that arise within particular regions, leading to distinctive literatures from Africa, South Asia, the Middle East, East Asia, and Southeast Asia, for example. Attending to local and civilizational modes of subjectivity, rather than to easy arguments about "the global," devising strategies for ethnographic research in this vein, and bringing regionally based discussions concerning subjectivity into conversation with each other are also important to the larger project.[21]

In the previous section of this introduction, on "disorders," we suggested three strands of writing on subjectivity and disorder—poststructuralist writing on agency, clinically influenced writing on trauma and other forms of psychopathology, and ethnographies of "social suffering." At the heart of the project we are proposing are efforts to both incorporate and move beyond these modes of analyzing subjectivity, to link the political and the psychological in more clearly theorized ways, and to reject rigid dichotomizing of studies of the social and the individual, with anthropology on the side of the former, psychology with its "methodological individualism" on the side of the latter and therefore beyond the competence of anthropologists.[22] The trope of "madness" to reference disordered states, the activities of terrorists, primitive and irrational social groups, and the dark forces operating behind the scenes to cause chaos, appear over and again in the essays of this volume, drawn from local discourses in such disparate settings as Spain, Brazil, Indonesia, and Haiti, challenging anthropological interpretation. Developing theories that allow us to analyze such claims as more than mere metaphor, and methodological approaches that facilitate close linking of studies of individual lives and subjectivity to social analysis, are important challenges for the project we are outlining. Many of the chapters in this collection provide innovative contributions to such an approach to the ethnography of subjectivity.

One of the themes recurring in this introduction is an argument that studies of subjectivity need to pay attention to that which is not said overtly, to that which is unspeakable and unspoken, to that which appears at the margins of formal speech and everyday presentations of self, manifest in the Imaginary, in dissociated spaces, and individual dream time and coded in esoteric symbolic productions aimed at hiding as well as revealing. This suggests close attention to memories and subjugated knowledge claims that are suppressed politically but made powerful precisely by their being left unsaid, to that which speakers strategically refuse to speak about in settings of surveillance and danger, to painful secrets and "poisonous knowledge" (Das 2000), and to traumatic memories and hidden transcripts, which may fade from everyday awareness but have explosive power when evoked. It suggests attention to forms of knowledge coded in highly symbolic art, in cartoons or in theatrical performances, as well as to that which is so embedded in everyday practices and assumptive worlds, shaped by contemporary assemblages of knowledge/power, that they become invisible to subjects, depending on their positions of power.

Obviously, these various ways of framing that which is hidden or left unspoken suggest diverse literatures and ethnographic methodologies as relevant to a project of investigating "postcolonial subjectivities" and "postcolonial disorders." They suggest the importance of an increasing body of writing on memory, traumatic memory, and memory politics and of methods aimed at observing or retrieving remainders of violence or traumatic historical events. Attending to the presence of the unspeakable points to the importance of what Derrida (1994: 10) calls "hauntology," an effort to understand specters and ghosts—the "specters of Marx" and the ghost that appears before Hamlet, but also the ghosts of those tortured and dead whose voices are heard in Haiti (see James this volume) and around the contemporary world. Derrida (1994: 9) suggests that analysis always requires attention to "mourning" ("attempting to ontologize remains"), to "language" and "the voice" ("that which marks the name or takes its place"), and the "work" of the specter ("whether it transforms or transforms itself, poses or decomposes itself"). Attention to the hidden also suggests the relevance of what Žižek calls the "veils" of fantasy. Žižek argues that "narrative ... serves to occult some original deadlock. ... It is not only that some narratives are 'false', based upon the exclusion of traumatic events and patching up the gaps left by these exclusions—Lacan's thesis is much stronger: the answer to the question 'Why do we tell stories?' is that narrative as such emerges in order to resolve some fundamental antagonism by rearranging its terms into temporal succession" (1997: 10–11).

But it is not only through the ghostly or apparitional that states and their disorders or traumatic memory or history shape subjective lives. It is also through the everyday. Jamie Saris argues in this volume that colonial encounters, resistances, and postcolonial contradictions need to be analyzed not only in periods of social breakdown but in relation to the "specific colonial apparatus in everyday life"—including old colonial institutions, such as the Irish asylum he studies, which have been domesticated in local communities and cultures. Veena Das (2000) also argues that subjectivity should not be studied exclusively in relation to past traumatic events—such as the Partition in India—but also in relation to "the new forms of subjectivity" inhabited by the women she studied. "It is not that older subject positions were simply left behind or abandoned," Das writes, "rather, there were new ways in which even signs of injury could be occupied" (2000: 210–11).

The interplay between the ordinary and the exceptional brings anthropological writing on subjectivity into conversation with the emerging literatures on "states of emergency," referring to Walter Benjamin,[23] and Giorgio Agamben's analyses of "states of exception" (1998, 2005). Although bringing clear attention to the "exceptional," Agamben's work does so through careful analysis of legal procedures and forms of sovereignty.[24] His description of those spatial and social domains formulated through the suspension of ordinary rights and the institution of "exceptional" legal regulations, both in the name of the emergency, have eerie resonance for Americans living in the age of the Patriot Act and Guantánamo. Agamben follows Benjamin in arguing that "in our age, the state of exception comes more and more to the foreground as the fundamental political structure and ultimately begins to become the rule" (Agamben 1998: 20), suggesting mechanisms by which everyday subjectivities and those subjectivities associated with these exceptional legal statuses are far from clearly separated. This is also true of the literature on subjectivity on the "borderlands" or the "margins of the state," as we will discuss below. In her essay in this volume, Mariella Pandolfi links this discussion explicitly to the "emergencies" used to mobilize interventions and the new "mobile sovereignties" associated with the global humanitarian complex. But these increasingly common sites of social breakdown and intervention suggest that "states of exception" can usefully be extended beyond totalizing institutions, like the Guantánamo prisons, to spaces of "indeterminacy, flux, extreme potency and vulnerability" (Abramowitz 2005).[25]

Finally, any discussion of the secret, the hidden, the unspoken, and the unspeakable as qualities of subjectivity have resonance with a wide range of psychoanalytic theories, bringing them into complex conversation with the issues discussed in this introduction. Perhaps one way to comment on the potential of the Lacanian tradition for the project outlined here is a brief review of the creative and subtle use of that tradition by Aretxaga in her essay in this volume. Aretxaga sets out to explore the "political madness," the virtually incomprehensible violence that a group of Basque ETA members loosed on their own population beginning during the 1990s, alienating those previously sympathetic to their cause and debilitating their own apparent nationalist aspirations. So self-defeating were their actions that a consensus grew that these radical nationalists were simply "out of their minds." "But what defined this state of insanity?" Aretxaga asks. On the surface, she suggests, the discourse on madness was linked to "an incomprehensible and traumatic excess, an eruption within the familiar order that defamiliarizes it." But Aretxaga argues that "the kernel of this madness is something much more problematic and secret, something that indeed must remain hidden. . . . The crazy violence of these young radicals might be less incomprehensible . . . if we see it as the manifestation of a phantom, the presence of an absence, the presence of a traumatic history that remains not altogether resolved."

To make this argument, Aretxaga draws on the analysis of Nicholas Abraham and Maria Torok (1959, 1986) of the phantom as a "secret that remains buried and can be passed from generation to generation, inherited as it were in an unconscious way." She pieces together the story of the *encapuchados*, the hooded youth who became the subjects of this new form of violence, and of the "uncanny character" of the family violence in which they engaged. In particular, she analyzes the story of Mikel Otegi, a radical youth who in "a lapse of consciousness" killed two members of the Basque police in 1995, and she references Lacan's definition of the unconscious as "the discourse of the other, which emerges precisely in the gaps, in the blanks, of personal and collective histories." Then, following this notion that madness is characterized by a "rupture . . . that finds itself patched over by fantasy," she explores how political culture "might function in ways analogous to that of a dream," amenable to analysis of the "hidden metonymic associations that trace a subjective structure present in nationalist violence and that articulate a knowledge that remains hidden, a knowledge that the political subject in question does not want to know."

We will leave the analysis and conclusion to the reader, but simply note that Aretxaga's questions, her willingness to pursue even that which may be hidden from the actors, and her assumption that a "subjective structure" revealed by this analysis is knowable suggests one promising theoretical and methodological frame for linking the political and the psychological. It suggests that it may be useful to move between trauma, memory, and commemoration at social and personal levels. It suggests further that in domains such as relations "between the sexes and within the family," as Sudhir Kakar says for the Indian subjectivity, *oneiros*—dream, fantasy—does not coincide with the cultural propositions on these relationships, "but consists of what seeps out of the crevices in the cultural floor," conveying a culture's versions of "the Impossible and the Forbidden" (Kakar 1989: 41). And it suggests that anthropologists remain at the level of "cultural propositions" at their peril if they are to explore subjectivity, the postcolonial, and disorder.

INTRODUCTION TO THE ESSAYS IN THIS BOOK

We have organized the essays in this book into three sections—"Disordered States," "Subjectivity in the Borderlands," and "Madness, Alterity, and Psychiatry." In what follows, we provide a rationale for this organization—given that many of the essays speak to each other in multiple ways and could be differently grouped—and discuss briefly how each essay speaks to the larger themes of this book.

Part I: Disordered States

The five essays in this section—by Begoña Aretxaga, Mary-Jo DelVecchio Good and Byron Good, John MacDougall, Erica James, and Mariella Pandolfi—explore the tension between our understandings of the dual meanings of "disordered states," referencing political states and disordered lives, the everyday and spectral or imaginary qualities of the state, as well as the dynamics of political subjectivity. The essays bring special attention to how the state becomes a subject in the everyday lives of its citizens (Aretxaga 2003: 395), imagined and at times fetishized as an actor, and how violent and rapacious states inflict anxiety, trauma, and suffering upon individuals. These authors engage disorders arising within five contemporary societies: postdictatorial, post-Franco Spain and the Basque Country autonomy movement; post–New Order/post-Suharto Indonesia, in particular, in Central Java and Lombok; post-Duvalier, post-Aristide Haiti; and the postcommunist collapsed states of the Balkans. Although the historical dynamics of colonial and neocolonial relations—of Spain to its far flung and internal "colonies," of Java to the Netherlands and to its own twentieth-century Indonesian expanse, and of Haiti to France and most importantly to the United States—are strikingly distinctive, a current, a resonance, runs across these essays and the analyses the authors bring to bear. This section concludes with Pandolfi's essay, which proposes an anthropology of intervention focusing on the politics of suprastate, humanitarian-military interventions in Albania and the Balkans.

The subjective fantasies of the state that appear in these essays are hardly those of the Weberian bureaucratic or democratic liberal state, but are rather imaginings and memories of experiences of states, past and present, linked to terror, insecurity, and betrayal—states like those described by Taussig (1992, 2003) in which "spaces of death" and hidden, secret forces of the state have for generations imbued daily life with collective anxieties, with an ambience of fear and terror (Indonesia and Haiti), oppression and resistance (Basque ETA), and an acute awareness of the fragility of normal life.

The haunting specter of the state in both memory and imagination and in everyday encounters with its agents are described and richly analyzed by each author, highlighting varieties of political and subjective experiences.[26] In each case, the political is characterized by what Aretxaga describes in her essay as a "metaphor" of postcoloniality—"a certain dislocation and often violent disarray of things . . . in which the logical order of Cartesian thinking doesn't quite work." Thus the "madness" of politics, a common theme in these essays, comes in the guise of ETA and the *cipayos* and "the phantom of dictatorship" (Aretxaga); the disrupted world of reformation politics represented as haunting figures and powerful, disturbing images by contemporary artists (Good and Good); "dark forces" and "moral militias" (MacDougall); and "haunting ghosts" and the "magico-paramilitary" (James). These highly contemporary albeit historically laden disorders of the state, with roots in colonial and neocolonial relations of power, dislocation, and disarray, are more than failures of the normative state or barriers to an idealized political life in which there is collective and personal freedom from insecurity, fear, terror, and daily "nervousness" (Taussig 1992). Each of these essays introduces us to the ways in which the state and its deformations, and even suprastate actors in the humanitarian-military intervention world of intergovernmental and nongovernmental organizations (IGOs and NGOs) (see Pandolfi this volume), loom large in the political subjectivity of citizens.

Begoña Aretxaga, in "Madness and the Politically Real: Reflections on Violence in Postdictatorial Spain," raises questions about the elements of postcoloniality that extend beyond what is normally considered the postcolonial world, notably marginal status within the "global political and economic order." Through the trope of political madness, Aretxaga seeks to understand the "incomprehensible logic" of the violence that arose in Spain's now-autonomous Basque Country, perpetrated by ETA against the Basque police. She pursues not only the contours and implications of the trope "madness" for describing political disorders and "altered states," but also its emergence at a particular point in time and history. Noting the bombings and killings of intimates—brothers, kin, friends, innocent compatriots—by ETA, which fostered a Basque Country fear of fratricide, and the curious labeling of the Basque police as *cipayo*, representing the police as intimate betrayers (*sipahi* was the name for Indian troops of British India), Aretxaga draws on a Lacanian analysis of the work of "displacement" in political culture to explore that which "the political subject does not want to know." The madness of violence of the radical nationalists, she argues, manifests a profound ambivalence toward the nation-state, a fear that the "unified sense of self as the colonized people" stands to be lost in a coming into nationhood.

This essay in particular explores the historical shape, structure, and feel of disorder as a sometimes unconscious process, recalling the memories of and reactions to the disordered dictatorial state of Franco's Spain—the phantom of the dictatorship from which the Spanish democracy was not fully divorced— as well as a far more contemporary set of dislocations characteristic of globalized political terrorism. Aretxaga presented this paper in December 2000 to the Harvard seminar, prior to the al-Qaeda attacks of September 11, 2001, on the World Trade Center in New York and the March 2003 train bombings in Madrid. ETA was initially suspected of the latter. Throughout her work, Aretxaga provided a model for demonstrating that political madness, disordered states, and the apparently "incomprehensible logic" of "crazy violence is not [necessarily] meaningless."

Mary-Jo DelVecchio Good and Byron Good, in "*Indonesia Sakit*: Indonesian Disorders and the Subjective Experience and Interpretive Politics of Artists in Post-Suharto Indonesia," explore how in the early period of post-Suharto reformation—characterized by an exploding and refreshing sense of cultural freedom and expression—citizen-artists creatively and critically engaged in subjectifying the state through pointedly political art, generating narratives and fantasies both visual and discursive, private and public, and images of past, present, and future. Good and Good discuss a genre of "reformation art" found in public exhibitions from 1999 to 2003, as well as in artists' private collections. Profoundly cynical images of the state abound, drawing on the artists' experiences of the waning days of the Suharto New Order: the state as "sick" with political, economic, and moral decay, internal ethnic strife, corruption, and national disintegration (Yulikodo's *Indonesia Sakit*); the state as "empty of value," its nationalist ideology disempowered, its core symbol of the Garuda transformed into a distorted pig head, "just a mascot," after a generation of rapacious abuse and corruption (Alex Luthfi's *Kado Reformasi*); the state, the nation, the archipelago as gone "amok" (Entang Wiharso's NusaAmuk series on mob violence, mindless followers, and the all-consuming world of global products); the global anxiety of weakened states and the corrupted misuse of religion to foster terrorism, and a visceral, screaming desire to reject any internalizing of the fear of terrorism (Entang's *Don't Touch Me*). The paintings reveal how the transformation of political engagements led to these artists' newfound subjectivity as post–New Order Indonesian citizens, capable of publicly critiquing the state as well as reenvisioning, through their paintings, imagined possibilities for a new democratic Indonesian state.

John MacDougall, in "The Political Dimensions of Emasculation: Fantasy, Conspiracy, and Estrangement among Populist Leaders in Post–New Order Lombok, Indonesia," explores an alternative type of political madness to that discussed by Aretxaga, one in which individual paranoia mirrors local and national political events. In the immediate post-Suharto breakdown of order,

Soleh, a lawyer and advocate for the ordinary people and a once-powerful local leader in Megawati's Democratic Party of Struggle, found his political star on the wane. MacDougall tells the story of how the complex evolution of subjectivity experienced by nationalist activists against the New Order dictatorship, the rise of moral militias in post–New Order Lombok, the co-opting of dissent and activism by anticrime militias, and local forms of organized surveillance became entwined with Soleh's psychological disintegration, filled with conspiracy theories of the dark forces of a spurned national military and the Suharto crowd, intent on destabilizing the postauthoritarian state and its reformation and democracy movement and "eager to see Indonesia fall into chaos." Soleh's fall into madness mirrored his fear and that of many of his compatriots—at that time, and even in 2006, after a direct presidential election—that Indonesia would fall into political chaos.

Erica James, in "Haunting Ghosts: Madness, Gender, and *Ensekirite* in Haiti in the Democratic Era," introduces readers to the harsh Haitian world of insecurity, fear, and collective anxiety in a profoundly disordered state. James argues that Haiti's case is "within the arena of geopolitics"—a postcolonial global politics that has not been generous to Haiti, its "fragile path toward democracy" fraught with organized violence and "haunting ghosts." James weaves her analysis around the complexities of the geography of trauma, fear, and insecurity—the domains of terror that Taussig (1992) refers to as "spaces of death." Through the story of "Danielle," who seeks justice from the police for the murders of her husband and sons in the mid-1990s, which left her to support her youngest five children through prostitution, James raises questions not only about the fragility of Haiti's political and civil institutions and processes, but about the international community's interventions and identification of what Haitians suffer from (PTSD and HIV) and what they need (condoms). James returns frequently to "insecurity," identifying it as a longstanding theme for Haitians, related to political turmoil, military rule, violence, natural disasters, personal psychic and bodily experiences, and the contemporary conditions of living through a political transition at the site of international humanitarian interventions. As in other essays, the sense of the uncanny breaks through James's ethnography and analysis as she leads us from the collective nervousness of a nation, which suffers frequent trauma and terror, the madness of internal violence, and geopolitical exploitation, to the personal and subjective experiences of contemporary individuals struggling to eke out a living, hoping to be buttressed from constant fear.

The final essay in this section, Mariella Pandolfi's "Laboratory of Intervention: The Humanitarian Governance of the Postcommunist Balkan Territories," is an ethnography of intervention. Pandolfi focuses attention on the politics of humanitarian intervention carried out by international and intrastate institutions in the crises in Bosnia, Kosovo, and Albania. When the postcommunist Balkan states disintegrated politically, devolving into ethnic genocide on Europe's margins, military-humanitarian intervention was mounted on a massive scale. Pandolfi's account is shaped by her own subjective experience as a global political actor and intervening anthropologist. She argues that over the past decade there has been a growth in the "gray zone" between humanitarian intervention, military humanitarianism, and the humanitarian war, of which collaborating academics are largely uncritical. Calling for anthropological analysis of interventions, Pandolfi focuses attention beyond the boundaries of specific states to disorders without borders and the obscuring of the true needs of civil society through the politics of intervention. "Without borders" becomes a rallying cry, the panache, the label for NGOs and local elites, "men without borders," brokers of intervention and humanitarian entrepreneurship. Although Pandolfi primarily addresses the Balkan cases, her theoretical and analytic arguments have relevance for understanding new forms of mobile sovereignties that transcend states, mimicking interventions of the colonial world.

Part II: Subjectivity in the Borderlands

The four essays in this section—by Sandra Hyde, Johan Lindquist, David Eaton, and Michael Fischer—explore subjectivity at the borderlands or margins of states and polities. The "borderlands" here refer not only to the geographical border areas of nation-states, but to the marginal spaces of governmentality, global economics, biopower, and moral politics.[27] These are spaces of contradiction and disorder, as well as sites of cultural fluidity, identity making, and diverse and marginal forms of citizenship.[28] They are settings of cultural, political, and economic traffic and border crossings, spaces through which laborers are moved and sites of "narratives of eviction" that shape subjectivity.[29] In this volume, multiple borders and overlapping, compounding marginalities are represented by HIV/AIDS among minority populations in a border region of China and in the Republic of Congo, itself a marginal polity; by young women and men who are migrant laborers in a free-trade zone on an island at the very edge of Indonesia, living at the edge of Islamic norms; and by the perpetual and constantly reworked boundaries and negotiations between Palestinians and Israelis.

Gupta and Ferguson (1997) initiated analysis of borderlands as critical domains for investigating processes of globalization—the opening, closing, and policing of massive flows of people, culture, capital, ideas, media, and images—and practices through which political centers and states are defined and managed. Borders, crossings, closures, and policing are integral to postcolonial dynamics of power, consciousness, and experience, just as in earlier eras they held relevance for colonial and precolonial states;[30] they locate persons in terms of markets, labor, citizenship, and sovereignty, based on state regulations of inclusion and exclusion and universalized rights; they accentuate difference and hierarchy, policing and restrictions (Chinese HIV minorities and Southeast Asian labor migrants), as well as historical fault lines (Israel/ Palestine), endless violence and insecurity, and failed states (Congo).

The four chapters in this section explore the relevance of such theorization of borderlands to the central themes of this book in two ways. They provide ethnographic analysis of disorders associated with marginal spaces—HIV/AIDS, trafficking, prostitution, exploitative labor practices—and the assemblages of state agencies, international organizations, and NGOs developed to manage, police, or treat them. And they provide rich explorations of *subjectivity* in these spaces, examining the complex and contradictory lives of bureaucrats and nongovernmental workers, activists, and afflicted communities, women whose unruly agency is not easily captured by global categories such as "trafficking" and "sex workers" or "women without morals" (Lindquist this volume), and soldiers and psychiatrists who over the years have tried uneasily to cross the diverse boundaries that define both Israel and Palestine.

Sandra Hyde, in "Everyday AIDS Practices: Contestations of Borders and Diseases in Southwest China," examines how in late-socialist China, HIV becomes a spatialized disease, identified with communities at the borderlands along China's multiethnic southern frontier. Hyde's analysis grows out of years of field research in the region of the former Tai kingdom that borders northern Thailand. She demonstrates, through the narratives of four state actors, how political subjectivity and everyday practices of surveillance and implementation of public health policies not only link local, national, and global interventions in China's HIV crisis, but how they also inscribe the sovereignty of the state onto subjects in the borderlands, labeling the population "at risk" through HIV discourses on "risky bodies" and "risky practices." Through the articulation of HIV/AIDS policies, individual state agents, such as police and public health bureaucrats, configure the state itself as an entity, thereby defining the hierarchical relationship between the Tai minority populations of the borderlands and the Han interior, identified with the central government. Hyde argues that "all over the globe associations with diseases [are] mapped onto certain places and people more readily than others," and in China this has occurred through the discursive construction of HIV disease and its geographical and ethnic borders through the everyday AIDS practices of state agents.

Johan Lindquist, in "Of Maids and Prostitutes: Indonesian Female Migrants in the New Asian Hinterlands," focuses on the space of migration of the

Growth Triangle, particularly Batam Island, at the borderlands between Indonesia and Singapore. Building on ethnographic research on Batam during and following the Asian monetary crisis, Lindquist privileges displaced narratives— "narratives of eviction"—of women trapped in the migrant labor markets of these hinterlands who have worked both as maids and prostitutes in search of economic success. These women are burdened with a nationalized cultural framing of migration (*merantau*), which includes romantic visions of new experiences, freedom, and risk but requires eventual success in accumulating new resources for family and future. Economic failure leads to intense embarrassment and shame (*malu*), an unwillingness to return home to family and village empty-handed, coupled with a fear of being lost and destitute in migration. In the face of these risks and the growing lucrative businesses in trafficking maids and prostitutes, Lindquist asks, "why do women go when they are called?" Critiquing the metaphors of channels and flows, Lindquist argues that "it is crucial to revalorize transnational labor mobility" in conversations about economic globalization and transformation, to acknowledge the moral tensions and contradictions of those who navigate these trajectories through affectively laden spaces of migration in the so-called borderless yet highly restrictive economic hinterlands.

David Eaton, in "Ambivalent Inquiry: Dilemmas of AIDS in the Republic of Congo," engages an alternative borderland in discussing the AIDS epidemic and the concomitant political and financial crises occurring in former French colonies of equatorial Africa. Eaton focuses on the postcolonial, postsocialist Republic of Congo prior to the 1997 civil war. Here the borderland is metaphoric and situational as much as geographic and postcolonial, a space where the HIV-afflicted lived in disordered settings, where treatments and interventions were virtually impossible, and where silence, denial, and refusal were constant, a space "complicated by the social disruption, insecurity, and violence associated with difficult political transitions in the region over the past two decades." The discourse on AIDS was "embedded within . . . larger systems of political discourse and historical consciousness." "*Le pays est malade* [the nation is ill]," Congolese say, asking "Is this country cursed?" AIDS is interpreted through the trope of national affliction and within a rich imaginary and symbolic order derived from colonial memories, colored with deep mistrust of the "foreigner" and global biomedicine through which AIDS literally becomes a postcolonial disorder. Eaton discusses local ways of managing and curtailing speech about and knowledge of AIDS, highlighting the role of sorcery as indexing global power relations, racism, and the politics of international health interventions as much as speaking for local culture.

In the final essay, "To Live with What Would Otherwise Be Unendurable, II: Caught in the Borderlands of Palestine/Israel," Michael Fischer presents new ethnographic work on Palestine and Israel and the "borderland of disorders (psychic and otherwise) where there is strong resistance to third-party intervention. . . ." Fischer draws our attention to the critical importance of subjectivity: "the payoffs and feedbacks among registers of the political, psychological, and bodily selves . . . as witnesses in situations of trauma, as agents in judgments of ethical action, as partners in creating elementary forms of social life." Invoking two ethnographic situations—conversations with a Gaza psychiatrist and an ethnographer of joint Palestinian-Israeli patrols—he contrasts the psychoanalytic and therapeutic discourses and the subtle choreography of emotion and gaming of the joint patrols with the seemingly thin responses and discourses of humanitarian intervention. Fischer urges anthropologists and the actors in these dramas to find folds in the borderlands, pores in the membrane, holes in the defenses, and modalities of border incursions in small intersubjective exchanges and talk, where "just gaming . . . is not just gaming but gaming toward justice." Fischer asks that we turn the mirror back upon subjectivity, returning to unstable grounds of witnessing and to performative rhetorics of subjectivity. He concludes this section of essays on the borderlands, challenging anthropologists by asking, what can the method of ethnography of social contexts do when using sites in this violent border war as crucibles? In general, this section of essays challenges ethnographers to attend both structurally and psychologically to borderlands and to the complex modes of contemporary subjectivity that evolve within them.

Part III: Madness, Alterity, and Psychiatry

The six essays in this final section—by João Biehl, Jamie Saris, Stefania Pandolfo, Sarah Pinto, Janis Jenkins and Michael Hollifield, and Kathleen Allden—address the subjective stakes of postcolonial disorder through the lenses of psychiatric models and "other" or "altered" mental states, as well as the negotiations and institutional entanglements associated with such states. These essays hold in tension the ways that categories of moral, mental, and emotional experience are at once spaces in which and techniques by which globalized power dynamics and postcolonial realities are grappled with. Ascriptions of madness, bestiality, fatalism, and disease are, on the one hand, addressed by these authors as means by which colonial and postcolonial "orders" are made and "disorders" pacified. On the other hand, it is in domains of emotional experience that fall along the margins, or that erupt into clinical, legal, and interventionist apparatuses, that the authors locate the intimate straits, the deep contradictions, and the often impossible stakes of transnational and transcultural structures of power and meaning.

It is worth recalling that major mental illness has long been a site for complex theorization of subjectivity by psychiatrists and anthropologists alike.[31] It is equally true that colonial and postcolonial psychiatry—knowledge structures, modes of practice, the colonial asylum, and contemporary postcolonial engagements within these institutions—have been settings for historical and ethnographic research.[32] Here, "disordered states" and "madness" are not metaphors but everyday realities. Investigations of subjectivity in these settings require special forms of listening, with an ear sensitive to the personal, cultural, and historical. The essays in this section indicate the value for the larger project of understanding postcolonial subjectivity of this work. Today, psychiatrists and anthropologists have increasingly been drawn into the globalized spaces linking mental health assessments with human rights work. In these settings, instrumental and moral issues challenge the theoretical and analytic in complex and interesting ways, as Allden's essay suggests.

João Biehl, in "The Mucker War: A History of Violence and Silence," examines the forging of a German Kultur in Brazil during the late nineteenth century, and the role of "a fratricidal war" and the colonial German bourgeoisie's use of natural and medical sciences, institutionalized religion, and contemporary media to stigmatize and eventually eradicate a millennial cult popular among poor German immigrants, called Mucker, which translates as "false believers" and "stubborn people." Biehl argues that the making of the Mucker as "Other," "as mad and bestial," was part of the larger Enlightenment project to transplant a rationalized scientific and enlightened German Self in the south of Brazil. His essay provides a reading of one of the traumatic foundational moments of this project, implicating the Brazilian German bourgeoisie's effort to constitute new, modern citizens in the colonial outposts of the time. He goes on to argue, provocatively, that the story of the Mucker war is "a continuous legend of the present," an "interpretative reservoir" of contemporary events, and the phantasm determining the course of reason and ethics.

Jamie Saris, in "Institutional Persons and Personal Institutions: The Asylum and Marginality in Rural Ireland," presents a detailed ethnography of a classic postcolonial institution—a state mental hospital built as a colonial asylum by the British in Ireland—through describing the daily life of a former mental patient of the hospital, who has become "the town character." Saris reflects on the life of this man, exploring Irish notions of being a "character" or "queer" and cultural margins between the respectable and unrespectable. He opens space for a modest understanding of the subjectivity of a man whose speech is apparently "crazy" but who is still quite effective in making assertions about local politics and community relations. Focusing on the quotidian, Saris argues that "colonial encounters and the resistances they provoke, postcolonial contradictions and the unsatisfactory results that they often inspire, need to be analyzed beyond moments of violence and in high literature. It is in the presence of specific colonial apparatuses of everyday life, the various changes that they effect, [and that are] wrought upon them that both colonial and postcolonial experience needs to be examined."

Stefania Pandolfo, in "The Knot of the Soul: Postcolonial Conundrums, Madness, and the Imagination," presents a single case study of a young Moroccan man experiencing the onset of psychosis, who was brought by police at the request of his mother to a psychiatric emergency department in Morocco, where the author met the patient. Her essay takes the form of a circumstantial commentary, in which she weaves observations of other patients and psychiatric ideologies with reflections on contradictions of the postcolonial era in Morocco. Pandolfo follows the complex language shifts of the patient as he speaks to the psychiatrist, as he speaks to and about his mother, and as patient and psychiatrist speak to each other. Arabic includes the mother; French provides dialogue between patient and psychiatrist that is exclusive, private, modern. In this Moroccan situation, French is the language of the former colonizers, the language of education and modernity. The indigenous is Arabic, the language of religion and magic, the nonmodern. The patient, Pandolfo tells us, finds his "cultural home" unlivable; he complains that his mother forced him "to consult with a Qur'anic healer against [his] will." He tells his psychiatrist in French that "he invents stories of jinns" and enacts them, practicing "literature in life." His mother exclaims of her son that "he is knotted"—an image of bewitchment from Moroccan magic and a term for the "complex" in modern psychology. Pandolfo explores how the personal subjective mirrors the "knottedness" of postcolonial Morocco, where the colonial and the indigenous live uneasily in this conflicted young man. Pandolfo's ethnography suggests that Fanon's original diagnosis of the subjectivity of the colonized may be of more continuing relevance than the diagnoses of many postcolonial theorists.

Sarah Pinto, in "Consuming Grief: Infant Death in the Postcolonial Time of Intervention," juxtaposes ways of addressing and coping with infant death in the context of rural poverty and transnational intervention in rural India, placing side by side the stories told repeatedly by grieving mothers and the universalized phrases associated with the pedagogies of health intervention. In juxtaposing ways of rendering causality in a region of India with high rates of infant mortality, Pinto identifies a structure similar to what Julia Kristeva (1989) calls "depressed speech," in which repressed or disavowed elements return as a "symptom of a larger disorder." The language of intervention, in particular, has roots in colonial representations that pathologize maternal reactions to babies' deaths and that locate the cause of such deaths in women's lack of affect. But women's stories of grief—especially those that link the complexities of everyday life to failed institutions and infrastructures, while referring to "the hands of God"—allow the persistence, rather than absence, of maternal grief to function as a sustained commentary on life and death on the margins. At the same time, Pinto shows the ways postcolonial structures and meanings articulate with and are refused by domestic and neighborly relations, in which intimate intersubjectivities are formed between women through talk about death.

Janis Jenkins and Michael Hollifield, in "Postcoloniality as the Aftermath of Terror among Vietnamese Refugees," address "the transformation of lived experience" and modes of subjectivity for Vietnamese refugees, primarily military men who have resettled to the United States. Focusing on the experiential themes of "alterity, trauma, and memory," the authors trace the experiential components of postcolonial forms of power and transformation, locating the conflicts of "fragmented selves" and the intrapsychic and intrasomatic "violence within" in the historical dynamics of the postcolonial nation-state's coming into being, as well as in the larger global and political contexts. Jenkins and Hollifield identify "the postcolonial problem of alterity," in which subjectivities "are transacted in relation to geography, religion, and political affiliation," as one of the key challenges to understanding postcolonial subjectivity.

Finally, Kathleen Allden, in "Cross-Cultural Psychiatry in Medical-Legal Documentation of Suffering: Human Rights Abuses Involving Transnational Corporations and the Yadana Pipeline Project in Burma," introduces the Istanbul Protocol, guidelines for documenting consequences of torture and other cruel, inhuman, or degrading treatment and severe human rights abuses, which was developed by seventy-five forensic physicians, psychologists, human rights monitors, and lawyers representing forty institutions and fifteen countries from 1996 to 1999. Allden considers the role of such guidelines, and of the medical and psychiatric disciplines that created them, in addressing human rights violations linked to activities of "corporate globalization and the new global economy." She recounts a legal suit brought by Burmese (ethnically Karen) villagers against the pipeline company Unocal. Allden discusses her own role as a psychiatrist in documenting human rights abuses against the villagers who were working on the pipeline project, and she explores supranational disorders and supranational/transnational agents of power.

In order to universalize human rights claims, the Istanbul Protocol and psychiatric evaluations of abuse emphasize diagnostic criteria and the biological components of trauma. Although medicalized criteria enable victims who are often among the most economically marginalized to make claims against powerful multinational corporations, Allden nonetheless questions the utility of PTSD diagnoses across cultures. Allden's essay captures the dilemmas of representing subjectivity in the language of medicine and universal human rights versus the experience-near language of suffering, suggesting the importance of multiple modes of investigating and framing the experiences of trauma and violence all too common in postcolonial settings.

CONCLUDING THOUGHTS

The essays of this volume are far from a neat and ordered whole. Reflecting current modes of subjectivity, they are an unruly lot, more provocative than prescriptive, opening up issues rather than providing closure, hinting at the hidden, at times intentionally subversive. The common thread—linking subjectivity to the political, and that to the disorders of the contemporary, postcolonial world—provides a sense of conversation more than conclusion. And the effort to grapple with a common set of theoreticians, few of whom are anthropologists, suggests a common enterprise. Together, the essays provide a sense of work at its beginning, the initiation of a project, as we indicated earlier in this introduction. We hope readers will experience a similar sense of freshness in the writing that the editors have felt in trying to bring together these authors and essays. And we hope that readers will take up the many challenges staked out in the essays, will respond to the provocations, and will join in this project.

NOTES

1. One only need reference Žižek's book, *The Ticklish Subject* (1999), to be reminded of the remarkably provocative ideas about political subjectivity found in the body of work drawn on by a number of the authors in this collected volume, and the difficulty of linking these ideas to the investigation of individual lives or to social analysis.

2. In Indonesia, individuals and mobs both "run amok" (*mengamuk*) (B. Good, Subandi, and Good 2001; B. Good and Good 2001). The resort to metaphorical language of psychopathology when attempting to understand the behavior of crowds of course has a long lineage. See Tambiah (1996: chap. 10) for a review of the history of ideas about the "political psychology of crowds."

3. This seminar has met on a weekly basis since 1984, supported by a National Research Scientist Award from the U.S. National Institute of Mental Health (MH 18006) focused on "clinically relevant medical anthropology" and "culture and mental health services research." The program has been directed by Professors Byron Good, Mary-Jo DelVecchio Good, and Arthur Kleinman.

4. Many of the papers from that seminar appear in *Subjectivity: Ethnographic Investigations* (Biehl, Good, and Kleinman 2007).

5. For example, see the discussions within the special issues of *Social Text* in 1992 and 2004. See in particular McClintock (1992) and Shohat (1992).

6. For example, Duran and Duran (1995), Brave Heart and DeBruyn (1998), Duran et al. (1998), and Whitbeck, Adams, and Hoyt (2004); cf. O'Nell (1996).

7. For reviews of relevant data on mental health disparities by race and ethnicity, see B. Good (1992, 1997) and M. Good et al. (2005).

8. For a set of papers that explore the emergence of distinctive "global assemblages" in contemporary technology, politics, and ethics, see Ong and Collier (2005). The colonial origins of many of these assemblages remain largely unexplored in this interesting collection.

9. Classic theories represented the nation-state as producing rational order, threatened by disorders at its margins or a return to "nature" and to primitive and uncivilized forms of violence not yet subdued by rationality, represented by civilization and the civilizing state. These classic formulations of the state and its relation to order, theorization of the "margins" of the state, and the relevance of these for anthropology are explored in Das and Poole (2004).

10. Such a listing presumes a set of literatures far too wide to reference fully here. Some examples include Fabian (2000), Mbembe (2001), Siegel (1997, 1998), Steedly (1999), Aretxaga (1997, 2003, 2005a, 2005b), Taussig (1992, 1997), Tambiah (1996), Daniel (1996), Warren (1993), Feldman (1991), Greenhouse, Mertz, and Warren (2002), Das and Poole (2004), Appadurai (1996, 2001), Csordas (1994a, 1994b), Stiglitz (2002), Marcus (2000), and Suarez-Orozco and Suarez-Orozco (2001).

11. See Werbner (2002) for a brief but cogent discussion of these distinctions.

12. See Okazaki (2002) and Lambek (2002) for examples of efforts to work through these issues ethnographically.

13. Examples include Caruth (1995, 1996), Antze and Lambek (1996), Young (1995), Hacking (1995), Leys (2000), and Robben and Suarez-Orozco (2000).

14. Examples include O'Nell (1992, 1996) and Khanna (2003).

15. Nancy Chodorow's book (1999) is a good introduction to this literature.

16. Kleinman, Das, and Lock (1997); Das et al. (2000); Das et al. (2001). This work builds on earlier phenomenological accounts, such as Kleinman (1973), B. Good (1994), Csordas (1994b), and Desjarlais (1992, 2003).

17. See Fanon (1967) in particular. The collection of essays on "the psychoanalysis of race" by Lane (1998) points to the ongoing relevance of Fanon's thought.

18. For example, Mitchell (2000), Gaonkar (2001a), and Chakrabarty (2002)

19. Mitchell's collection (2000) both reviews and contributes to a critical analysis of evolutionary theories of modernity and the modern subject, while providing a fascinating set of studies from India and North Africa indicating the diverse histories of "modernity" in these civilizational and colonial settings. Gaonkar's collection (2001a) provides both critical theoretical essays and ethnographic accounts of modernity from diverse societies. See also Rabinow (1996), Kolakowski (1990), and Habermas (1987) for relevant theoretical and philosophical reflections, and Cohen (1998) and Langford (2002) for ethnographic examples.

20. Stoler's critique (1995) of Foucault is notable in this regard (cf. Stoler 2002, 2006).

21. Again, it is worth noting the Mitchell volume (2000) and the project of bringing South Asianists and Middle East specialists with interests in subjectivity and multiple modernities into conversation with each other.

22. Byron Good has expressed this as follows: "Rather than juxtaposing the individual to the social or cultural, linked to a series of binary oppositions (the social, cultural, public, symbolic, cognitive, and conscious *rather than* the physiological, personal, private, psychological, affective, and unconscious), with anthropology on the side of the former, reductive psychology on the side of the latter, investigations of the social life of emotions should incorporate studies of individuals. . . . A new anthropology of the emotions . . . will have to be crafted through a serious confrontation with more diverse theorists of subjectivity, theorists who link the individual to the social and make psychological processes relevant to both" (2004: 532).

23. "The tradition of the oppressed teaches us that 'the state of emergency' in which we live is not the exception but the rule" (Walter Benjamin, from "Theses on the Philosophy of History"); see chapter 2 of Taussig (1992), "Terror as Usual: Walter Benjamin's Theory of History as State of Siege," for an ethnographic reflection on Benjamin.

24. See Agamben (1998, 2005); see also Das and Poole's discussion (2004) of Agamben in relation to their explication of the margins of the state.

25. In an unpublished commentary on Agamben, Sharon Abramowitz (2005) calls for analysis of how "social processes are enacted with (and outside) this anomic normative and extra-legal space," and for an approach that "decenters Agamben's static representation of the state of exception as universal and totalizing, and re-situates the state of exception as a space of indeterminacy, flux, extreme potency and vulnerability, and most certainly as a power and violence-ordered space of contestation, with varying degrees of totalization."

26. See Steedly (1999), Aretxaga (2003), and Das and Poole (2004) for examples of a new anthropology of the state to which the chapters in this section contribute.

27. There is a broad literature that addresses borders, border zones, frontiers, and hinterlands. While the following is not an exhaustive list, it highlights some of the scholars whose work first addressed these concepts: Sahlins (1989), Hastings and Wilson (1994), Alvarez (1995), Lavie and Swedenburg (1996), Flynn (1997), Spener and Staudt (1998), Smith et al. (1998), Wilson and Donnan (1998), and Castillo and Cordoba (2002).

28. See, for example, Lefebvre (1991), Gupta and Ferguson (1992, 2002), Anzaldua (1999), Berdahl (1999), Hyde (2002), Winichakul (1994), and Das and Poole (2004).

29. W. Fisher (1997), Appadurai (1996, 2001), Aneesh (2001), Sassen (1998).

30. In the works of Eric Wolf, Janet Abu-Lughod, and Sidney Mintz.

31. See Jenkins and Barrett (2004) for a fine recent example. The introduction to that volume has a rich review of issues of "subjective experience" in studies of culture and schizophrenia.

32. See, for example, L. Fisher (1985), Kleinman (1986), McCulloch (1995), Pandolfo (1997), Mills (2000), Bhugra and Littlewood (2001); cf. Rhodes (2004) for a critical ethnography linking these issues to psychiatry in the American prison system.

REFERENCES

Abraham, Nicholas, and Maria Torok. 1959. *The Shell and the Kernel*. Chicago: University of Chicago Press.

———. 1986. *The Wolf Man's Magic Word: A Cryptonomy*. Trans. Nicholas Rand. Foreword by Jacques Derrida. Minneapolis: University of Minnesota Press.

Abramowitz, Sharon. 2005. States of Exception. Unpublished ms.

Abu-Lughod, Janet. 1989. *Before European Hegemony: The World System, AD 1250–1350*. New York: Oxford University Press.

Abu-Lughod, Lila. 1993. *Writing Women's Worlds: Bedouin Stories*. Berkeley: University of California Press.

Agamben, Giorgio. 1998. *Homo Sacer: Sovereign Power and Bare Life*. Trans. Daniel Heller-Roazen. Stanford, CA: Stanford University Press.

———. 2005. *State of Exception*. Trans. Kevin Attell. Chicago: University of Chicago Press.

Alvarez, Robert R., Jr. 1995. The Mexican-US Border: The Making of an Anthropology of Borderlands. *Annual Review of Anthropology* 24:447–70.

Aneesh, Aneesh. 2001. Skill Saturation: Rationalization and Post-Industrial Work. *Theory and Society* 30:363–96.

Antze, Paul, and Lambek, Michael. 1996. *Tense Past: Cultural Essays in Trauma and Memory*. New York: Routledge.

Anzaldúa, Gloria. 1999. *Borderlands/La Frontera*. San Francisco: Aunt Lute Press.

Appadurai, Arjun. 1996. *Modernity at Large: Cultural Dimensions of Globalization*. Minneapolis: University of Minnesota Press.

———, ed. 2001. *Globalization*. Durham, NC: Duke University Press.

Aretxaga, Begoña. 1997. *Shattering Silence: Women, Nationalism, and Political Subjectivity in Northern Ireland*. Princeton, NJ: Princeton University Press.

———. 2003. Maddening States. *Annual Review of Anthropology* 32:393–410.

———. 2005a. *Empire and Terror: Nationalism/Postnationalism in the New Millennium*. Reno: Center for Basque Studies, University of Nevada.

———. 2005b. *States of Terror: Begoña Aretxaga's Essays*. Ed. Joseba Zulaika. Reno: Center for Basque Studies, University of Nevada.

Behar, Ruth. 1993. *Translated Woman: Crossing the Border with Esperanza's Story*. Boston: Beacon Press.

Berdahl, Daphne. 1999. *Where the World Ended: Re-Unification and Identity in the German Borderland*. Berkeley: University of California Press.

Bhabha, Homi K. 1994. *The Location of Culture*. New York: Routledge.

Bhugra, Dinesh, and Littlewood, Roland, eds. 2001. *Colonialism and Psychiatry*. New York: Oxford University Press.

Biehl, João, Byron Good, and Arthur Kleinman. 2007. *Subjectivity: Ethnographic Investigations*. Berkeley: University of California Press.

Bosniak, Linda. 2000. Citizenship Denationalized. *Indiana Journal of Global Legal Studies* 7 (2): 447–509.

Brave Heart, Maria, and Lemyra DeBruyn. 1998. The American Indian Holocaust: Healing Historical Unresolved Grief. *American Indian and Alaska Native Mental Health Research* 8 (2): 60–82.

Butler, Judith. 1997. *The Psychic Life of Power*. Stanford, CA. Stanford University Press.

Castillo, Debra, and María Socorro Tabuenca Córdoba. 2002. *Border Women: Writing from la Frontera*. Minneapolis: University of Minnesota Press.

Caruth, Cathy, ed. 1995. *Trauma: Explorations in Memory*. Baltimore: Johns Hopkins University Press.

———. 1996. *Unclaimed Experience: Trauma, Narrative and History*. Baltimore: Johns Hopkins University Press.

Chakrabarty, Dipesh. 2000. *Provincializing Europe: Postcolonial Thought and Historical Difference*. Princeton, NJ: Princeton University Press.

———. 2002. *Habitations of Modernity: Essays in the Wake of Subaltern Studies*. Chicago: University of Chicago Press.

Chatterjee, Partha. 1993. *The Nation and Its Fragments: Colonial and Postcolonial Histories*. Princeton, NJ: Princeton University Press.

———. 1998. Beyond the Nation? Or within? In *Social Text* 56 (Autumn): 57–69.

Chodorow, Nancy J. 1999. *The Power of Feeling*. New Haven, CT: Yale University Press.

Cohen, Lawrence. 1998. *No Aging in India*. Berkeley: University of California Press.

Cohn, Bernard. 1996. *Colonialism and Its Forms of Knowledge*. Princeton, NJ: Princeton University Press.

Copjec, Joan, ed. 1994. *Supposing the Subject*. New York: Verso.

Csordas, Tom. 1994a. *Embodiment and Experience*. Cambridge: Cambridge University Press.

———. 1994b. *The Sacred Self: A Cultural Phenomenology of Charismatic Healing*. Berkeley: University of California Press.

Daniel, E. Valentine. 1996. *Charred Lullabies: Chapters in an Anthropology of Violence*. Princeton, NJ: Princeton University Press.

Das, Veena. 1995. National Honor and Practical Kinship: Unwanted Women and Children. In *Conceiving the New World Order: The Global Politics of Reproduction*, ed. F. D. Ginsburg and R. Rapp, 212–33. Berkeley: University of California Press.

———. 2000. The Act of Witnessing: Violence, Poisonous Knowledge, and Subjectivity. In *Violence and Subjectivity*, ed. Veena Das, Arthur Kleinman, Mamphela Ramphele, and Pamela Reynolds. Berkeley: University of California Press.

Das, Veena, Arthur Kleinman, Margaret Lock, Mamphela Ramphele, and Pamela Reynolds, eds. 2001. *Remaking a World: Violence, Social Suffering, and Recovery.* Berkeley: University of California Press.

Das, Veena, Arthur Kleinman, Mamphela Ramphele, and Pamela Reynolds, eds. 2000. *Violence and Subjectivity.* Berkeley: University of California Press.

Das, Veena, and Deborah Poole, eds. 2004. *Anthropology in the Margins of the State.* Santa Fe, NM: School of American Research Press.

Derrida, Jacques. 1994. *Specters of Marx.* Trans. Peggy Kamuf. New York: Routledge.

Desai, Gaurav. 2001. *Subject to Colonialism: African Self-Fashioning and the Colonial Library.* Durham, NC: Duke University Press.

Desjarlais, Robert R. 1992. *Body and Emotion.* Philadelphia: University of Pennsylvania Press.

———. 2003. *Sensory Biographies.* Berkeley: University of California Press.

Dirks, Nicholas B. 1998. In Near Ruins: Cultural Theory at the End of the Century. In *In Near Ruins: Cultural Theory at the End of the Century,* ed. Nicholas B. Dirks, 1–18. Minneapolis: University of Minnesota Press.

Driscoll, Mark. 2004. Reverse Postcoloniality. *Social Text* 22 (Spring): 59–84.

Duran, Eduardo, and Bonnie Duran. 1995. *Native American Post-Colonial Psychology.* Albany: State University of New York Press.

Duran, Eduardo, Bonnie Duran, Maria Brave Heart, and Susan Yellow Horse-Davis. 1998. Healing the American Indian Soul Wound. In *International Handbook of Multigenerational Legacies of Trauma,* ed. Yael Danieli, 341–54. New York: Plenum Press.

Eagleton, Terry. 1996. *Literary Theory: An Introduction.* 2nd ed. Minneapolis: University of Minnesota Press.

Edwards, Brent Hayes. 2004. The Genres of Postcolonialism. *Social Text* 22 (Spring): 1–15.

Fabian, Johannes. 2000. *Out of Our Minds.* Berkeley: University of California Press.

Fanon, Frantz. 1963. *The Wretched of the Earth.* Trans. Constance Farrington. New York: Grove Weidenfeld.

———. 1967. *Black Skin, White Masks: The Experiences of a Black Man in a White World.* New York: Grove Press.

Feldman, Allen. 1991. *Formations of Violence.* Chicago: University of Chicago Press.

Fisher, Lawrence. 1985. *Colonial Madness.* New Brunswick, NJ: Rutgers University Press.

Fisher, William. 1997. Doing Good? The Politics and Antipolitics of NGO Practices. *Annual Review of Anthropology* 26:439–64.

Flynn, Donna K. 1997. We Are the Border: Identity, Exchange, and the State along the Benin-Nigeria Border. *American Ethnologist* 24, no. 2 (May): 311–30.

Foucault, Michel. 1997. *Ethics: Subjectivity and Truth.* Ed. Paul Rabinow. New York: New Press.

———. 1998. *Aesthetics, Method, and Epistemology.* Ed. James D. Faubian. New York: New Press.

———. 2000. *Power.* Ed. James D. Faubian. New York: New Press.

Gaonkar, Dilip Parameshwar, ed. 2001a. *Alternative Modernities.* Durham, NC: Duke University Press.

———. 2001b. On Alternative Modernities. In *Alternative Modernities,* ed. D. P. Gaonkar, 1–23. Durham, NC: Duke University Press.

Gates, Henry Louis. 1987. *Figures in Black.* New York: Oxford University Press.

Gilroy, Paul. 1993. *The Black Atlantic: Modernity and Double Consciousness.* Cambridge, MA: Harvard University Press.

Good, Byron J. 1992. Culture, Diagnosis and Co-morbidity. *Culture, Medicine and Psychiatry* 16:1–20.

———. 1994. *Medicine, Rationality, and Experience: An Anthropological Perspective.* Cambridge: Cambridge University Press.

———. 1997. Studying Mental Illness in Context: Local, Global, or Universal? *Ethos* 25:230–49.

———. 2004. Rethinking "Emotions" in South East Asia. *Ethnos* 69 (4): 529–33.

Good, Byron J., and Mary-Jo DelVecchio Good. 2001. Madness and Violence in Indonesian Politics. *Latitudes* 5 (June): 10–19.

———. 2005. On the "Subject" of Culture: Subjectivity and Cultural Phenomenology in the Work of Clifford Geertz. In *Clifford Geertz by His Colleagues,* ed. Richard Shweder and Byron Good, 98–107. Chicago: University of Chicago Press.

Good, Byron J., Subandi, and Mary-Jo DelVecchio Good. 2001. Le sujet de la maladie mentale: Psychose, folie furieuse et subjectivité en Indonésie. In *La maladie mentale en mutation: Psychiatrie et société,* ed. Alain Ehrenberg and Anne M. Lovell, 163–95. Paris: éditions Odile Jacob.

Good, Mary-Jo DelVecchio, Anne Becker, Cara James, and Byron J. Good. 2005. The Culture of Medicine and Racial, Ethnic and Class Disparities in Healthcare. In *The Blackwell Companion to Social Inequalities,* ed. Mary Romero and Eric Margolis, 396–423. Oxford and Malden, MA: Blackwell Publishing.

Good, Mary-Jo DelVecchio, and Byron J. Good. 1988. Ritual, the State and the Transformation of Emotional Discourse in Iranian Society. *Culture, Medicine and Psychiatry* 12:43–63.

Graubard, Stephen. 1996. Preface. In "Social Suffering," *Daedalus* 125 (1).

Greenhouse, Carol. 1999. Commentary (in an issue of PoLAR on citizenship and its alterities). *PoLAR: Political and Legal Anthropology Review* 22 (2): 104–9.

Greenhouse, Carol J., Elizabeth Mertz, and Kay B. Warren, eds. 2002. *Ethnography in Unstable Places.* Durham, NC: Duke University Press.

Guha, Ranajit. 1983. The Prose of Counter-Insurgency. In *Subaltern Studies,* vol. 2, ed. Ranajit Guha, 1–42. New Delhi: Oxford University Press.

———. 1999. *Elementary Aspects of Peasant Insurgency in Colonial India.* Durham, NC: Duke University Press.

Gupta, Akhil. 1996. *Postcolonial Developments: Agriculture in the Making of Modern India.* Durham, NC: Duke University Press.

Gupta, Akhil, and James Ferguson. 1992. Beyond Culture: Space, Identity, and the Politics of Difference. *Cultural Anthropology* 7 (1): 6–23.

———. 1997. *Anthropological Locations: Boundaries and Grounds of a Field Science.* Berkeley: University of California Press.

Habermas, Jurgen. 1987. *The Philosophical Discourse of Modernity.* Trans. Frederick G. Lawrence. Cambridge, MA: MIT Press.

Hacking, Ian. 1995. *Rewriting the Soul.* Princeton, NJ: Princeton University Press.

Hansen, Thomas Blom. 2001. *The Wages of Violence: Naming and Identity in Postcolonial Bombay.* Princeton, NJ: Princeton University Press.

Hansen, Thomas Blom, and Finn Stepputat. 2001. Introduction to *States of Imagination: Ethnographic Explorations of the Postcolonial State.* Durham, NC: Duke University Press.

Hardt, Michael, and Antonio Negri. 2000. *Empire.* Cambridge, MA: Harvard University Press.

Hastings, Donnan, and Thomas M. Wilson. 1994. *Border Approaches: Anthropological Perspectives on Frontiers.* London and New York: University of America Press.

Herzfeld, Michael. 2002. Absent Presence: Discourses of Crypto-Colonialism. *The South Atlantic Quarterly* 101 (Fall): 899–926.

Hyde, Sandra. 2002. The Cultural Politics of HIV/AIDS and the Chinese State in Late-Twentieth Century Yunnan. *Tsantsa* (Review of the Swiss Society of Ethnology) 7:56–65.

Jameson, Frederic. 1991. *Postmodernism, or, the Cultural Logic of Late Capitalism.* Durham: University of North Carolina Press.

Jenkins, Janis Hunter, and Robert John Barrett. 2004. *Schizophrenia, Culture and Subjectivity: The Edge of Experience.* Cambridge: Cambridge University Press.

Kakar, Sudhir. 1989. *Intimate Relations.* Chicago: University of Chicago Press.

Khanna, Ranjana. 2003. *Dark Continents: Psychoanalysis and Colonialism.* Durham, NC: Duke University Press.

Kleinman, Arthur. 1973. Medicine's Symbolic Reality: On the Central Problem in the Philosophy of Medicine. *Inquiry* 16:206–13.

———. 1986. *Social Origins of Distress and Disease.* New Haven, CT: Yale University Press.

Kleinman, Arthur, Veena Das, and Margaret Lock. 1996. Introduction. In "Social Suffering," *Daedalus* 125 (1): 11–20.

Kleinman, Arthur, Veena Das, Margaret Lock, Pamela Reynolds, Mamphela Ramphele, eds. 1997. *Social Suffering.* Berkeley: University of California Press.

Kleinman, Arthur, and Joan Kleinman. 1996. The Appeal of Experience; the Dismay of Images: Cultural Appropriations of Suffering in Our Times. In "Social Suffering," *Daedalus* 125 (1): 1–24.

Kolakowski, Leszek. 1990. *Modernity on Endless Trial.* Chicago: University of Chicago Press.

Kristeva, Julia. 1982. *Powers of Horror: An Essay on Abjection.* New York: Columbia University Press.

———. 1989. *Black Sun: Depression and Melancholia.* Trans. Leon S. Roudiez. New York: Columbia University Press.

Lavie, Smadar, and Ted Swedenburg. 1996. *Displacement, Diaspora, and Geographies of Identity.* Durham, NC: Duke University Press.

Lambek, Michael. 2002. Nuriaty, the Saint, and the Sultan: Virtuous Subject and Subjective Virtuoso of the Post-Modern Colony, in *Postcolonial Subjectivities in Africa,* ed. Richard Werbner, 25–43. New York: Zed Books.

Lane, Christopher, ed. 1998. *The Psychoanalysis of Race.* New York: Columbia University Press.

Langford, Jean M. 2002. *Fluent Bodies.* Durham, NC: Duke University Press.

Lefebvre, Henri. 1991. *The Production of Space.* Oxford: Blackwell.

Leys, Ruth. 2000. *Trauma: A Genealogy.* Chicago: University of Chicago Press.

Limon, Jose E. 1998. *Dancing with the Devil.* Madison: University of Wisconsin Press.

Luhrmann, Tanya. 1996. *The Good Parsi.* Cambridge, MA: Harvard University Press.

Marcus, George E., ed. 2000. *PARA-SITES: A Casebook against Cynical Reasoning.* Chicago: University of Chicago Press.

Mani, Lata. 1990. Contentious Traditions: The Debate on Sati in Colonial India. In *Recasting Women: Essays in Indian Colonial History,* ed. K. Sangari and S. Vaid, 88–126. New Brunswick, NJ: Rutgers University Press.

Mbembe, Achille. 2001. *On the Postcolony.* Berkeley: University of California Press.

McClintock, Anne. 1992. The Angel of Progress: Pitfalls of the Term "Postcolonialism." *Social Text* 10 (2–3): 84–98.

———. 1995. *Imperial Leather: Race, Gender and Sexuality in the Imperial Conquest.* New York: Routledge.

McCulloch, Jock. 1995. *Colonial Psychiatry and the African Mind.* Cambridge: Cambridge University Press.

Mignolo, Walter. 1995. *The Darker Side of the Renaissance: Literacy, Territoriality, and Colonization.* Ann Arbor: University of Michigan Press.

Mills, James H. 2000. *Madness, Cannabis and Colonialism.* New York: St. Martin's Press.

Mintz, Sidney. 1985. *Sweetness and Power: The Place of Sugar in Modern History.* New York: Viking.

Mitchell, Timothy, ed. 2000. *Questions of Modernity.* Minneapolis: University of Minnesota Press.

Mohanty, Chandra Talpade. 1988. Under Western Eyes: Feminist Scholarship and Colonial Discourses. *Feminist Review* 30 (Autumn): 61–88.

Nandy, Ashis. 1983. *The Intimate Enemy: Loss and Recovery of Self Under Colonialism.* Delhi: Oxford University Press.

———. 1995. *The Savage Freud, and Other Essays on Possible and Retrievable Selves.* Princeton, NJ: Princeton University Press.

Okazaki, Akira. 2002. The Making and Unmaking of Consciousness: Nuba and Gamk Strategies for Survival in a Sudanese Borderland, in *Postcolonial Subjectivities in Africa*, ed. Richard Werbner, 63–83. New York: Zed Books.

O'Nell, Theresa. 1992. "Feeling Worthless": An Ethnographic Investigation of Depression and Problem Drinking at the Flathead Reservation. *Culture, Medicine and Psychiatry* 16:447–70.

———. 1996. *Disciplined Hearts.* Berkeley: University of California Press.

Ong, Aihwa. 1999. *Flexible Citizenship: The Cultural Logics of Transnationality.* Durham, NC: Duke University Press.

Ong, Aihwa, and Stephen J. Collier. 2005. *Global Assemblages.* Oxford and Malden MA: Blackwell Publishing.

Pagden, Anthony. 1986. *The Fall of Natural Man: The American Indian and the Origins of Contemporary Ethnology.* New York: Cambridge University Press.

Pandey, Gyan. 1992. In Defense of the Fragment: Writing about Hindu-Muslim Riots Today. *Representations* 37:27–55.

Pandolfo, Stefania. 1997. *Impasse of the Angels.* Chicago: University of Chicago Press.

Prakash, Gyan. 1990. *Bonded Histories: Genealogies of Labor Servitude in Colonial India.* New York: Cambridge University Press.

Prakash, Gyan, ed. 1995. *After Colonialism: Imperial Histories and Postcolonial Displacements.* Princeton, NJ: Princeton University Press.

Rabinow, Paul. 1996. *Essays on the Anthropology of Reason.* Princeton, NJ: Princeton University Press.

Robben, Antonius G. G. M., and Marcelo M. Suarez-Orozco. 2000. *Cultures under Siege: Collective Violence and Trauma.* New York: Cambridge University Press.

Rhodes, Lorna. 2004. *Total Confinement: Madness and Reason in the Maximum Security Prison.* Berkeley: University of California Press.

Sahlins, Peter. 1989. *Boundaries: The Making of France and Spain in the Pyrenees.* Berkeley: University of California Press.

Said, Edward W. 1993. *Culture and Imperialism.* London: Vintage Press.

Sartre, Jean-Paul. 1963. Preface to *The Wretched of the Earth,* by Frantz Fanon. Trans. Constance Farrington. New York: Grove Weidenfeld.

Sassen, Saskia. 1998. *Globalization and Its Discontents: Essays on the New Mobility of People and Money.* New York: New Press.

—. 2000. *The Global City: New York, London, Tokyo.* Princeton, NJ: Princeton University Press.

Shohat, Ella. 1992. Notes on the "Postcolonial." *Social Text* 10 (2–3): 99–113.

Siegel, James T. 1997. *Fetish, Recognition, Revolution.* Princeton, NJ: Princeton University Press.

—. 1998. *A New Criminal Type in Jakarta: Counter-Revolution Today.* Durham, NC: Duke University Press.

Smith, Graham, Vivien Law, Andrew Wilson, Annette Bohr, and Edward Allworth. 1998. *Nation-Building in the Post-Soviet Borderlands: The Politics of National Identities.* Cambridge: Cambridge University Press.

Smith, Linda Tuhiwai. 1999. *Decolonizing Methodologies: Research and Indigenous Peoples.* New York: Zed Books.

Spener, David and Kathleen Staudt. 1998. *The US-Mexico Border: Transcending Divisions, Contesting Identities.* Boulder, CO, and London: Lynne Reiner Publishers.

Spivak, Gayatri Chakravorty. 1988. Can the Subaltern Speak? In *Marxism and the Interpretation of Culture,* ed. C. Nelson and L. Grossberg, 271–313. Urbana: University of Illinois Press.

—. 1999. *A Critique of Postcolonial Reason: Toward a History of the Vanishing Present.* Cambridge, MA: Harvard University Press.

Steedly, Mary Margaret. 1999. The State of Culture Theory in the Anthropology of Southeast Asia. *Annual Review of Anthropology* 28:431–54.

Stiglitz, Joseph E. 2002. *Globalization and Its Discontents.* New York: W. W. Norton and Co.

Stoler, Ann. 1995. *Race and the Education of Desire: Foucault's "History of Sexuality" and the Colonial Order of Things.* Durham, NC: Duke University Press.

—. 2002. *Carnal Knowledge and Imperial Power: Race and the Intimate in Colonial Rule.* Berkeley: University of California Press.

————2006. *Haunted by Empire: Geographies of Intimacy in North American History.* Durham, NC: Duke University Press.

Stavrakakis, Yannis. 1999. *Lacan and the Political.* New York: Routledge.

Suarez-Orozco, Carola, and Marcelo M. Suarez-Orozco. 2001. *Children of Immigration.* Cambridge, MA: Harvard University Press.

Tambiah, Stanley J. 1996. *Leveling Crowds.* Berkeley: University of California Press.

Taussig, Michael. 1987. *Shamanism, Colonialism and the Wild Man: A Study in Terror and Healing.* Chicago: University of Chicago Press.

————. 1992. *The Nervous System.* New York: Routledge.

————. 1997. *The Magic of the State.* New York: Routledge.

————. 2003. *Law in a Lawless Land.* New York: The New Press.

Taylor, Charles. 2001. Two Theories of Modernity. In *Alternative Modernities*, ed. D. P. Gaonkar, 172–96. Durham, NC: Duke University Press.

Todorov, Tzvetan. 1984. *The Conquest of America: The Question of the Other.* Trans. Richard Howard. New York: Harper Perennial.

Visvanathan, Gauri. 1989. *Masks of Conquest: Literary Study and British Rule in India.* New York: Columbia University Press.

Visveswaran, Kamala. 1994. *Fictions of Feminist Ethnography.* Madison: University of Wisconsin Press.

Warren, Kay B., ed. 1993. *The Violence Within: Cultural and Political Opposition in Divided Nations.* Boulder, CO: Westview Press.

Werbner, Richard, ed. 2002. *Postcolonial Subjectivities in Africa.* New York: Zed Books.

Whitbeck, Les. B., Gary Adams, Dan R. Hoyt. 2004. Conceptualizing and Measuring Historical Trauma among American Indian People. *American Journal of Community Psychology* 33 (3/4): 119–30.

Wilson, Thomas, and Hastings Donnan. 1998. *Border Identities: Nation and State at International Frontiers.* Cambridge: Cambridge University Press.

Winichakul, Thongchai. 1994. *Siam Mapped: A History of the Geo-Body of a Nation.* Honolulu: University of Hawaii Press.

Wolf, Eric. 1982. Europe and the People without History. Berkeley: University of California Press.

Young, Allan. 1995. *The Harmony of Illusions: Inventing Post-Traumatic Stress Disorder.* Princeton, NJ: Princeton University Press.

Žižek, Slavoj. 1997. *The Plague of Fantasies.* New York: Verso.

————. 1998. *The Ticklish Subject: The Absent Center of Political Ontology.* New York: Verso.

————. 1999. *The Ticklish Subject: The Absent Centre of Political Ontology.* London: Verso.

PART I: DISORDERED STATES

Reflections on Violence in Postdictatorial Spain

Begoña Aretxaga

When I was invited to take part in this seminar I was happy to have an opportunity to discuss some of my current work with former colleagues and friends. I have been increasingly preoccupied with the problem of madness as it plays and as it is displayed in the theater of politics. This is for me the beginning of a dialogue about this issue that one could broadly call "politics and madness." In this sense what I am speaking about today is more the beginning of a formulation than a crafted thesis.

One of my worries as I started to think about this seminar was that I know close to nothing about postcolonial psychiatry except perhaps for the work of that major and wonderful theorist of coloniality, Frantz Fanon. And to make matters worse I am not properly speaking about questions of postcoloniality either, even though I know a bit more about this issue, having worked for a long while in Ireland, the land of "Saints, Scholars and Schizophrenics" as Nancy Scheper-Hughes (1979) dubbed it, and known most recently as the land of crazy violence and terrorism.

But it is not about Ireland that I want to speak today but my current research in the Basque Country of Spain. The Basque Country is not a colonial or

Begoña Aretxaga contributed this chapter—a slightly revised version of her initial seminar presentation—for publication in Postcolonial Disorders in June 2002. The editors thank Michele Levine for assistance with bibliographic edits and Sarah Pinto for minor copy editing. Overall, very few changes have been made to the submitted manuscript and to Professor Aretxaga's original talk, delivered on December 1, 2000, at the Friday Morning Seminar on Medical Anthropology and Cultural Psychiatry.

postcolonial setting, although some Basque radicals think of the Basque Country in these terms. Yet one could argue that after thirty-six years of dictatorship Spain has gone through a veritable change of status that transformed the country into another state of being. One could say that the series of issues that arise out of this transition and transformation from a totalitarian to a democratic polity have a family resemblance to at least some issues arising out of the postcolonial setting. At the risk of using postcoloniality here as a metaphor of a particular existential state let me say nevertheless that something that characterizes the postcolonial state and the transitional state of countries like Spain or those of the former socialist bloc is a marginal status within the global political and economic order. The second related characteristic is a certain dislocation and often violent disarray of things. It is a state in which the logical order of Cartesian thinking doesn't quite work and yet doesn't quite not work either. It is a state in which things are a little off where they should be and sometimes very much off, so that the state of things seems crazy. And it is frequently through the trope of madness that these "altered states" are made sense of. It is this discourse on madness, national identity, and statehood that I am trying to think about here. What does this discourse say about both the lived experience of politics in these altered states (transitional, changed states) and about the changing nature of the state in our postmodern global world (Fabian 2000; Siegel 1998; Bhabha 1994; Fanon 1967; Geertz 1973)?

I have been thinking about the question of political madness because it has become a privileged trope in the current discourse on Basque violence, particularly since the guerrilla organization ETA called off a year-and-a-half-long cease-fire in December 1999 and initiated an all-out campaign for independence, NOW, that has reached the toll of twenty assassinations so far as well as a high number of arsonist attacks and widespread intimidation. Many of the victims are politicians, some journalists, some of them with leftist histories. None of the targets are particularly salient in the apparatus of power. There is something profoundly difficult to understand about this kind of violence, an incomprehensible logic that seems out of sync with the reality of the majority of the population in the Basque Country and falls into the space of unreason and the out of control called madness. ETA has emerged after the cease-fire as a particularly callous and radical force that seems to have disposed of its usual parameters for legitimate targets. Although the political organizations that are associated with ETA continue to demand a political negotiation to end the violence, the virulence of the violence unleashed by ETA seems to cancel any possible negotiation. Furthermore, ETA's violence has not spared former nationalist allies, creating the puzzling result of reinforcing the Spanish right wing in the Basque Country and debilitating the social fabric of the country. In other words, rather than strengthening, the violence of ETA and of young activists has the effect of debilitating nationalist aspirations and the possible avenues to achieve them. So paradoxical are their politics that many have suspected that ETA must have been infiltrated by the Spanish state, which would like to see the end of Basque nationalism, not only its radical side but its conservative and democratic sector as well. The reaction of commentators is that radical nationalists have gone mad. But why should the political discussion about the meaning of violence in the Basque Country be situated in the field of rationality versus madness? What exactly is insane about it? What is the structure of this madness? This discourse of madness is not arbitrary; it makes its appearance during the 1990s at a moment when a Basque police force enters the scene of Basque politics and a moment when a new youth movement emerges as an aggressive nationalist force.

BACKGROUND

First let me situate very briefly what I am talking about by giving you some sociological background: ETA was born in 1959 as a response to brutal political and cultural repression by the military regime of Francisco Franco. It did not begin its armed operations, however, until 1969, a decade later. ETA's ultimate goal was the unification of the French and Spanish Basque provinces into an independent Basque Country. In practice, however, its actions were antidictatorial. Most of ETA's targets from 1969 to 1975, when Franco died, were members of the security forces. The most spectacular of such actions was the assassination of Admiral Luis Carrero Blanco in 1974, right hand and only possible successor of General Franco in the military regime. With Carrero Blanco out of the way the small possibility of continuation of the military regime in Spain was eliminated. After the death of Franco in 1975 Spain undertook a period of reform, called not very originally La Reforma (The Reform). In the Basque Country, La Reforma was met with a great deal of resistance and suspicion on the part of a radicalized population with a strong nationalist consciousness. The Basque Country, one of the most industrialized and densely populated areas of Spain, was also one of the most politicized. It had a strong labor movement, a potent nationalist movement, and a variety of active social movements emerging in the political arena. In the Basque Country the population was divided between a reform of the former regime that would transition the country to a parliamentary democracy and a ruptura, a firm rupture with the structures of the former regime. I don't have the time to get into this; suffice it to say that the reform strategy won, but not without trouble, and thus the constitution of the current democratic regime was endorsed by the Spanish people in a referendum held in 1977, but was rejected in the Basque Country because it did not contemplate the right to self-determination for the *nationalidades* or ethnic regions within the Spanish state, that is, Catalunya, the Basque Country, Galizia, and so on. Still, it did contemplate a process of increasing regional autonomy, and during the following decade the Basque Country developed what could be considered the embryonic structures of a state, a government and parliament and even its own police force, judicial, and educational apparatuses. True, all of them were still subordinated to the Spanish constitution and legislation, but they enjoyed a considerable degree of autonomy. In this scenario, where the goal of an independent Basque Country could be pursued through the conventions of democratic politics, ETA's armed strategy was expected to stop. But it did not. In fact during the first decade of the reform it escalated and radicalized. Its rationale was that the regime had not really changed. Under the appearance of democracy there was still a dictatorial state that manifested itself in the practices of unwarranted arrest, torture, and paramilitary assassination, not to mention the existence of over five hundred Basque political prisoners dispersed throughout Spain. This rationale was aided by the succession of emergency legislation in the Basque Country, which permitted the infringement of civil and human rights of those accused of having any kind of relation with Basque terrorism. The repressive legislation and tactics were now specifically directed to people and organizations associated with radical nationalism and sympathetic to ETA. In spite of the hard blows suffered by radical nationalists during the period of the dirty war, ETA survived and seemed to attract the sympathy of an emerging, vibrant youth movement. These radical nationalist youth became during the 1990s the stars of the Basque political theater. Known as *encapuchados* because they wore hoods to cover their heads, these youths became the subjects of a new kind of violence—characterized by arson attacks on public buildings and services as well as on police vehicles, and rioting—a violence that transgressed the moral boundaries of local communities by intimidating and attacking neighbors and peers who opposed their politics, including other nationalists. The novelty of this violence, in addition to massive use of arson, was that it was directed mostly to those persons, institutions, and symbols associated with the Basque government and that by association were linked to a figurative and potential Basque state. Prominent among them was the *ertzaintza*, the Basque police. Let me say few words about them.

The development of a Basque police force was considered crucial in resolving the problem of terrorism, which had received so much support from the repressive tactics of the state police forces. The Basque police force is young, just above a decade old. The first year that officers graduated from the Basque police academy was 1988. The Basque police were intended to be the trusted civil police that the Basque Country never had. Unlike the officers of the Spanish police forces who were born and raised in other parts of Spain and were in the Basque Country only for a transitory service period, the young members of the Basque police were local men and women. Unlike the Spanish police forces who lived in their own headquarters at the outskirts of the community, the *ertzaintza* lived interspersed with the local population in towns and cities, had their families and friends within the Basque geography, and thought of themselves as an integral part of a local and (Basque) national community. The Spanish police forces identified as Spanish, the Basque police officers identified as Basque. As the new Basque police developed in numbers and in the complexity of functions they assumed, they also were called for riot control and antiterrorist struggle. These more specialized interventions entailed the deployment of violence against Basque people, mostly Basque radical nationalists, who were the main actors in political demonstrations, riots, and of course terrorist violence.

The police work of the Basque police has had a profound effect in reorganizing the "scene of violence" in the imaginary of radical nationalists. Until the introduction of the Basque police, radical nationalists conceptualized the scene of violence in the Basque Country as a liberation struggle in which Basques defended themselves and fought against the oppressive forces of the Spanish state. At a metonymic level this transcendental national struggle was represented by the riots in which Basque radicals confronted Spanish police. With the *ertzaintza* assuming the labors formerly performed by the Spanish police, the scene of violence took a more complex form. Now the confrontation was one between Basques: radical nationalists and Basque government. In towns and villages this confrontation between political projects and definitions of Basqueness translated into a confrontation between neighbors, those Basques supporting the radical politics and violence of the armed group ETA and those supporting the Basque government and against ETA. The confrontation between the Spanish state and Basque radicalism had not disappeared but was complicated by the emergence of a more troublesome conflict among different kinds of nationalists.

In September 1998, ETA, facing increasing hostility and isolation, called a cease-fire as part of a new coalition agreement with conservative nationalists (PNV and EA) dominant in the government. Radical nationalist political fate changed overnight with the cease-fire. Their cessation of violence and coalition with the other major nationalist parties won them an increased number of votes in the following elections, placing them as the second-largest nationalist force. Their support made possible a nationalist government in the Basque Country that could govern without the support of Spanish parties, socialist and conservative. This was the first time that such a configuration was achieved in the Basque Country. From night to day, the radical nationalists had passed from a marginalized force to a growing central player. Political possibility was in the air and the end of violence triggered within the political culture of the Basque Country a new excitement. The Spanish government stalled on the negotiations for a definite peace, using as an excuse that youth violence and intimidation—now called low-intensity terrorism—had not disappeared. Frustrating popular expectations in the Basque Country, the Spanish state seemed to do everything possible to indeed deter the peace process.

After more than a year of lack of progress on a possible negotiation between ETA and the Spanish government, ETA called off the cease-fire on the third of December, 1999. A few months later ETA published a *communicado* explaining that the cease-fire did not have as a goal the achievement of peace but the building of a sovereign Basque state. They said that they ended the cease-fire because *el proceso*, "the process" (raising Kafkaesque echoes), was stalled by the PNV, their nationalist allies who wanted to transform it into a mere peace process. They also said that the time was ripe to act as de facto sovereign. This action seemed to be so much against their own political rationale of advancing toward Basque independent sovereignty that it created puzzlement and prompted madness as an explanation. After the cease-fire, ETA emerged radicalized and intransigent in its actions, targeting politicians, journalists, and former state officials. The moral controls that seemed to have bound political violence to certain targets were dissolved. Anybody who spoke or campaigned against Basque independence or radical nationalism seemed to be a legitimate target. Radical nationalists were out of their minds.

But what defined this state of insanity? The discourse of madness in relation to Basque nationalist violence is linked to an incomprehensible and traumatic excess, an eruption within the familiar order that defamiliarizes it. One example will be the petrol bombing of a van of *ertzaintza* by radical nationalists. The van caught fire and the policemen trapped inside suffered major burns. One of the policemen was the brother of one of the assailants. It is also linked to loss of touch with reality as exemplified in ETA's attempt to assert the sovereignty of the Basque Country against the majority of the population. What I would like to argue is that the madness of radical nationalists does not reside in an excess of violence in the pursuit of an independent nation, nor in the distortion of a political reality that demands the end of nationalist violence rather than the intensification of it. Their madness does not reside in believing that they are the true embodiment of the Basque nation and that the conditions for their liberation are all set for it to happen now. My argument is that the kernel of this madness is something much more problematic and secret, something that indeed must remain hidden: the madness of radical nationalists in my country is the manifestation of a profound ambivalence toward the nation-state form they are pursuing so ferociously. I would argue that the crazy violence of these young radicals might be less incomprehensible if we see it as the manifestation of a phantom, the presence of an absence, the presence of a traumatic history that remains not altogether resolved. I am speaking here of the phantom of the dictatorship—recurrently invoked as a permanent present by young radicals who believe the Spanish democracy is fascist at its core. The specter of the dictatorship is invoked too by those who oppose the violence of ETA and young radicals who see them as the embodiment of the fear and authoritarianism experienced under Franco. In either case it would be difficult to miss the recurrent allusion to this past that has not completely disappeared and that the violence of radical nationalists (and the state) pushes to the surface as something one would like to ignore but cannot cease to feel.

Nicholas Abraham and Maria Torok (1959) have written extensively about the phantom as a secret that remains buried and can be passed from generation to generation, inherited as it were in an unconscious way, making its presence felt even when there is no conscious knowledge of it. I find this notion of the phantom as a secret extremely helpful in thinking about certain political dynamics and political effects that remain bewildering, if not incomprehensible—needless to say the area of nationalist violence and the state is permeated by secrets and phantomic presences. You might be wondering what kind of secret this phantom represents. I cannot go fully into this question, which I began to analyze in two other pieces, but I would suggest, because I think it is important for the argument, that this secret has to do with the tainted birth of democracy in Spain. I will be more explicit: the secret that the whole political system endeavors to suppress is that the Spanish democracy was the result of a pact with Francoist forces that did not dispose of the former structures but used them in its favor. The monarchy itself, today a symbol of the democracy, was deposed by Franco and precluded the possibility of a return to a republic, which was after all the legitimate political form popularly elected before Franco's military coup overthrew it. This sense of continuity has triggered anxiety at various moments in the short life of the democracy and marks a point of uncertainty and vulnerability, a sense of not being totally separate from the former regime. Perhaps there is here a family resemblance to what we have come to know as a postcolonial condition, one that Homi Bhabha (1994) describes as characterized by ambivalence. I will come back to this ambivalence from a different angle later. But now I would like to return to the question of madness in relation to Basque political violence, which was the question that led us to the issue of the phantom in the first place.

The question of madness is linked to forms of violence that defy comprehension and produce shock. It is also linked to a discourse in which the relation to reality seems fractured. In relation to radical nationalism, madness begins to figure prominently in association with the development of practices of *kale borroka* (street fighting or urban guerrilla) by an increasingly radicalized youth. These *encapuchados*, mentioned earlier, emerged as political actors after 1992, when the leadership of ETA was arrested. By the second half of the decade it had become a quotidian scene in towns and cities to see a group of youngsters coming into the central streets and plazas, their faces covered with hoods and kerchiefs and their hands full of Molotov cocktails destined to burn public buses and telephone booths, attack Law Court buildings, ATMs, head-quarters of opposing political parties, and police vehicles—permanently sta-tioned in the centers of public space—and disappear as swiftly as they had appeared. The *encapuchados* call this form of violence sabotage, in contraposition to the mass media, which has characterized the violence as vandalism. For the *encapuchados* it is sabotage against the state. During 1995 and 1996, there were 408 and 440 sabotages performed according to the counts of the provincial attorney's office, and they increased 25 percent during 1997 and continued during the ETA cease-fire. During my fieldwork in 1997, the violence of the *encapuchados* was impossible for most people to understand, and it still is. It rep-resented a block, an epistemological rupture in the political culture of the Basque Country, or as my friend Juana said, "it shatters your mental schemes," provoking an apprehension, an eerie feeling triggered not so much by the actual actions of violence but by their ghostly and uncontrolled character, the simultaneous feeling of close familiarity and utter estrangement evoked by the young *encapuchados*. The uncanny characteristic of the *encapuchados* is that their targets are not so much obvious Spanish institutions or personalities but those within the sphere of nationalism that are considered associated with the enemy state. Thus, for example, the Basque police became a favorite target, but so did institutions that, while associated with the state (such as local judicial build-ings), remain under the jurisdiction of the Basque government. Similarly, members of the moderate PNV became objects of intimidation. This is signifi-cant because in spite of their ideological and political rivalry they remain part of what is often described as "the nationalist family." So, indeed, the violence of the *encapuchados* has the uncanny character of family violence, of violence per-petrated by a familiar turned stranger.

Several events have become emblematic of this madness and the rupture in the structure of the external world that they seem to represent. In March 1995 a group of *encapuchados* attacked a van of the *ertzaintza* with Molotov cocktails. The van caught fire and five officers were seriously wounded. The van lost control and hit two bystanders who were also seriously wounded. The attack was trau-matic and the councilor of the interior declared the situation created by these youngsters "dramatic and incomprehensible" (*DiarioVasco*, 3/26/95). The editorial of the *Diario Vasco* (the most widely read newspaper) speaks of "a maddening strategy of urban warfare" (3/26/95), while the mayor of the town (Renteria) speaks of a war paranoia suffered by radical nationalists (3/26/95). Radicals accuse the *ertzaintza* of constant harassment and say they are crazy. Many talked to me about the madness of the *ertzaintza*.

The most shaking and emblematic case of these mirroring positions of violent madness was that of Mikel Otegi, a radical youth from a small village in the Basque Country who, in December 1995, killed two *ertzaintzas* in "a lapse of consciousness," an act that the jury considered the product of transitory insanity and thus an act for which he was not responsible. It was a crime that received heightened attention in the mass media, a traumatic action that rippled social life with a wave of panic and anxiety about identity, about terrorism, about reality, about the future. In his deposition to the judge, Otegi could only remember that at some point he "lost it" (*se salió de sus casillas*). He said that he saw the two *ertzaintzas* on the side of the road, less than a mile from his farmhouse, when he was driving home in the morning. He said that when he arrived home he went to bed. Then he heard the dogs bark, came out of the house to see what was happening, and saw the two *ertzaintzas*, one of them near his car. According to his testimony, the *ertzaintzas* asked for his identification and told him to go with them. Otegi told them to go away but the *ertzaintzas*, he said, did not pay attention to him. He then "lost it," went inside the house and does not remember what happened next. Two years later Otegi testified at the trial that one of the policemen had drawn a gun in the course of the discussion and he became very frightened and went back to his house, got his hunting gun, and came out again. It was at that point when he and the policemen were facing each other that he lost consciousness (*Diario Vasco*, 2/25/97). Otegi is also strangely absent from his own actions, having killed literally in a lapse of consciousness. It is this absent presence that haunts the social imagination in the Basque Country, for it seems not only to pervade the whole case, infusing it with phantasmagoric and uncanny qualities, but to pervade the whole domain of political violence in the Basque Country as well. The shocking effect of Otegi's killing was articulated in the language of madness. "He is mad" was the first thing my sister said. Juana, who was born and raised in the same town as Otegi, also thought him crazy and links his madness to hidden domestic violence:

> Everybody knew that youth, so did I, since I was a kid because my father
> sold his family hay for the animals. His farmhouse is behind my house. His
> father was very authoritarian, one of those who beat the children quite
> often, and Mikel was one of those who was in the first line of riots and he
> was always imprecating the *ertzaintza*. He hated the *ertzaintza*. He was the kind
> that throw stones, break things, the kind that when something appeared

broken in the town everybody suspected that Mikel had something to do with it. I can understand that one has a moment of madness and kills somebody, but what I don't understand is that the same day there is a demonstration in my town of people demanding "*Mikel askatu*" [Mikel free], *that is mentally shattering [te rompe los esquemas*], you say . . . but what is happening here?! Are we all crazy? Is this happening here? In my town? Not in the USA or some remote place that you see in the television news, but my town!

In Juana's narrative the discourse of madness is both asserted and problematized. For if Juana links Otegi's craziness to the intimacy of family violence, she also links political violence to a kind of collective madness, one that de-realizes reality all the more for occurring within the boundaries of the socially familiar. Thus, in Juana's narrative, family violence and nationalist violence are linked by multiple associations. First in the person of Otegi, who partakes of both, second in the identification of the radical nationalist movement with Otegi's predicament, third in the social intimacy that renders Otegi's killings and nationalist violence a shock—like a family murder. These associative links complicate the attribution of the crime to individual insanity. For if Otegi's madness could be understood, it was more difficult to understand the apparent madness of the people who identified with him and demanded his freedom. And more threatening too. For Juana, individual madness does not threaten the premises of the social order; collective madness, however, blurs the very distinction between madness and sanity and thus turns reality upside down.

Juana's associations are significant because the family has been a recurrent metaphor of the Basque nation in the rhetoric of both moderate and radical nationalists—law-abiding and law-transgressing nationalists. If the intimacy of family is linked to the nation in both Juana's narrative and the rhetoric of nationalism, so is political violence tied to the intimacy of family in the discourses following Otegi's killing. While Basque newspapers emphasize the fear of fratricide, Spanish newspapers emphasize the link between radical nationalism and madness. *El País*, for example, wrote under the headline "fertile ground for paranoia" that "the killings in Itsasondo suggest the existence of a relation between the individual paranoia suffered by the killer and the paranoia collectively practiced by those who since long ago have incited to attack the officers of the *ertzaintza*" (12/11/95). *El Mundo* reported, "the presumed assassin, who had been arrested as a result of a confrontation with the Basque police, had just had a conflict with an *ertzaintza* whom he called '*zipaio*' [an insult signifying betrayer by which the *ertzaintza* is habitually addressed by radical nationalists]" (12/11/95). For *El Mundo* "the event is the last expression of the conflict that has pitted radical youth against the *ertzaintza* since ETA [the nationalist armed group] made the *ertzaintza* a target of its violence" (12/11/95). Experts and politicians reinforced this idea of madness: Javier Elzo, a well-known sociologist, noted that "the crime points to two societies increasingly estranged from each other," fearing "the possibility of confrontation between two parts [of Basque society]" (*El País*, 12/11/95). For a professor of psychiatry at the Basque University, the killing expressed "a pathology of delirious ideas" among radical nationalists. Underlying the opinions and comments of scientific experts and political authorities there is an opposition between reason and madness—the reason of democratic coexistence against the madness of nationalist violence. The Councilor of the Interior of the Basque government, for example, affirmed that the killing "does not have an explanation other than the madness of the youth in the radical movement, so fanatic that they have lost reason." The crime was also interpreted in the discourse of mainstream newspapers as the logical consequence of a climate of violence unleashed by Basque radical nationalists against the Basque police: "The double assassination cannot be abstracted from the context of hostility against the *ertzaintza* promoted by the current strategy of the MLNV [Movimiento de Liberación National Vasco/Basque Movement of National Liberation] and it has devastating consequences for peaceful and civilized coexistence. The danger is that this seed of hate, appealing to some psyches that then degenerate into paranoid pathology, will be justified by attributing to it a political motivation." For radical nationalists, Otegi's killings are also the result of madness, but of the madness of the *ertzaintza*, which is to say the madness of the Basque government, which by association is the madness of the Basque state: "they should be in the hands of a psychiatrist for sending 7,000 *cipayos* [a derogatory name for the *ertzaintza*] to act brutally."

The villagers are quoted saying that the boy was a normal boy, just like any other, and his friends said that he was suffocated by the harassment of the *ertzaintza*. The discourse of madness articulates itself around polarized and mirroring positions within the nationalist family. Otegi was as absent from the narrative about his crime as he was from the scene of the crime, the killings being in his own words "an unconscious act." Jaques Lacan (1977: 54) has defined the unconscious as the discourse of the other, which emerges precisely in the gaps, in the blanks, of personal and collective histories. If Otegi's double crime is the effect of an agency produced in the gap of (political) consciousness, then one could say that this speechless murder—and much of the current violence—constitutes, in fact, a discourse, the discourse of the unconscious in the field of Basque politics. Something is being said through Otegi's double murder, but what is it that is being said? I want to take seriously this figure of madness not as a language of dismissal of what defies comprehension within political culture, but as a domain of knowledge. I want to suggest that, contrary to what many people think, this crazy violence is not meaningless. It has a structure and what is at stake in it pertains to the order of knowledge, a knowledge that the subject (the political subject) does not want to know. Johannes Fabian (2000) has made a related argument, namely that the knowledge produced in the colonial encounter was not the product of rational epistemologies but was the outcome of various states of insanity. So, in which way can we begin to approach this knowledge?

Here I would like to focus on a term, a signifier, a metaphor that appears to organize (and disorganize) the whole scenario of this nationalist madness. This is the term *cipayo*, used to address Basque policemen, a term whose significance goes far beyond that of a simple insult. In this analysis I assume two things: (1) that madness is characterized by a fault, a point of rupture in the structure of the external world that finds itself patched over by fantasy (Lacan 1977); and (2) that culture (and political culture specifically) might function in ways analogous to that of the dream. That is, the articulation of the struggles and anxieties that characterize it might well follow the principles of condensation and displacement (Obeyesekere 1990). In the field of language and cultural discourse these major mechanisms of symbolization are translated as metaphor and metonymy (Fernandez 1974, 1986; Lacan 1977). For Lacan, metonymic articulation—the work of displacement—is at the base of figuration, of the dream work and of course of the work of political culture. For him "the emergence of this always hidden substrate that is metonymy" is a condition for the investigation of both the psychosis and the neurosis. The remainder of this paper is an attempt at tracking those hidden metonymic associations that trace a subjective structure present in nationalist violence and that articulate a knowledge that remains hidden, a knowledge that the political subject in question does not want to know.

During the 1990s the *ertzaintza* proved itself as a police force that could violently repress demonstrations, gather intelligence, and conduct antiterrorist operations. In other words it proved capable of conducting the same functions as the Spanish police. This meant that the *ertzaintza*, this metonymy of a desired Basque state, used violence against other Basques, and more specifically against radical nationalists, the very people who most intensely desired an independent Basque state. In acting as metonymy of the state, the *ertzaintza* introduced a threatening shift in the culture of Basque nationalism, which like other nationalisms rests on the fraternal unity of the imagined Basque nation (Anderson 1983). The rhetoric of a unitary national subject—Basque people—against the oppressive Spanish state was seriously threatened by the existence of a national police acting against nationalists.

At the beginning of the 1990s the special antiterrorist unit of the *ertzaintza* killed one member of ETA while attempting an arrest. The killing had the effect of a shock for Basque radicals, for it meant that the political conflict in the Basque Country could not be articulated as one existing between a national self and a dominating Other, but as one existing within the national self itself. In performing as state (Basque state), the *ertzaintza* had introduced an unbearable ambiguity at the core of the nation. Moreover, this ambiguity was compounded by the fact that this (Basque) "state" was enforcing Spanish law and thus it could be seen as Spanish as well as Basque. It was at this point that the metaphor *cipayo* appeared on the scene. This metaphor had the mission of covering up this ambiguity, best articulated as the problematic character of national identity, riddled as it is with unrecognized difference. It was to do so by redrawing the boundaries of identity in a rigid manner so that difference was strictly positioned outside the boundaries of national identity and not within it.

CIPAYO: THE INTOLERABLE AMBIGUITY OF BEING

I first encountered the term *cipayo* in 1993 when I was spending part of the summer in the Basque Country. It was part of graffiti painted on the wall of a public building that read "*cipayos asesinos.*" I remember my puzzlement, for the graffiti pointed at something and somebody that seemed important to Basque political culture and about which I knew nothing in spite of my intimate knowledge of that culture. I asked the friend who was accompanying me at the time, "Who were these mysterious *cipayos?*" I learned from her that *cipayos* was the name given to the *ertzaintza* by radical nationalists. *Cipayos*, she said, was the name for the soldiers of Indian origin serving in the British colonial army (*sipahi*). The graffiti began to make sense. Radical nationalists were accusing the *ertzaintza* of violent betrayal. I was still unaware of the motivations triggering such metaphoric predication, much less the train of its complex associations. But after I saw its accusatory presence for the first time, it was suddenly all around me. I realized that radical nationalists habitually referred to the *ertzaintza* as *cipayos* in their everyday speech. This, I thought, was more than a passing accusation. The transmutation of identity operated by metaphoric predication appeared to be taking root, if not already encrusted, in the everyday political culture of radical nationalists. Then I saw them. It was in Renteria, an industrial town close to San Sebastian, where I had gone to have dinner with a group of women at one of the many local *sociedades*, a mixture of bar/restaurant and social club organized as a cooperative of members. It was not far from the *sociedad* that I saw a gathering of policemen in what looked to me like Spider-man outfits. Their uniforms were different from those of the familiar Spanish police. They were dressed in full riot gear: red and black uniforms, boots, helmets, bulletproof vests, riot arms, and faces covered with black balaclavas. They were the *cipayos*, I was told, and the reason they were there was because there was a demonstration by radical nationalists scheduled to take place that evening. My only image of the *ertzaintza* until that moment was that of harmless men and women dressed in a rather folkloric fashion with white shirts and Basque berets, bereft of arms and standing in front of local government buildings. I had obviously missed some important developments during my stay out of the country. Equally interesting was the talk that was following my inquiries about the *ertzaintza*. My friends were preoccupied with what they thought to be a growing animosity between radical nationalists supporting the violence of ETA and other nationalists who supported the established autonomous institutions. The fabric of social life, so tight in the Basque Country, was dangerously rupturing and my friends feared what they called a Balkanization of the Basque Country. *Cipayo* was associated now with another metaphor of Balkanization.

In the political culture of the Basque Country, the metaphor of *cipayo* appears as both a manifestation of an anxiety about the rupturing of identity and an attempt to repair it. In this sense, a metaphor can also be a form of concealment. In this case what *cipayo* conceals are different thoughts and feelings people have about what it means to be Basque. This alterity at the core of ethnic identity translates into divergent political projects. The metaphor of *cipayo* negates that alterity and symptomatizes a profound social anxiety about it. By predicating the identity of traitor onto the Basque police, radical nationalists are suggesting that the Basque police are not truly Basque. By extension, those who support it are not truly Basque, including the Basque government, which is directly responsible for the actions of the *ertzaintza*. What is being affirmed is a unitary dogmatic vision of Basque identity that denies the appearances, contradictions, or practices of power. But in so emphatically denying difference, radical nationalists reproduced it by making it a constant presence.

NATIONALIST AMBIVALENCE:
THE COLONY WE NEVER WERE

There are two dimensions to the image of *cipayo* that require further exploration if we want to understand what this metaphor *does* in the field of Basque political culture. One is the image itself, the other is the predication of betrayal. Here I move to what Jane Gallop has called "a metonymic reading": "whereas a metaphoric interpretation consists in supplying another signifier which the signifier in the text stands for [e.g., *cipayo* represents *ertzaintza*, in our case] a metonymic interpretation supplies a whole context of associations" (1985: 129). Let's then look more carefully into this context. Radical nationalists could, of course, call the Basque police simply "traitors" or simply "assassins," as the Spanish police were called in response to outrageous acts of violence. Or they could predicate on them the metaphor of *txakurra* (dog), long used to debase the police to the category of the subhuman, thus legitimating the use of violence against them.[1] Instead of direct accusations or familiar metaphors that could have equally legitimized violence against the *ertzaintza*, they chose the new, rather obscure image of *cipayo*.

What the image of *cipayo* does that the other images do not is to frame the political conflict in the Basque Country in colonial terms. By predicating on the *ertzaintza* the identity of *cipayos*, radical nationalists are not only casting on them the identity of betrayers, they are also positing a relation of analogy between the Basque Country and colonial India. In so doing they are stating that the Basque Country is a part of the Spanish state by virtue of a colonial relation. By virtue of its inherent domination, this colonial relation is one of polarized opposition between colonizers and colonized that admits no middle ground. In the argument constructed by these images, the Basque Country remains colonized as long as it remains part of the Spanish state, regardless of how autonomous its autonomous institutions might be. In this logic, the Basque government and Basque parliament are not truly Basque as long as they remain part of Spain. The *ertzaintza* are betrayers because they act in the interest of a colonizer state when they suppress the resistance of radical nationalists. The metaphor of *cipayo* establishes a colonial scenario by establishing a metonymic link between the Basque Country and Spain. In this fantasy scenario, national identity is delineated along a polarized line—Basque/Spanish—that does not admit mediation. In this situation, violence is legitimized by the identification of Basque with the colonized who must use any means to get rid of the colonizer. In this polarized scenario, the predication of betrayal legitimizes violence against the Basque police, who by virtue of their subordination to the Spanish state are not Basque anymore. And yet the predication of betrayal reasserts the Basqueness of the *ertzaintza*, for one cannot betray those with whom there is no intimate connection.

The associative chain described above has led to a political and social situation of increasing polarization, hostility, and violence within the Basque Country since the 1990s. In some ways, this revival of colonial logic is a regression to the political logic predominant in the radical nationalism of the late 1960s and early 1970s when Spain was still under a dictatorship and the Basque Country was the site of a brutal cultural and political repression. What is ironic is that this logic would surface at a moment when the Basque Country enjoys a great deal of freedom in organizing its cultural, social, and political affairs. But this is also a moment when the meaning of Basqueness is not taken for granted but is subject to debate and contestation, a moment of rearticulation of what it means to be Basque in an increasingly globalized world. What the metaphor of *cipayo* conceals is the anxiety and uncertainty that such rearticulation produces, the fear that in developing a flexible and multiple identity the line between self and other might be blurred and one's identity might disappear altogether.

For radical nationalists the existence of autonomous institutions such as Basque government, parliament, and police within the boundaries of the Spanish nation-state poses a threat because, while they are a metonymy of the Basque state that radical nationalists are fighting to achieve, they are also part of the Spanish state, indeed a salient trait of Spanish contemporary identity. Radical nationalists find threatening the ambiguity of institutions that represent at once the imagined Basque nation and the law of the Spanish state. It is this ambiguity that radical nationalists have tried desperately to erase through the colonial scenario arising out of the metaphor of *cipayo*. But it could be also that what is really feared and resisted is the dissolution of a phantasmic unity of identity, bound to occur with the disappearance of an outside enemy.

The colonial scenario evoked by the metaphor *cipayo* is also linked by metonymic contiguity to the scenario of the independent nation. This is a scenario where the unity of the anticolonial struggle gives rise to internal division, struggles of power, and violence. (India is a good example, and it is telling that the chosen image to accuse the *ertzaintza* would be taken from that context.) One could argue that the actual political reality of the Basque Country, with its autonomous institutions, political parties, and force relations, constitutes a preview of the independent nation. The violent resistance of radical nationalists to this scenario of nationhood by predicating a colonial situation would suggest that a resistance to achieving an independent nation coexists with a desire to form it. Thus, if *cipayo* attempts to dispel political ambiguity it also manifests profound ambivalence toward the national object. This would explain why the growing indiscriminate violence of radical nationalists threatens to destroy the very nation it purports to construct. During the last years this violence has not only damaged the fabric of social relations considerably, it has also played in favor of antinationalist parties who have notably risen in the last elections.[2] Let me explore the play of ambiguity and ambivalence a bit further by returning to the treacherous identity that *cipayo* predicates.

NATIONAL INTIMACY

I have said that *cipayo* attempts to dispel the ambiguity of a Basque "state" that is simultaneously Spanish. It does so by effecting a move that divests the *ertzaintza* (metonymy of the Basque state) of Basque identity by accusing them of betrayal and placing them firmly on the Spanish side of the Basque/Spanish boundary. Once this is done the *ertzaintza* become a legitimate target of nationalist violence and the boundaries of national identity are clearly reestablished. During the last years the *ertzaintza* have indeed become ritualized targets of radical nationalists' harassment and violence. And yet, as I said before, the notion of betrayal that *cipayo* conveys suggests a bond, a (national) intimacy that cannot quite be shaken out. Unlike the invader, or the stranger, the traitor retains a trace of us. It was one of us and his/her betrayal has separated us. But this separation is not complete; if it were there would not be betrayal. The betrayal itself ties us together, it makes the betrayer part of me, a wounded part to be sure, but still a part that cannot be extricated until the betrayal itself has disappeared, forgotten. The image of the *cipayo* contains the traumatic residue of an imaginary unity that has not been given up, while it signals the fact that it no longer exists. It is thus an ambivalent object, a threat and an object of identification. This ambivalence complicates the relation between radical nationalists and the Basque police with an excess of affect that is absent in the relation with the Spanish police. This excess manifests itself in practices of disclosure such as the public uncovering of individual *ertzaintzas* in towns and villages, ritualized attacks, and riots. Such practices are de facto policing practices aimed at enforcing the boundaries of ethnic identity by punishing those who are considered to threaten them. They suggest a movement where the trauma of difference is repeatedly played out without resolution. The *cipayo* is thus a threat and a necessity, the despised object that challenges their fantasized ethnic community and the that which by virtue of evoking the Basque state is an object of desire; the despised object that stands in the way of unity and the one that, by suggesting a colonial setting, legitimizes nationalist violence.[3]

This ambiguity and ambivalence of an image representing at once national betrayal and nationalist identification can be tracked in the metonymic traces contained in the signifier *cipayo*, as it shifts etymologically from a representation of the colonial British army in India (*sipahi*), to a representation of anticolonial force emerging with the mutiny of *sipahis* against the British in 1857, to a representation of the police (*sipahi*) in the postcolonial nation.[4] This etymological history points to the ambiguity of the *sipahi* as a threat not only to national liberation but to colonial rule as well. This ambiguity is disguised yet present in the trope of the Basque *cipayo*, which acts simultaneously as a metonymy of the Basque nation and a metonymy of the hegemony of the Spanish state. Such ambiguity and its concomitant ambivalence manifest themselves in the distrust periodically expressed by the Spanish government in relation to the *ertzaintza*, and the suspicion voiced by radical nationalists that the *ertzaintza* are infiltrated by the secret services of Spain.[5]

To recapitulate, then, there is a kind of madness in the violence of Basque radical nationalists. But this madness is not defined by the belief that they are the voice of the people who can achieve national independence now. That is the fantasy that hides something unspeakable and rather shameful; that is the belief that the goal of nation-state would entail the loss of an idealized unified nation with which they deeply identify. Such belief engenders a deep ambivalence toward the possibility of a nation-state. Thus, while they strive madly indeed to obtain their object of desire, a Basque nation-state, they do everything possible to ensure that it will not happen. And thus we have this ongoing state of paralysis characterized by increasing violence on the part of ETA, young radicals, and the state that seems geared to perpetuate itself ad infinitum. Why? Because, while the nation is an object of desire, they can maintain a unified sense of self as the colonized people and continue to figure as main characters in a story that, to quote Samuel Weber, "is split into a present that never comes full circle and a future that is always oncoming but never fully here" (2000: 16). It is perhaps this repetition, this continuous present that the uncanny reveals. And isn't it this uncanny sense, too, that characterizes the profound ambivalence that defines the colonial situation of which Homi Bhabha (1994) speaks?

NOTES

1. See, in this respect, Zulaika (1988).

2. The well-known politician and former mayor of Barcelona explicitly affirmed that (Basque) terrorism had benefited the right wing Partido Popular currently in government, helping them achieve an absolute majority in the last parliamentary elections. The Partido Popular government is virulently antinationalist and has systematically refused to negotiate a cease-fire with ETA. It would seem that radical nationalists are doing everything possible not to achieve their goals.

3. There are many examples of the ambiguity associated with the Basque police. The latest appeared in the form of a communiqué published by all major newspapers May 24, 2000. In the communiqué radical nationalist youth accuse the *ertzaintza* of being *cipayos* for arresting a group of youths charged with arsonist activities. The communiqué accuses the *ertzaintza* of acting against the Basque people and of being "a servant of Spanish parties," ending by threatening the *ertzaintza* if they stand in the way of national sovereignty (El País, 5/24/2000; Gara, 5/24/2000).

4. See Lewis (1997), Metcalf (1964), and Mukherjee (1984) for more extensive etymology of the word *sipahi* and for a history of the rebellion of 1857 in India.

5. See, for example, *El Mundo* (1/15/1997) and *Egin* (1/15/1998, 4/22/1997, 4/20/1997).

REFERENCES

Abraham, Nicholas, and Maria Torok. 1959. *The Shell and the Kernel.* Chicago: University of Chicago Press.

Anderson, Benedict. 1983. *Imagined Communities: Reflections on the Origin and Spread of Nationalism.* London: Verso.

Bhabha, Homi. 1994. *The Location of Culture.* New York: Routledge.

Fabian, Johannes. 2000. *Out of Our Minds: Reason and Madness in the Exploration of Central Africa.* Berkeley: University of California Press.

Fanon, Frantz. 1967. *A Dying Colonialism.* Trans. Haakon Chev. New York: Grove Press.

Fernandez, James. 1974. The Mission of Metaphor in Expressive Culture. *Current Anthropology* 15 (2): 119–46.

———. 1986. Persuasions and Performances: Of the Beast in Everybody and the Metaphors of Everyman. In *Persuasions and Performances: The Play of Tropes in Culture,* 3–27. Bloomington: Indiana University Press.

Gallop, Jane. 1985. *Reading Lacan.* Ithaca, NY: Cornell University Press.

Geertz, Clifford. 1973. *The Interpretation of Cultures.* New York: Basic Books.

Lacan, Jacques. 1977. *écrits: A Selection.* Trans. Alan Sheridan. New York: W. W. Norton.

Metcalf, Thomas R. 1964. *The Aftermath of Revolt: India, 1857–1870.* Princeton, NJ: Princeton University Press.

Mukherjee, Rudrangshu. 1984. *Awadh in Revolt, 1857–1858: A Study of Popular Resistance.* New York: Oxford University Press.

Obeyesekere, Gananath. 1990. *The Work of Culture: Symbolic Transformation in Psychoanalysis and Anthropology.* Chicago: University of Chicago Press.

Scheper-Hughes, Nancy. 1979. *Saints, Scholars, and Schizophrenics: Mental Illness in Rural Ireland.* Berkeley: University of California Press.

Siegel, James T. 1998. *A New Criminal Type in Jakarta: Counter-Revolution Today.* Durham, NC: Duke University Press.

Weber, Samuel. 2000. *The Legend of Freud.* Stanford, CA: Stanford University Press.

Zulaika, Joseba. 1988. *Basque Violence: Metaphor and Sacrament.* Reno: University of Nevada Press.

2

INDONESIA SAKIT

Indonesian Disorders and the Subjective Experience and Interpretive
Politics of Contemporary Indonesian Artists

Mary-Jo DelVecchio Good and Byron J. Good

I painted *Indonesia Sakit* [Indonesian Disorders] in early June
[2001]. I finished it in a week. I expressed all the ideas I had,
they were immediately there. I had this vision about what
would happen in the future. I meditated, reflected, to get buried
ideas out. At that time, Indonesia was in transition. The New
Order entered the reform era [*masuk reformasi*]. There were many
problems. As soon as Suharto resigned, there were people who
wanted to take over the presidential post, they wanted to be the
national leader. Well, that is why I painted the tiger, then the
map of Indonesia, and the symbol of a woman, although it is
only an image. At that time, the strongest party rising up was
the PDI-P, the Indonesian Democratic Party of Struggle, with Bu
Mega as the leader.[1] When I painted it, she was not yet in power.
The presidential chair seemed very promising for those who
were trying to grab it. Someone could be president because the
people elected him or her. So I represented in these little sup-
ports, the unity of people required to get the presidential chair.
Actually, the chair is very shaky.

The danger at that time was the rebellion in Aceh—it had begun
but not exploded.[2] Therefore I put the tiger in this corner—it
meant "gobble up" Aceh, to show the danger in Aceh. The sepa-
ratists appeared there; this movement endangers the unity of
Indonesia. The tiger symbolizes anger, dissatisfaction, the people
who are disappointed. The white pigeon symbolizes love and
compassion; [the umbrella is a symbol of protection, the naked
running man is people's desire for freedom]. The naked people
are the people's simplicity and honesty—we have many people
in Indonesia who are like that. Hypocrisy and greed—these are
symbolized in the spots. Here are the diseases, disorders and
pain of Indonesia—in the many spots.

> Yulikodo, Yogyakarta artist, January 2004

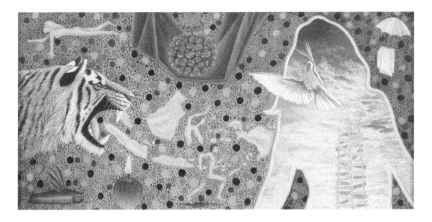

FIGURE 1.
Indonesia Sakit (Indonesian Disorders). 2001. Artist: Agus Yuliantara "Yulikodo."
Photo: Karen Philippi.

Artists—painters, playwrights, musicians—imagined and re-imaged the state and Indonesian society as Suharto's New Order regime unraveled after thirty-three years of autocratic rule. At the heart of this chapter are the work and reflections of three contemporary Indonesian painters and their efforts to constitute a space and visual language for critical engagement with their society. The chapter draws on our conversations about their subjective experiences of producing art and describes their ongoing efforts to carve out distinctive modes of subjectivity as artists and intellectuals during the period of *reformasi*, or reform, that followed the fall of Suharto.

The chapter's title, "*Indonesian Sakit*," is from an evocative painting by Agus Yuliantara "Yulikodo," one of Yogyakarta's young generation of artists. The image of Indonesia as *sakit*—as "sick" or "disordered" or "in pain"—resonates with the experience of many of Indonesia's leading contemporary artists that resulted in an outpouring of vivid political paintings during the immediate post-Suharto era. In this chapter, we explore creative responses to the world of *reformasi* Indonesia by three artists, all based in Yogyakarta: Yulikodo, a graduate of the Art Institute of Indonesia in Yogyakarta (ISI—Institut Seni Indonesia), who specializes in super-realist and surrealist paintings; Alex Luthfi R., a nationally known painter and senior member of the faculty at ISI; and Entang Wiharso, an innovative leader of contemporary Indonesian artists who has exhibited his work in Indonesia and around Asia, Europe, and the United States. Their critical portrayals of Indonesia and its place in the global order at the end of the Suharto era are conveyed through paintings and commentaries upon making art.[3] We examine in particular the role these artists and their contemporaries played in "subjectifying" the state, exploring how they imagined and positioned themselves as critical citizens, fearful yet risk taking, by making political art and placing it on public exhibition.[4]

Begoña Aretxaga suggests the importance of the "subjective dynamics that link people to states" (2003: 395). "The question of desire as well as fear becomes most crucial in rethinking the kind of reality the state might be acquiring at this moment of globalization," she argues, asking "how does it [the state] become a social subject in everyday life? This is to ask about bodily excitations and sensualities, powerful identifications, and unconscious desires of state officials," as well as the "discourses, narratives, and fantasies generated around the idea of the state. . . . The state cannot exist without this subjective component, which links its form to the dynamics of people and movements" (395).

The artists we discuss were, and remain today, deeply involved in generating narratives and fantasies of the state, visual and discursive, private and public. Their paintings provide profoundly disturbing imagistic responses to the Indonesian state—images of a "sick" state, as those in Yulikodo's *Indonesia Sakit*; of the state "empty of value," abused for a generation by the corrupt and rapacious cronies of the Suharto regime, its nationalist ideology of unity in diversity, Pancasila, lost, as in Alex Luthfi's *Kado Reformasi* (Gift of Transformation); or of the nation, its bureaucrats, politicians, and populous "run amok," as in Entang Wiharso's exhibition collection, NusaAmuk. These artists and their contemporaries provided graphic images of a weakened and disordered state, of the state gone awry.

Political "reformation," or *reformasi*, and steps toward democratic reforms brought a dynamic albeit incremental shift in political experiences and in the artists' newly found subjectivity as post–New Order kinds of citizens, allowing for a flourishing of highly charged and politically critical art displayed in "freedom" at public exhibitions. Mary Steedly, a long-time student of Indonesia, responding to shifts in public media and political culture in post-Suharto Indonesia, has challenged anthropologists to provide ethnographic investigations focused explicitly on the state and its powers. "Might it not be worthwhile," she asks, "to reflect on the internal mechanisms, limits, contradictions and failures of state power?" (1999: 444). Indonesian artists making reformation art took up just this task with vigor in 1999.

FESTIVAL OF FINE ARTS, YOGYAKARTA, 1999

In July 1999, we happened upon the Festival Kesenian Yogyakarta XI (FKY XI 1999—the Eleventh Fine Arts Festival of Yogyakarta) held in the Benteng Vredeburg Museum, a nineteenth-century colonial-era wooden structure of many rooms, sheds, and courtyards. The Vredeburg has a heavy political history as a prison for nationalists fighting the Dutch during Indonesia's war for independence and as a holding center for leftist prisoners in 1965–66, many of whom were executed or left to die. In contemporary life, it is the center for Yogyakarta's yearly art exhibition. As a collection, the juried paintings, titled Three Generations of Yogyakarta Artists, were astonishingly critical of the former New Order and Indonesian society, state, and politics. And although the varied techniques resonated with the work of earlier Indonesian masters (see Spanjaard 2004), including teachers of the newest generation of contemporary artists, and global images and painting styles, including American pop art, super-realist painting, and German expressionism, the exhibition clearly marked a turning point for political art in Yogyakarta and the rise of a genre of *reformasi* painting.[5]

The year 1999 was an extraordinary time for Indonesians. Economically, Indonesia continued to suffer the consequences of the 1997 Asian monetary crisis (*krismon*) and the 1998 political crisis (*krispol*). After nearly a year of a cascading collapse of the Indonesian currency, in which the rupiah's value fell precipitously against the dollar (from 2,500 to 15,000 R per US dollar), the simmering political crisis and public disaffection with President Suharto's New Order government exploded in May 1998. A tumultuous month of rioting and assaults against Indonesian Chinese communities in Jakarta and Solo, military killings of Trisakti student demonstrators calling for democracy, and state-linked thuggery against civilians led to President Suharto's forced resignation. Thirty-two years of New Order "national discipline" was replaced by a heady, democratic reform movement. By 1999, *reformasi* found its way into daily popular discourse. Many Indonesians experienced an intense sense of freedom— an ability to criticize publicly what they perceived to be the social, economic, and political ills of Indonesia's past and present and to imagine influencing the nation's future through democracy movements. Caution and cynicism about deeply rooted "corruption, collusion, and nepotism" (KKN), fear of "dark forces" associated with the old regime, and anxiety over military collusion in fostering social unrest balanced optimism about possibilities for serious reform. Yet, artists, playwrights, and musicians throughout the country joined public intellectuals in exercising their new freedom to critically address Indonesian society. Our artist friends engaged in a kind of "reformation bravado," overcoming fear of political repression and possible imprisonment even as they made and exhibited art that appealed to a newly burgeoning Asian and international art market.

What led these artists to paint as they did? How did they represent the disorders of the late New Order and post-Suharto Indonesia and interpret and act out emergent forms of political subjectivity and critical citizenship? What do we learn about political subjectivity via a reading of graphic artworks and images, linked to artists' reflective conversations on their work, and from our ethnographic engagements with these artists?[6] Michael Fischer opens an essay on film with a subheading "Truth in Painting," a play on Derrida's commentary on the artist Cezanne's promise, "I owe you truth in painting and I will tell it to you" (Fischer 2003: 61) The following sections on the FKY XI 1999 and on Alex Luthfi, Yulikodo, and Entang Wiharso, are devoted to the "truths" Yogyakarta artists evoked in their words and paintings.

Painting the Post-Suharto Reformation

The paintings exhibited at the Eleventh Fine Arts Festival of Yogyakarta (FKY XI 1999) enthusiastically celebrated *reformasi* freedom. Ranging from the humorous to the cynical and from the romantic to the despairing, incorporating images from Javanese *wayang* (shadow puppets) and international pop culture, and contrasting the desire for globalized products[7] with states of poverty caused by the monetary crisis, the juried paintings expressed an intense emotionality and energy, experienced by Indonesian and foreign viewers alike.[8] Artists juxtaposed ancient Javanese script and *ketoprak*-carved wooden masks of traditional Javanese theater with pop-art images—particularly variations on the American art of Roy Lichtenstein, James Rosenquist, Andy Warhol, and Robert Indiana with corporate products' ad art, including the 1970s album cover notably titled *Crisis? What Crisis?* (by Stomp, a rock band). Super-realist images of Javanese children peering yearningly into the world of capitalist production and city life, material products, white faces, and Texas-sized Marlboros intensified ironic commentary on the "global flows" of cultural products and politics and on the irrationalities and volatility of international currency markets, implicating global inequalities in Indonesia's plight—and its crises—in the late modern era. Making *reformasi* art, such as that displayed in the FKY XI 1999, placed many of Yogyakarta's artists at the heart of political debates on globalization that engaged university students, academics, and public intellectuals in Indonesia as in similar circles around the globe—debates about corrupt states and empires and the nature of postcolonial societies, about crises, emergencies, and international interventions, and more broadly about economic globalization and postmodern capitalism. The FKY XI 1999 became for many artists an exercise in fantasizing the state, in all its weaknesses, flaws, and raw power, in past, present, and future.

The appearance of overtly political art in the FKY XI 1999 was no accident. The exhibition catalog opens with a manifesto by its editor, Sumbo Tinarbuko: "We are entering a new era for Indonesia. In this new time, power can no longer remain in the hands of the government, but in the grasp of the people [masyarakat], who are independent and democratic" (Sutejo and Luthfi 1999).[9] The curators, Alex Luthfi and Godod Sutejo, organized the exhibit under the theme Three Generations of Artists in part to highlight the creativity, energy, and political activism of the younger artists of Yogyakarta.[10] Writing about the youngest generation of artists, the selection coordinator, Edi Sunaryo, noted that "the reformation theme is of one breath with the restlessness which still howls in their young souls" (13); and Luthfi wrote that "they want to say something that has a provocative and disturbing message and meaning. . . . We look for the emotions which explode with the themes of actual freedom for the young painters" (13, 16).

The FKY XI 1999 clearly appealed to Indonesian collectors and investors as well, and many impressive paintings were purchased prior to or during the exhibit, according to gallery staff. Astri Wright, historian of Indonesian twentieth-century art, identifies the development of an Asian modern art market through the 1980s and 1990s as encouraging a "contemporary art culture in Indonesia characterized by great pluralism" (2000: 96–97). She credits the New Art Movement of the 1980s "with partial success in reestablishing artists' right to draw on the whole spectrum of social experience, including the political" (2000: 96).

Despite the dynamic contemporary art world of Indonesia of the 1990s, the FKY XI 1999 was clearly a political and emotional turning point for many who contributed to the exhibit. Artists spoke about their psychological struggles to overcome the deep personal sense of fearfulness and insecurity experienced in response to the abuses of the late-Suharto regime. Yulikodo's visions of state violence (real and envisioned) made him physically and psychologically ill. Alex Luthfi joked about "being taken away by security forces." Entang Wiharso fled the country in response to an ominous threat. All recalled the ubiquity of the secret police during the New Order regime. Artists worried about censorship, even as they tried to reason that in reformasi Indonesia they should not need to fear. They worried about repression and the possibility of imprisonment in retaliation for their politically critical paintings. Nevertheless, being berani (brave) and painting explicitly political images as social critique were at least partially behind the social, emotional, and visual power of the 1999 exhibition and sources of an artists' fame. Art made in the then-giddy days of a newly experienced personal freedom, the early post-Suharto reformation period, appeared to many observers to have a quality of energy and joy, even when the topics were socially weighty.

Yogyakarta artists represented at the FKY XI 1999 debated the more guildlike "truths" of their art as well (e.g., Is surrealism contemporary art? What should be the relationship between commercialism and idealism, or between art and politics?), even as they reflected on the social precariousness of previous artistic movements and cooperatives such as Lembaga Kebudayaan Rakyat (LEKRA —The Institute for People's Culture). LEKRA, a cultural organization supportive of leftist artists founded in the Sukarno era, was labeled "communist" by the New Order regime; many of the artists associated with LEKRA were imprisoned, dating from the 1965–66 massacres of the left.[11] Most of the artists with whom we spoke had a deep sense of historical connectedness to social movements within Indonesian fine arts, from the nationalist and LEKRA artists to contemporary movements (Ruwantan Bumi, or Earth Exorcism 1998) and the "cultural fever" and "insurgent consciousness" (Friend 2003: 322) that ultimately contributed to the collapse of the Suharto regime. The FKY XI 1999 and subsequent exhibitions from 2000 to 2003 exhibited work painted prior to Suharto's fall from power, and many of the Yogyakarta artists were part of the wider national democracy and reformation movements that predated Suharto's resignation in the spring of 1998. Nonetheless, the FKY XI 1999 would come to mark a new turn in the arts movement in Yogyakarta into the next decade.[12]

Reformation Artists: A New Critical Citizenship, "Emotions Exploding with Themes of Freedom"

The public identity of the new reformation artist as critical citizen was at least partially framed by the FKY XI 1999 curators in their search for young artists "whose emotions [and art] explode with themes of actual freedom" (Sutejo and Luthfi 1999). The development of a critical subjectivity resonates with the earlier personal journey of Indonesian/Acehnese artist Abdul Djalil Pirous, recounted by Kenneth George (2005).[13] George explores the tensions between establishing a unique aesthetic vision and creating a national or "Indonesian" art that modern Indonesian artists faced (cf. George 1999, 2004).

> The pull between pursuing an autonomous and unique subjectivity and serving as a representative of a people and a nation has been the principal (if normative) tension for most Indonesian artists and art critics in the post-independence period (1945–present). In short, searching for a distinctive national identity has been as crucial to locating postcolonial aesthetic projects as it has been to asserting political autonomy. . . . Being subject to a nation, then, meant acknowledging a set of imagined political and social differences that when refracted through the discourses and techniques of art production would yield a recognizable "Indonesian" art. (George 2005: 193)

Although the painters we discuss in this chapter are clearly Indonesian in their aesthetic vision and imagery, the work that emerged in the *reformasi* era was less focused on establishing a postcolonial, national identity than on exploring the positioning of the artist as critical citizen in Indonesian political life and addressing the disorders that emerged at the end of the Suharto regime—the violence between ethnic and religious groups, often organized by shadowy elements of the state, in a nation "run amok"; the loss of Indonesian spirituality and culture in the face of globalized consumerism and materialism; and the permeation of the very grammar of Indonesian political thought and political subjectivity by the pervasive, hegemonic New Order ideology. (Pirous, during this period, also began to openly criticize the horrid violence of the Indonesian military and central government in his native Aceh [George 2005].) These artists participated in a broad struggle to reflect on these processes critically and to establish alternative modes of political subjectivity appropriate for a new democratic era and a newfound freedom of expression.

Yogyakarta artists were engaged in the daring adventure of political art in the late New Order years. Alex Luthfi, Yulikodo, and Entang Wiharso are three painters who were deeply engaged in representing the end of the New Order regime and the emergent forms of democratic consciousness in the years following 1998. Each uses his own subjectivity, and at times bodily experience, to constitute a space for critical reflection on the state. Each represents the state as "social subject" through creation of a distinctive artistic imaginary and emotionally powerful, although rarely beautiful, visual images. Their paintings from this period represent a moment in the exploration of the place of political subject or citizen vis à vis the state, which shifts through various paintings and eras.

Painting the State: *Kado Reformasi* by Alex Luthfi

Displayed prominently across from the entrance to the FKY XI 1999 gallery, *Kado Reformasi* was the first painting one viewed upon entering the exhibit. Thick with paint, it is a deeply black, white, and red image of the mystical Garuda, the bird symbol of the Indonesian state, surrounded by large, glittering yellow stars. But it is a distorted Garuda. A wild pig's head has replaced the head of the mystical bird. A necktie, "the mark of the power of the executive" (as Alex Luthfi told us), dripping in red, lies on the Garuda's chest.[14] The painting is imposing, at once compelling and ominous. We were struck by the shaped texture of the black paint on the Garuda's uplifted wings and by the richly painted yellow stars, textures reminiscent of Jasper Johns's American flag paintings (*Flag*, 1954–55; *Three Flags*, 1958) (Phillips 1999). Luthfi's painting was very strong, a fantasy of distorted state power.

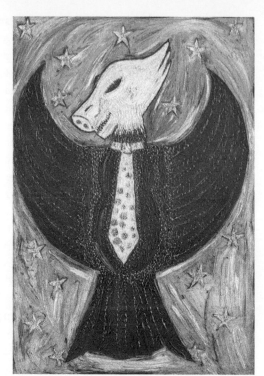

FIGURE 2.
Kado Reformasi (Gift of
Reformation). 1999.
Artist: Alex Luthfi R.
Photo: Karen Philippi.

"Pak" Alex, born in Surabaya in 1958, has been painting since his early twenties. A nationally renowned contemporary artist who exhibits in Jakarta and Yogyakarta, he is on the faculty of ISI, the Art Institute of Indonesia in Yogyakarta. He studied for his BFA (STSRI-ASRI) in Yogyakarta from 1979 to 1983 and received his masters degree from the Institute of Technology in Bandung (ITB) in 1992. During his student days in Yogyakarta, he worked in the studio of Affandi, Indonesia's first famous modern artist.

The title of his painting, *Kado* (gift) *Reformasi* (reformation), was interpreted by our Indonesian friends in Yogyakarta as a strong proreformation sign, despite the ominous image of the Garuda with the head of a pig. We showed pictures of the painting in 2000 to politically active friends in Bali, who excitedly saw in the painting the power of the people. The stars they said are the people rising up to take over the Garuda from the failed New Order regime. Some saw Shiva, the Hindu god of destruction, in the painting of the pig head, replacing the rapacious and corrupt capitalists associated with the New Order (and the bloodied tie); others identified the thick red drips of paint around the pig's neck as symbolizing the death of New Order rule, of military

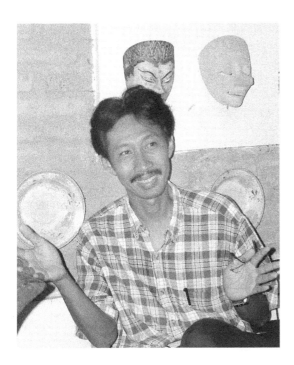

FIGURE 3.
Alex Luthfi at home, 2004. Photo: M.-J. D. Good.

corruption, nepotism, and exploitive capitalism. Our Balinese friends, who were middle-class employees of the tourist industry—one was a PDI-P (Democratic Party of Struggle) provincial assembly member, the other was from an island whose residents had been forced to relinquish rights to the village's beachfront land at rifle point so that developers from "Jakarta" could begin a now abandoned marina and casino hotel project—enjoyed the puzzle of interpretation. Perhaps because of the title and a continuing sense of political optimism in 2000, they viewed the painting as a positive statement about the future for popular democracy and governmental reform. The greedy pigs would be defeated.

In January 2004, we visited Pak Alex again several times to talk at length about his art. His elegant home was filled with his paintings of pig-headed figures. Masks of pig heads decorated the tables and hung from the ceilings, gifts from his artist friends from Bali and Yogyakarta. "I want people to think of me when they see pigs," he said, smiling. Because *Kado Reformasi* had stimulated considerable controversy when viewed by our academic colleagues, we asked Pak

Alex if he would give us an extended interpretation of his painting. He began with a discussion of a turn in his work, and his interest in pigs.

> All right, so it's like this. Actually, the first painting I made of a pig was this one, and I keep it. [Pak Alex pointed to a painting of a standing pig with a floppy, jokerlike crown.] So here we see the power, the painting tells the story about power. There are three points on the crown—this means it is the king. And this is a necktie; the tie is a symbol of people who feel they hold power and authority. At that time I figured three people felt they were in power, at least more than two. So there were many people in power, but they were like pigs. Why pigs? Because in Indonesia, pigs multiply very rapidly. . . . New Order people multiplied themselves to be people who held power; they were abusive, corrupt, and they kept multiplying and spreading. Therefore the pig is the most fitting symbol, and the pig is the symbol of reproduction. And what's interesting is that when I started to have an interest in the symbol of the pig, I spent time at a pig farm. Coincidently, it is just south of my house—next to our village. The shape, the smell . . . I wanted to immerse myself in pig characters.[15]

He elaborated on the meaning of the image of "pig":

> I use the pig as a symbol about what we don't like in Indonesia. And Indonesians have a tradition about pigs, they are hunted, hunted. I am not saying that the authorities have to be hunted, it is too direct. Too rough, too rude. Not human. I prefer to portray a phenomenon—but I can be rough too. For instance, this painting is The King of Corruption [E Raja Korupsi]. This first painting was made in 1995. It was before there was a reformation movement; I painted it then. In 1995, I saw that Indonesia had reached a point where it obviously was in need of reformation, so even before Amein Rais and his friends, I had thought about this and put it on the canvas.
>
> When I was making decorative art [before 1995], there was something bothering and depressing me. I was not reading the situation in Indonesia— not attending to its many problems. I came to feel I had to start thinking about Indonesia, to think about something more contextual and linked to our life, and to our social and political problems. I thought Indonesians should start caring about this too, and it turned out that after 1995 there was reformasi—a reformation movement. So actually, we all thought similarly, Indonesians who cared, who knew, we all grew up together. It was like that.

Pak Alex then discussed the sketches of pig figures playing golf on rice land that were published in the *Jakarta Post* newspaper in 1995; he had previously given us copies in our first conversation in August 2000. He explained:

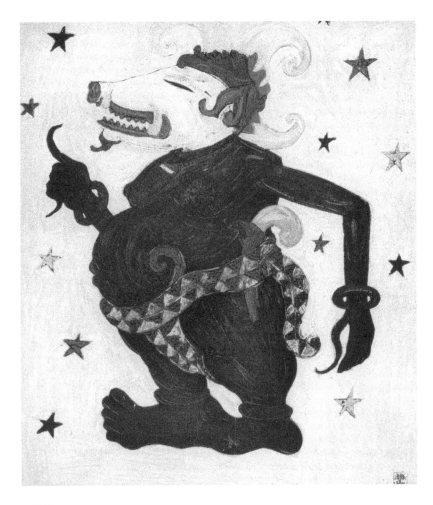

FIGURE 4.
E Raja Korupsi (The King of Corruption). 2001. Artist: Alex Luthfi R.

The drawings in the *Jakarta Post* were very provocative. Very provocative. My friends told me, "Watch out, don't sleep early because they may come to get you" [*Awas kamu, jangan tidur sore, sebab biasanya diambil oleh aparat*]. During the New Order, there was . . . a tendency for those who were political and in opposition [to the government] to be picked up late at night [*malam-malam*, by the authorities].

We turned our discussion back to *Kado Reformasi* and asked, "Why the pig's head?" He replied, "When I exhibited this painting at FKY, there were many people who asked me: Why? Why make the Garuda with a pig head? Why? Everybody! The collectors, the Chinese collectors were all afraid and questioned me. It made me think that well, they did not understand."

And what, we asked, is the meaning of *kado*, in *Kado Reformasi?* Alex's reply startled us. "Well, so now, as I see it, when I painted it, it [referring to but not using the word Garuda] had become like a mascot. It was no longer a symbol. They are different, right!" "Mascot?" we queried, a bit confused. This was the first hint of this powerful image of the Indonesian state being a mascot. "Mascot is mascot, the same [as in English]. Mascot, just a mascot, the value is different, it is no longer a symbol, just a mascot."

And so what does *Kado Reformasi* mean? Pak Alex hesitated; he finally used Garuda's name.

> It is like this. When it no longer is the fundamental powerful principle, when it no longer is a principle . . . it no longer has symbolic power, it . . . it . . . the Garuda, consequently, the Garuda becomes just a mascot. A mascot is like a souvenir. So the value shifts. It becomes a mascot, like a souvenir, to be given away or to be reproduced. Therefore, Garuda Pancasila no longer has any power[16]. And it was given away to the people of the reformation. Like a gift. Here—here is this gift. Like that.

"Why the pig?" we asked him to go on. "Why the stars?"

> If we look at pigs closely they are the symbol of power, the executive, and the tie is the symbol of the executive power. And in this painting, the Garuda is in the hands of the people with pig heads. So I see, I always put stars—like this one here and here, and behind these shining stars there is a hidden evil.

"Behind the stars, what do you want people to see, Pak Alex?" He replied, "I want to warn them not to become enchanted by the figure, by the physical thing, but to look behind." And what is behind?

> And behind, to look at what are its values—morals, ethics, spirit. It seems to me that this Garuda hasn't shown evidence for a long time that it still has those values. What is left is just the sparkle—it has the character of the sparkle, it shines, but the values that were there, the ethics, morality, spirit, they are gone.
>
> Well in this case, this Garuda [*Kado Reformasi*] is given to the reformation people. "Here is Garuda Pancasila, please, please fix it." Now the problem is that as soon as it's given to the reformation people, Garuda remains a phe-

nomenon, just a discourse. Just a discourse, an expression (*wacana*). So these people—they can't see Pancasila either. The Garuda no longer embodies these values—it only views them from afar.

We asked him if he thought there would be a return to Pancasila, with the reformation people. "Up to now, I haven't seen it. It remains a phenomenon only, just a phenomenon, a discourse, just talk." So the real values of Pancasila have already been lost? "They have already gone. " Have already gone? "Not really gone. The values are no longer the focus of their thoughts. Therefore, Garuda becomes just a decoration, right? This bull, this banyan tree, this gold chain [*rantai*], this rice and cotton, these are no longer in him, they are out of him, they no longer have a connection with Garuda. That is the problem." (Alex pointed to these images in another painting.)

When we told of the more hopeful interpretation of the painting by the Balinese, Pak Alex exclaimed, "But I like it, I like the interpretations. So there are multi-interpretations" (*Tapi saya senang. Saya senang itu. Jadi, e multi interpretasi ya!*).

Pak Alex showed a small painting at the FKY XIII 2001. The field was divided into four boxes, with two military officers with pig heads, one opposite corn, one opposite a gun. We asked his intention. Pak Alex cheerfully responded, "Sometimes I just want to make fun of them, to make a joke—what if I replaced the gun with an ear of corn?"

When we asked Alex to compare subsequent shows with FKY XI 1999, he remarked, yes there was growing pessimism. Pessimism about the state pre- and post–New Order continues to be represented in his work. Other paintings from this period show pig-headed military shooting student demonstrators, a response to the May 1998 student killings. He also creates physically beautiful paintings that collectors initially desire. One recently completed painting features a beautifully elaborated *wayang kulit* (a shadow puppet) as its central figure, surrounded by the five symbols of Pancasila, the national ideology. The colors are deep and rich, reds and whites. He said about his own pessimism: "Now I see the new corruptors wearing the clothes of *reformasi*—they are just like puppets—red and white—many kinds. This is the painting with the *wayang kulit* images—I made it so nicely and using nice colors, because their orientation is so materialistic." The collector who intended to purchase the painting turned it down after his wife said it made her fearful. Other paintings too are beautiful art, if harsh ideology. Many, such as *E Raja Korupsi* (The King of Corruption), or *Kerasnya Pistol–Lemahnya Jagung* (Gun and Corn), harbor deep cynicism, lurking behind the humorous images. All suggest a political pessimism and are haunted by hidden evil behind the sparkle, the artistic power, and the beauty.

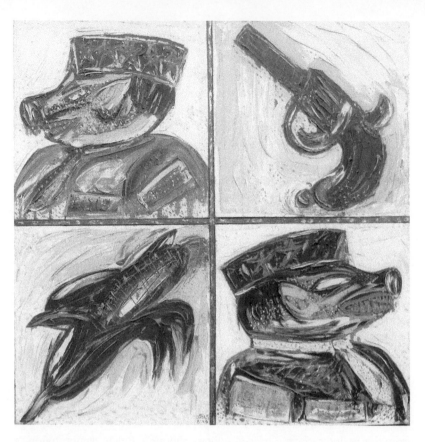

FIGURE 5.
Kerasnya Pistol–Lemahnya Jagung (Gun and Corn). 2001.
Artist: Alex Luthfi R.

During our visits in January 2004, we asked Alex if he was ever afraid to keep his own paintings. His reflections are sensitive to the New Order and post–New Order state. He responded: "Oh no. No, it's not dangerous. So far I have never been afraid to keep my paintings. It is just the collectors in Indonesia who don't have the courage to keep them. That is because they want to sell them. Coincidently my works don't have high economic value. So only those people who have an awareness of the social context and a high level of appreciation have the courage to possess them."

Concluding our most recent conversation, Alex spoke about his role as a humanist in the future of Indonesia, noting that he would be preparing new works on the coming election for an exhibit in Jakarta. He remarked that his

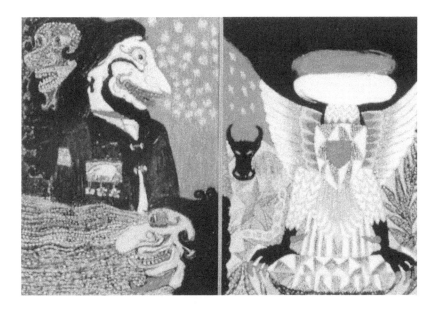

FIGURE 6.
Fatamorgana / "Pancasila." 2001–02. Artist: Alex Luthfi R.

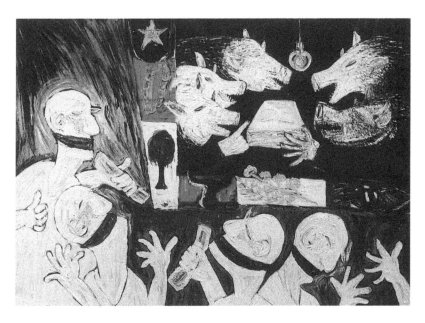

FIGURE 7.
Rapat (Meeting) 32 Years of Corruption. 1999–2000. Artist: Alex Luthfi R.

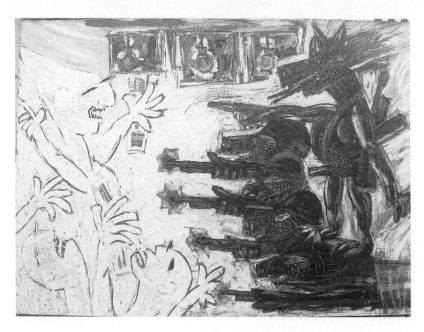

FIGURE 8.
White September Trisakti Shootings. 1999–2002. Artist: Alex Luthfi R.

paintings were not influential nor to be feared because he was a loner, not part of a politically active group. In reflecting on the importance of ideology in painting and on his concern about humanism in Indonesia's future, he remarked: "I don't know how we realize it [humanist government] politically because I am not a politician. What I can do is portray events, to help those who are in politics, to make people realize that when the New Order was in power, here is what happened, here is the portrait of what they did while they were in power. That's what I can do."[17]

Alex Luthfi's paintings directly and vividly address the "subjectification" of the state, the imagining of the state as a particular kind of subject, a distinctive set of actors with particular characteristics, motives, and behind-the-scenes actions, as well as the fantasies generated around the state during the Suharto era. His *Kado Reformasi* brings together his reflections on the New Order elite, symbolized as pigs, with the national image of the Garuda. This juxtaposition provides a harsh commentary on the current status of the Indonesian state and the dark and ironic fantasies these images evoke. In the process of creating this imagery, Luthfi elaborated a position for artists engaged in critically reimagining the state, while establishing himself as political subject responsive to his ideals of humanism and the social demands of his time.

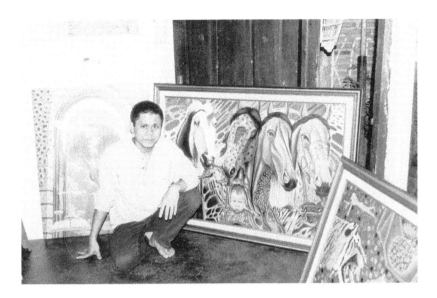

FIGURE 9.
Agus Yuliantara in his studio, 2001. Photo: M.-J. D. Good.

Painting the "Sick" State: Yulikodo

In July 2001 we sought out Agus Yuliantara "Yulikodo," a thirty-three-year-old artist, in his densely populated neighborhood of traditional houses within the *kampung* of the Sultan of Yogyakarta. Yulikodo "was not surprised," he "expected us," and had "seen" us in a recent dream, and we were coming to talk about his painting *Indonesia Sakit* then on exhibition at the Thirteenth Fine Arts Festival of Yogyakarta (FKY XIII 2001). Being in Yogyakarta, where many cultivate Javanese forms of spirituality and exchanges with the spirit world, Yuli's comments were not particularly exceptional. On a return visit, we asked Yuli to explain once again what led him to paint *Indonesia Sakit*. He began by explaining what he meant by the title. In English, *Indonesia Sakit* may be roughly translated as "Indonesia is sick" or "Indonesia in pain," but Yuli's references are broader, entwining personal sensibility—and the sensation of intense illness arising from political chaos—with subjectivization of the nation state. Yuli exclaimed— I will tell you "forthrightly!"

> Well *sakit* [sick] here actually refers to the situation and condition at that
> time. It was the transition era from Pak Harto [Suharto] to his successors. We
> all experienced this feeling, from university students to the little people.
> Especially, all of Indonesia was like that. Including the economy, which also

suffered; it was *sakit* outside [physically] and inside [mentally/spiritually]. So its [Indonesia's] mind [*pikiran*], emotions, conscience, all were sick. That's what *sakit* is all about. And I express it in the form of those painted spots and those symbols. Like the apple, which represents the IMF, but there is fire on it [like a bomb].

In a later interview, Yuli explained again the meaning he was giving to *sakit*: "The chair [or throne] of leadership was also sick, the people were sick, all the systems were sick, that's what I mean by *Indonesia Sakit*. Consequently, the people had to deal with the suffering. You know I had painted it before it happened. I was sick for three years."

Social disorders and personal pain are entwined in Yulikodo's artistic creation. He has visions of the ills of Indonesia; he mirrors the sickness of the state, its leadership, the political system and economic systems, and the people with his own bodily and psychological "sickness." He paints through his sickness, making order and story through painting. He went on to describe his experiences and feelings that preceded the painting of *Indonesia Sakit*.

In 1992, I wanted to start painting social phenomena. I was fearful. I told myself, hold it for the time being. At that time, the surveillance police were everywhere. Everything developing was immediately uprooted [ideas, political movements]. I was confused, fearful. I had many visions, sad, fearful, disturbing. Even before the Trisakti incident [when students were killed in May 1998], my mind was filled with that kind of thing. I didn't put it on canvas yet; I just put it into symbols, like the four horses.[18] When I started to get visions, they were not vulgar; and, well, I had fear. At that time many students and activists disappeared. Even before the PDI [PDI-P] case exploded, July 27 [1996].[19] I had this vision clearly, ooo . . . this is happening—like watching a 3-D film; it was like I was there joining it; it was sick, I felt sick. My heart ached, my body felt sick [*sakit*] and weak; my thoughts felt sick. My vision exploded into shootings, [with] blood everywhere.

"You felt as if you saw it?" we asked. "Yes," he replied. "Are you like a paranormal?"

I don't know. I am just a normal person. I don't want people to think of me as a paranormal. It felt to me as if I was undergoing a transition. I live in this material world, but something supernatural was revealed to me. I tried to forget it, to prevent it from capturing my memory; I tried to get rid of the stress, of being entrapped in the memories of the visions, by reading, hanging out with friends, going to the beach, the mountains, to lighten the bur-

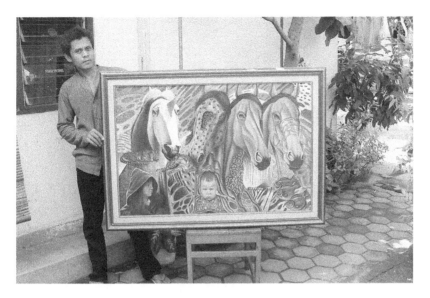

FIGURE 10.
Agus Yuliantara "Yulikodo" with *Yang Kuat Tidak Lagi Perkasa*
(Those Once Strong Are No Longer Powerful). 2001.
Photo: M.-J. D. Good.

den [of these visions of the future] in my mind. We all have our own ways
for self protection, right? If we challenge "the trap" it breaks, it disappears.

Yulikodo's visions found their way into his surrealist paintings—the corrupt
Suharto regime illustrated by the four diseased horses, the attempt of "the common people" to rise up against nepotism polluting the reformation movement
symbolized by a powerful bull, with fire and snakes on his horns, the fists of the
people raised against the hummingbird (the honey suckers of corruption) dis-
tracting the bull. Yulikodo's paintings are filled with passion, he speaks with a
cool anger, he paints his own young son's face into many of his works, with furrowed brow—representing children's futures compromised by the state apparatus of corruption, collusion, and rapacious rampant global capitalism.

Yuli's own suffering and his anxieties and anger over the uncertain fortunes
of his child's generation characterize his relationship with the state, with its
surveillance, corruption, and lack of commitment to the "people." He paints
General Sudirman, against a red horizon, as the popular hero, a hero of the
independence struggle and of a simpler Indonesia. Conversations with Yuli are
also dispiriting, in a certain sense. Hope is limited. Yet *Indonesia Sakit* features a

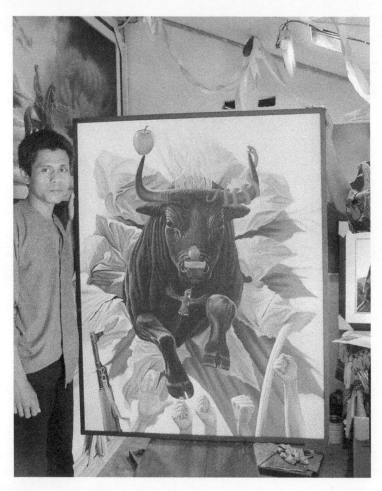

FIGURE 11.
Agus Yuliantara with *KRIS (T) IS* (Raging Bull). 2002. Photo: M.-J. D. Good.

political angel, an idealized woman, painted in heavenly clouds and sky blue, a fantasied Megawati Sukarnoputri, who would look after the ordinary people (*rakyat*). Yuli works in construction to earn a living, but his foreign patrons from Holland appreciate his surrealist and passionate images.

Yulikodo's subjective response to the Suharto regime and the *reformasi* era is more classically *kejawan*, or Javanese, than that of Alex Luthfi. Yuli is not a member of the academic art community or a public intellectual. His visions, which often come to him in dreams, warn him of dangers and tell him of future events. His deep intuitions and clear visual images provide him esoteric knowledge and an uncanny sense of Indonesian politics. All of these appear as powerful images in his paintings. At the same time, his paintings reflect both a common stylistic tradition—rooted in Yogyakarta surrealism—and an understanding of Indonesian politics that is widely shared across social classes in urban Indonesia. He too paints to take a moral stand and to represent a distinctive vision of Indonesian society and political life.

Painting a Nation "Run Amok": Entang Wiharso

Although the paintings displayed in the Fine Arts Festival of Yogyakarta in 1999 touched on diverse themes, critical reflections on the oppressive Indonesian state dominated the work of the younger generations of artists. The "explosion" of emotions, described by Alex Luthfi in the show's catalog, arose from pent-up anger at the arrogance and corruption of the military and the state *aparat*, and at the economic crisis that dramatized Indonesia's dependence on global economic institutions and heightened the gap between rich and poor. However, 1999 was also a time of optimism. Suharto had been swept from power, and a new election was called. Much of the public participated vigorously in the 1999 campaigns, with diverse political parties fielding candidates and Megawati's reorganized party expressing the aspirations of the "little people," the *wong cilik*, for real change. Despite the violence associated with the end of the Suharto order, there was hope for a new democratic era.

By 2001, the mood was far less optimistic. The Suharto family had not been held accountable; few of those accused of human rights abuses had been brought to trial, and corruption continued unabated. Insecurity resulting from political and civil turmoil destabilized the state and civil society. The military unleashed terrible violence in East Timor, following the 1999 referendum vote for independence. Muslims and Christians who had long lived in peace in Ambon turned on each other, loosing communal violence that threatened to spread throughout the eastern islands of the archipelago. The bitter civil war in Aceh between the military and the guerilla fighters of the Free Aceh Movement (GAM—Gerakan Aceh Merdeka) intensified again, and villagers became the object of the military's campaign to destroy GAM "at its very roots" (Good et al. 2006).

When in 1997, with Suharto still in power, the popular magazine *Gatra* devoted an issue to the question "*Mengapa massa gampang mengamuk?*" (Why do the masses so easily run amok?), the phrasing of the question reflected the New Order regime's fear of the democracy movement and its paranoia about outbursts of violence that had erupted sporadically during the 1997 election campaigns (B. Good and Good 2001; Good, Subandi, and Good 2007).[20] Journalists, covertly critical of the regime, used the question to suggest that violence was a natural response by the masses to the corruption and failures of the New Order. By 2001, the same question (*Mengapa massa gampang mengamuk?*) was more widely asked in disappointment. Why had the democratic forces and the *reformasi* movement failed to produce a new basis for order and stability? Why were ethnic and religious conflicts continuing to multiply? Were the "dark forces" of the old order still responsible for destabilizing society in an attempt to drive *reformasi* Indonesians back into the fold of the ruling clique and the army? These were the questions debated by public intellectuals and artists, as well as by the reformist parlimentarians, as they impeached Gus Dur (Abdurrahman Wahid), removing him from the presidency, and elected as president Megawati Sukarnoputri, who had been the winner of the largest number of popular votes in the 1999 election. In July 2001, "Ibu Mega" assumed the presidential chair, fulfilling Yulikodo's earlier vision, and faced the challenging task of quieting communal strife and reinstating civil security.[21]

It was in this context that our attention was drawn to a banner announcing an exhibition of paintings by artist Entang Wiharso titled NusaAmuk, "the archipelago/nation run amok," being held in the cultural center, Purna Budaya, of the University of Gadjah Mada Yogyakarta in June–July 2001. We caught the exhibition on its last day and entered Entang's political and emotional landscape. It was an astonishing collection, at once amusing and startlingly bizarre. To engage Entang's world was a deeply moving and intensely visceral experience. The two-story exhibition hall, designed for exhibitions of large paintings, was completely filled with over eighty oil paintings—a few as small as 3-by-5 feet, many 8-by-12 feet, with one remarkable seven-panel painting measuring nearly 9-by-40 feet.

Entang's images mesmerized, pulling us into his fantasies: huge grotesque figures, some headless, questioning their own open-mouthed screaming heads. Ominous figures clad in dark gowns; partial bodies of all sizes, distorted, floating in primary colors—brilliant red, black, white, and yellow. Techno-industrial culture and "global products" (televisions, guns, an operating table, an IV drip, a remote control for electronic devices, a red/yellow/green traffic signal) mixed with symbols of traditional Javanese culture (the *keris*, a ceremonial knife, which serves as an object of power in Java; the placenta, which is ritually treated as an infant's double and protector at birth; human figures in traditional Javanese meditation). Bodies split open, blood spewing from mouths; a small figure urinating on a man's head; a torso defecating on the double head of a male figure. Entang's paintings mixed humor with the strangely ominous (Bart and Homer Simpson figured prominently, Superman appeared here and there, a mouse nibbled on a watermelon), and these mingled uneasily with religious symbols (floating angels and cherubs). We had an immediate and overwhelm-

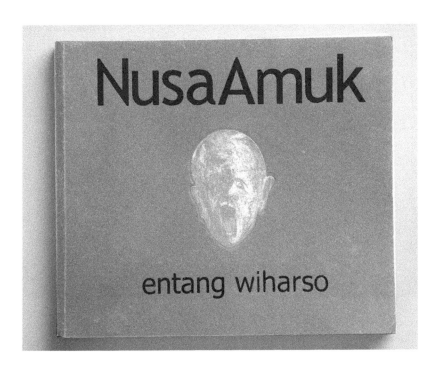

FIGURE 12.
NusaAmuk catalog cover, 2000. Artist: Entang Wiharso. Photo: Karen Philippi.

ing sense of a powerful artistic presence, harkening back, in some ways, to the German expressionist paintings of post–World War II, but distinctively Indonesian. The scope of the paintings and the title of the exhibit, which focused explicitly on *amuk* and issues we were writing about at the time, led us to look for this enormously creative painter. We would eventually meet him, first in Rhode Island, then in Yogyakarta, in 2003.[22]

Born in 1967 into a Muslim family in Tegal, a small town on the north coast of Java, Entang spent his adolescence between Tegal, where he lived with his father and went to school, and Jakarta, where his mother ran a small cafe (*warteg*, or *warung Tegal*). In 1987 he began to study painting at the Art Institute of Indonesia in Yogyakarta (ISI), receiving a BFA in 1994. Yogya surrealism, the dominant style among his ISI teachers, had developed in reaction to decorativism, which had been supported by the Suharto regime (Entang 1999). Entang initially painted within the Yogya surrealism mode, winning student prizes. After being ridiculed by a senior staff member for attempting to break out of the surrealist mode in 1992, he stopped painting for a short time. He

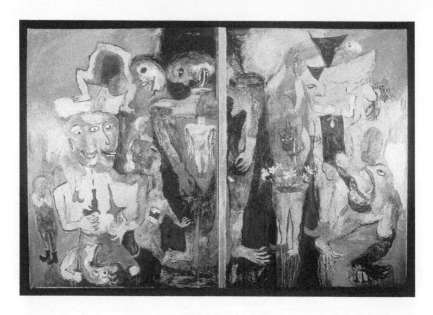

FIGURE 13.
Shit on the Head. 1998. Artist: Entang Wiharso.

then painted *Hug*, which loosed a torrent of paintings in his own style of abstract expressionism (Entang 1999). Conflicts, Dreams and Tragedy, a 1995 solo exhibition at the Purna Budaya Art Center in Yogyakarta, established Entang as a leading contemporary artist in Indonesia. In 1995 he received the Sultan's Best Artist Prize and was named to the top one hundred Indonesian artists; in 1996 he was named among the top ten Indonesian artists by the Phillip Morris Group and Indonesian Art Awards program. Since then, Entang has mounted nonstop solo and group exhibitions in the United States, Canada, Europe, China, Hong Kong, and Singapore, as well as in Indonesia, creating an extraordinary range of paintings and installations.[23]

Entang in Exile   Entang first moved to the United States in 1996, after an Indonesian journalist published confidential comments he made during an interview, in which he explained how one of his paintings was a symbolically coded representation of the July 27 (1996) tragedy.[24] Warned that the interview placed him in danger, Entang moved to Rhode Island, where he married his fiancé Christine Cocca, whom he had met while she was a Fulbright scholar in Yogyakarta. He did not return to Yogyakarta to set up his household and studio until 1999, after Suharto was forced from power. He watched—from a self-imposed exile—the rioting, burning, looting, and military violence associated with the end of the Suharto regime, as well as the ethnic, religious, and political violence that followed. These events unfolded on CNN and American television, giving Entang a view of Indonesia and its disorders from outside the country. He also experienced being "different" in the United States, and his critical reflections on globalization, consumerism, and international media were framed by his bicultural experiences. Although conversant in English, Entang was separated from his cultural and intellectual environment. His deeply critical, philosophical perspective and thoughtful engagement with current events in Indonesia were expressed primarily through his paintings. The NusaAmuk collection, which includes paintings made in the United States and after his return to Indonesia from 1998 through 2001, represents this engagement.

The NusaAmuk Exhibition   Although the title NusaAmuk was given after the fact to paintings displayed in three smaller exhibits—the New God Series, Melting Souls, and Community Storage[25]—the title reflected Entang's efforts to respond to the violence and loss of moral cohesion that he observed in Indonesian society. "*Amuk*," Entang told us, is "uncontrolled and unpredictable," actions in which individuals "melt into, you know, the big groups or collective action . . . it's like unconscious, ya, uncontrolled, unpredictable." Although referring to specific incidents of political violence, he said, "I'm also talking about the bigger picture. . . . I have the opportunity to see Indonesia from a distance, from outside Java, from the US or Europe when I'm traveling there," and "see more, I think, more, even with distance, more clearly, . . . like a bird sees directly what is happening on land. So it's a bigger picture. So that's why I think NusaAmuk is good for me, it really fit well with my works."

The paintings can be read as a rich, sustained set of reflections on the classic Malay and Indonesian category "amok," in which an individual was said to explode into violence in a kind of dissociated state of consciousness, later awakening with little awareness of what he had done (B. Good and Good 2001). One set of paintings and installations, grouped under the name *Jiwa Larut* or *Melting Souls*, explored the nature of individual consciousness when in the presence of mass violence. In an exhibition catalog, Entang recalled an experience he had in Jakarta, after returning to Indonesia, that triggered this set of paintings.

"Once when I was on a bus, something happened that made everybody start
yelling and get really angry and aggressive. I don't know why, but I also
started yelling and was furious." Entang wondered, if the people on the bus

were to attack a thief—something which was often reported in the mass media and frequently resulted in death—was it possible that he would eventually be pulled into this current of savagery and join the crowd? Then he would witness what his own restrained desires, soul, mind and hands could do in a situation that could quite possibly enable him to cause a human death. He suddenly became deeply anxious. (Supangkat and Wisetrotomo 2001: 29–30)

Entang told us a less "edited" version of this story, describing his fear of mob violence and the possibility of being personally swept up and implicated in *amuk*. He recalled talking with people who had participated in the looting during the 1998 riots in Jakarta, in which they "just went crazy, blindly stealing whatever they could get their hands on and returned home with all kinds of things including TVs, refrigerators, mattresses, and other breakable items." Later, some told him they felt guilty and attempted to return the items they had stolen, suggesting how easily it was to melt into the mass consciousness of the crowd.

Fears such as these are obliquely represented throughout the Melting Souls collection, particularly in a set of paintings titled *Run: Seri Kepala-kepala yang Hilang* (Run: Lost Heads Series). One painting portrays a partially distorted figure of a man with jacket and tie, mouth opened in a scream, half of his face red with a large eye, half white with a closed eye. He wears shorts, is barefooted, holds a bag in a red-painted right hand, a black *keris* in a raised, white left hand. Heads and distorted bodies, some white, some black, some bodies with, some without heads, float about this central figure. One distorted body is urinating on the head of a dark blue figure. Painted in 2000, the images seem to suggest the threat of losing one's head, of "melting" into the collective, and allowing what Julia Kristeva (1982) calls "abjection" to flood social life.

These themes are extended to the more general case of individuals becoming a part of mass consciousness in a set of life-sized installations Entang titled *Membebek*. *Bebek* means "duck," *membebek* "to follow unthinkingly" or "to imitate" or "to quack." Twelve men with gold-colored bald heads, uniformly large smiles on their faces, eyes wide open, clothed in shirts, ties, and jackets but wearing no pants or shoes, stand in a line, all facing forward. Each figure's stomach is an epoxy-encased cavity containing a severed duck head. Each wears a brass name tag, inscribed with titles such as lawyer, tax official, senior official, art worker, or curator.[26] In front of each, in the shape of a microphone, is a speaker that plays the sound of ducks quacking. The installation is a commentary on government bureaucrats and the elite having merged their identities or spirits with that of the regime (and thus *jiwa larut*, or "melting souls"). It embodies a saying from Entang's hometown of Tegal, "On the top you are dressed, but below you are

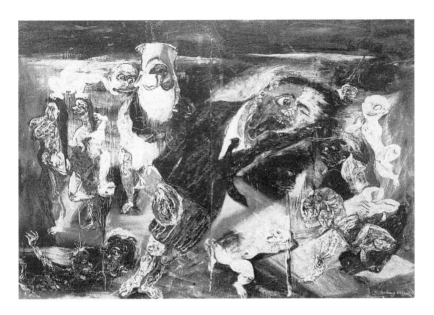

FIGURE 14.
Run: Seri Kepala-kepala yang Hilang (Run: Lost Heads Series). 2000.
Artist: Entang Wiharso.

naked,"[27] implying that someone is a hypocrite (Spanjaard 2002: 15). It also suggests that the abject is never completely invisible.

The *bebek* theme is elaborated in other exceptional installations. A group of twelve unclothed resin women, each wearing one red shoe, stand in a circle, holding in their hands a duck egg. Encased in their stomachs is an image of meat, representing the placenta. The installation is named, ironically, *Kulahirkan Untuk Tidak Menjadi Bebek* (I Gave Birth [to You] Not to Be Ducks, or "to not become a duck" or a mindless follower). The Melting Souls collection is not meant simply to suggest the behavior of individuals in violent crowds, but to point to broader phenomena in which individuality and personal responsibility are handed over to a larger entity—to the state, the party, the ethnic group, or the crowd—leading individuals to act in ways that are out of character and that cause shame.

These themes are further explored in a set of paintings that are part of the Community Storage collection in NusaAmuk. The image of "community storage" grew out of a trip Entang took to the secondhand market near the *kraton*, the sultan's palace in central Yogyakarta, to find a roller-skate wheel, he told us.[28] Fascinated with the collection of community objects, circulating because

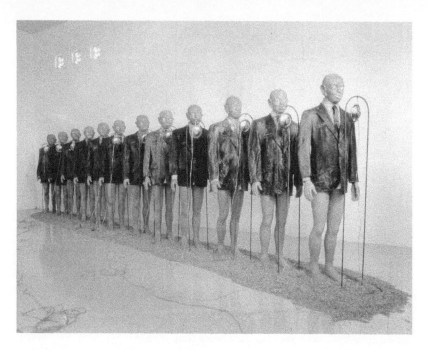

FIGURE 15.

Membebek. 2000–01. Artist: Entang Wiharso.

emotions and memories are attached even though they have little intrinsic value (a form of "collecting memories," he told us), Entang began exploring ideas of the relation between objects and collective experience. *Display Window: Community Storage* is a version of the displays of these Yogya *klithikan* merchants, with odds and ends of objects—from guns and military insignia to bits of electronic gadgets to parts of human bodies—strewn about. These represent forms of community consciousness, which may be specific to ethnic groups, religious communities, or social classes, and which may lead to the kinds of confusion and disorder Entang was observing in the newly democratic Indonesia.

Political ideology may become a particularly insidious element in group consciousness—an idea Entang explored in a remarkable series of paintings on "yellow sperm." A man's face dominates one of these paintings, titled *Forgotten Yellow Sperm.* Half is shaded white and blue, cool colors Entang associates with calm and purity, half is shaded black with touches of red, denoting darker forces. A white figure of a woman floats across the man's forehead. Above his open left eye is a blob of bright yellow color. The title makes clear its meaning. Yellow is the symbolic color of Golkar, Suharto's political party that dominated

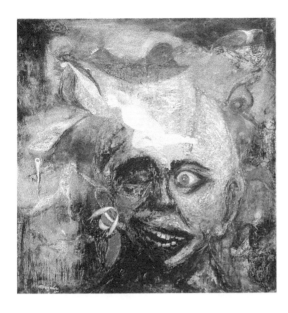

FIGURE 16.
Forgotten Yellow Sperm. 2000.
Artist: Entang Wiharso.

both the ideological and institutional structures of the New Order. The image of the yellow sperm daubed onto the foreheads of members of the community suggests how New Order ideology infused mentality and collective life, a masculine force reproducing itself and infecting social reproduction. Such processes are largely "forgotten," ensuring that New Order ideologies will remain a part of the hidden order, embedded insidiously in consciousness and social organization, long into the future.

Leaving the Yellow Sperm Community, another painting in the series, suggests the wide range of social forces mounted to prevent escape, by using the image of a floating naked man, a yellow mass rising above his body, surrounded by men shouting, wearing jackets and ties, striving to block his escape as they sit on other naked souls. *Self Portrait with 1000 Yellow Sperm* shows Entang, bare chest, white pants, his face chalked in white, his mouth open in a scream, surrounded by a bright yellow aura, with gold-colored sperm filling the canvas, swarming toward him. Everyone becomes "part of the system," Entang told us; "[even if] I "disagree with what the government does . . . or about corruption, it's hard to get away, because [I become] part of the system."

Placed in the context of the Community Storage collection, the yellow sperm series takes on special resonance. The New Order ideologies enter community consciousness, infiltrating affects and memories that are stored in the collective consciousness and that circulate around a community, providing the

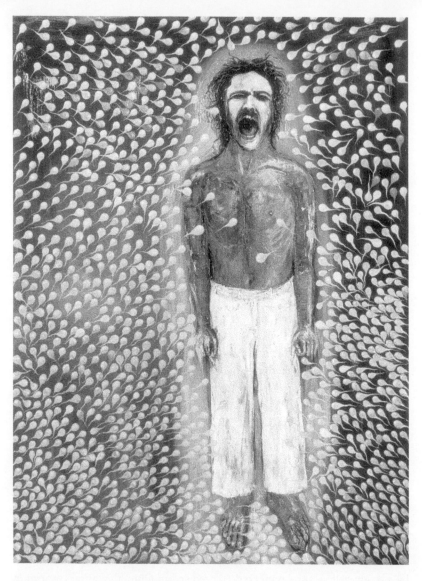

FIGURE 17.
Self Portrait with 1000 Yellow Sperm. 2001. Artist: Entang Wiharso.

deep causes for the masses "running amok." And these ideologies, as other community objects and memories, are circulated by "mass marketing . . . by television . . . or electronic devices, television or radio, something like that."

This idea, that media and mass marketing structure the objects and affects that make up group and individual consciousness, provides the basis for a third collection folded within NusaAmuk, the New God Series. Entang introduces the theme: "The New God Series . . . explores the idols we are now worshipping in our global community: wealth, violence, consumerism, standards of beauty, and fame. These works are inspired by our 'physical culture'; a culture that is concerned with what is seen rather than what is unseen" (Entang 2001: 52). Entang suggests that the media and consumerism have produced common "globally accepted images. . . . We are intoxicated by physical pleasures and are increasingly dependent on mass marketed notions of success and happiness . . . unable to escape from the images that have become our new gods" (22). He juxtaposes the visible world of external realities to the invisible world of spiritual forces and inner spirituality, an important distinction, drawn from Javanese culture and religiosity, arguing that images purveyed through global media have an intoxicating or indoctrinating effect, asking "Can we control or change the influence of the New Gods?" His answer suggests his vision of art and the artist in society: "The New God Series is intended to create a ceremony for our Soul. It will be a bridge—allowing people to see what is invisible becoming visible" (55).

Entang's statements are eloquent; being in the presence of his paintings, however, produces quite a different effect. *Global Products,* one of the New God Series, is a predominantly red painting, with several key figures. A television with the words "global products" on its screen has a thin, dark tube emerging from its side, leading directly to the stomach (or umbilicus) of a rather obscure, large figure, all red in color except for a white face. In a similar image, a male figure wearing only underpants and a white helmet and blindfold has a tube attached to his mouth, leading off to a round, flesh-colored image Entang indicated is a "brain" into which a black *keris* is stuck. The upper half of an angel figure, gold in color with white wings, has a tube leading out of its stomach or umbilicus. The powerful impression is of the media being piped directly into the stomach, the Javanese seat of emotions, or into the mouth of a blindfolded man, forcibly ensuring the internalization of the images associated with global products, the media, and the new gods.

The visual images of Entang's work contrast with the catalog commentaries (Entang's and his curators') on the paintings. The published text is often quite clear, the visual figures far less explicit, even when Entang personally provides a key to the vocabulary and coding he has developed. Together, these images,

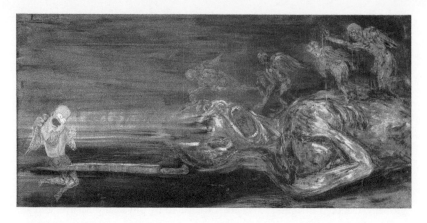

FIGURE 18.
Don't Touch Me. 2002. Artist: Entang Wiharso. Photo: Karen Philippi.

writings, and conversations constitute an extended, critical reflection on the nature of subjectivity in this period of Indonesian history.

During our 2004 conversations about NusaAmuk, Entang seemed to be weary of turmoil and of NusaAmuk's ominous story of melting souls. He remarked, after discussing the themes and the exhibition: "Well before September 11, it was different. After September 11 happened, it brought paranoia and trauma, and people were more sensitive, melting into a bigger picture. I think it is time now to get away from trauma." Nonetheless, he retrieved his 2002 painting, *Don't Touch Me,* from museum storage. It is a painting that extends his reflections on *Amuk* and communal violence to the global arena, and sets the stage for new directions in his work.

Painting Terrorism: Don't Touch Me *by Entang Wiharso*   We were looking at *Don't Touch Me* in Entang's studio garden in Yogyakarta in January 2004; the cobalt blue paint glistened in the bright sun. *Don't Touch Me* pulsed with a particularly poignant spiritual energy.[29] The screaming figure, the cherubs making offerings of grapes, Homer Simpson in cherub wings, dodging a sword splitting between his legs,[30] were a dizzying mix of images. The head and body of the screaming figure are distorted in visceral revulsion. No commentary appeared in the catalog for Hurting Landscape, the exhibit in which the painting was shown. The painting was intriguing, not only for its images, but for the intense, brushed cobalt blue, so different from the dominant red and yellow of the NusaAmuk projects. We asked Entang what led him to this particular creation. "I painted this painting after September 11." It was, he told us, his reaction to 9/11. The following story is drawn from our taped conversations in November 2004.

> It was 9/11. I was in Spain [for an exhibit]. I could not get hold of Christine [who was in Rhode Island]. I had been out and had returned to my hotel, and the desk clerk said, "You have a message from your wife—your wife and family are OK." I did not know why he was telling me "Your wife and family are OK." I had talked to Christine the day before about my plans, when I was coming home. I did not know anything happened. And then I looked at the TV. I did not realize what I was seeing. I went out into the street. People were watching this huge screen—this huge screen TV, in the street, with the images of the World Trade Center burning. People were crying, they were overwhelmed, deeply sad. I remember when I walked in the street, people everywhere were crying. [He haltingly described an overwhelming emotionality, exuded by the crowds on the street.] It was unreal. I thought at first the TV was showing a movie, a very vivid good movie, and I was unconnected. At first, I could not believe this was really happening, a real event.

Entang traveled from Spain to the airport in Amsterdam, where he was to board his flight to the United States. He described what happened when he went through security:

> The security were checking people; every one was paranoid at that time. They looked at my sketchbook, saw the knife and gun sketches. "So you are an artist?" they asked. "I am an artist," I said. I had the sketchbook—something like this one, with an image of a knife. . . . The guard asked me, "What is this?" Security began asking me more and more questions, and I got more and more nervous. They asked: "When did you get married?" I could not remember the date. I became extremely nervous. They checked my sketchbook. Then they took me to another room. They interrogated me for several hours. I had to open my shirt. Undress. It's kind of a funny story. Everybody was waiting in the airplane. It was sad. I understood at that time everyone was in the airplane, waiting for me. I was the last to board. Everyone was paranoid. I flew in on Northwest, from Amsterdam to Boston, a week after 9/11. In Boston, there was just a little screening. Christine was there to meet me at the airport. This is my experience.

And this is the experience that generated Don't Touch Me.

We looked closely at the painting together. Entang began describing the painting's dynamic life and his interpretations of the work, both prior to and beyond when it was painted. Don't Touch Me refers not only to Entang's present experiences but to those of the past and the imagined future, to inner and outer experiences, to spiritual and visceral responses, to Indonesian and American disorders, to global insecurities and paranoia. It portrays—he told us—his personal revulsion, his protest against being tainted with fear and terror, the desire to escape being emotionally overwhelmed by the war on terror, the desire to discover "the sublime." As we stood in front of *Don't Touch Me*, Entang discussed its various meanings.

> This painting is about my experience during Suharto's time. It is about when Suharto used religion for the [regime's] goals, for their political sins. It's what's behind those sins, screaming people, like me, in a dream, experiencing an intense physical discomfort.

And what of Homer Simpson and the sword? "Outside America, people see Americans going to war, and this painting is painted after September 11." And the sword?

> It can be a knife, a sword, and it can get into the wrong hand, and it can hurt people.
> The *malika*, the angels, are icons, church cherubs—like those you see in the Catholic churches. They are the good things about religion. . . . They are carrying the grapes for peace offerings, like in church, making offerings— religion is very peaceful. Religion should be like this, very peaceful. But religion can be distorted by groups or governments—misusing religion for the purpose of disorder.

He suggested that the Suharto regime was behind the church bombings and mosque burnings that occurred in the latter half of the 1990s. Religion "by government" could be used for political ends and for creating disruption, terror, evil. He described how when people like himself disagreed with the former regime and its actions, they were repulsed and felt this repulsion as a visceral "discomfort."

The painting's image of the body being stretched, the screaming head, mouth wide in protest, is meant to elicit in the viewer Entang's repulsion and visceral reaction to terrorism and the unrelenting media bombardment.

> You live surrounded with the media, and you cannot ignore it. And you get nervous, or stressed. For me I get nervous. Especially when you watch TV about terrorism. So one experiences more stress. The body screaming is how your own body reacts against the discomfort—the body is protesting.

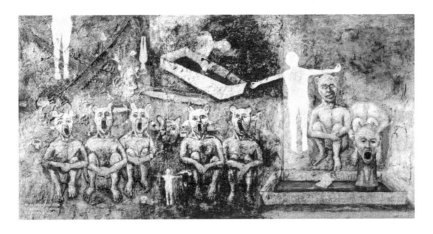

FIGURE 19.
Me as Teddy Bear. 2004. Artist: Entang Wiharso. Photo: M.-J. D. Good.

We asked why the boundaries of the body in this and in many of his paintings are often torn apart, with the interior exposed, like bodies in an anatomy lab.

> Actually it is not a recent technique. I have used it before. People can be thinking inside your body. . . . I use color to build the body up like a sculpture. I build it with the color scheme. It is not just the physical body. Initially, when I began to paint, I wanted to do something very different from that clean, nice aesthetic [referring to his earlier discussion of the dominant decorative art, even art with hidden political symbols]. If people wanted to understand—if you wanted to see how things really are—you needed to see inside, the bad and the good, and to see deep. I used this technique in my other work. In all my other work, I used earthier colors black and red. But now, things have changed mentally and psychologically changed.

And, we then asked, "The blue? It's so different from your reds." Entang: "Ah yes. Blue—blue because I want peace. Blue is a meditative color, a calm color. Sublime."

At the conclusion of our day together in November 2004, Entang declared: "So it's done [the making of NusaAmuk and similar protest paintings]. I don't want to do it over and over. I want to be making new art." He has begun to move on, he told us, from focusing on the crises of democracy. "In the reformation era, people were so angry and pissed off that it was like an explosion. When people feel hurt, you scream, you cry. And through that expression you stimulate each other, [and that energy would fill] the community storage. 'So

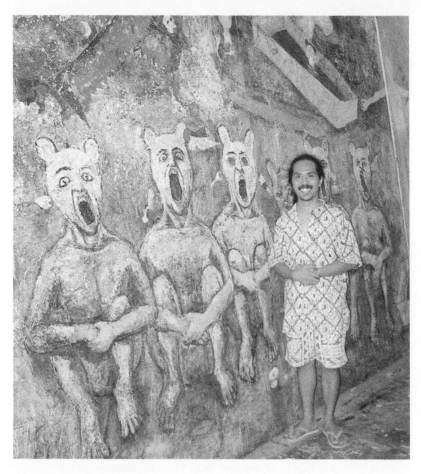

FIGURE 20.
Entang with *Me as Teddy Bear*. 2004. Photo: M.-J. D. Good.

what do you feel? Are you still hurt or looking for something else?' That is my question. My answer is 'stay quiet' [calm]. I am looking for something sublime. Something that is not transcendental but something to build anew with one's own mentality and heart."

Entang had already turned to his next project, which was titled *Sublime Tunnel*.

A RETURN TO "TRUTH IN PAINTING"

Michael Fischer (2003) explores the philosophical and anthropological debates on visual genres, the relation between subject and frame, artwork, and context, and idioms of painting and explanations of artists—and the place of "truth in painting."[31] Discussing the emergence of moral narratives, searing social critiques, and "the everyday as anthropological and philosophical work space[s] with multiple registers or cultural resource levels, filled with hybrid symbols," fantasies and desire, Fischer concludes that by "externalizing the complexities of subjectivities," Iranian film can "reorient ethics and religion" and "write life anew, renew life" (88–89).

Fischer's argument resonates with our own project concerning Indonesian art and artists. The art of Alex Luthfi, Yulikodo, Entang Wiharso, and many of their peers "externalize the complexities of subjectivities," making public their own personal moral stances and emotional registers, their anxieties, uncertainty, and fear, and their resolute and creative responses to these feelings as they seek to make "truth in painting." Each has created complex visual images in multiple registers, filled with hybrid symbols, fantasies, and desire. Each has engaged in "searing" social and cultural criticism of the Suharto regime and the reformation period, as well as wide commentary on "the broader picture," as Entang phrases it, of the social and the personal, of NusaAmuk; of violence and terrorism in Indonesia and in America; of the personal, visceral, and soul-tainting experiences of trauma, terror, and fear, and the corrosive effects of terror on one's humanity; and of the cynical manipulation of religion to produce civil strife. Each artist has also begun work on new anxieties of democracy, worrying about compromised idealism. Alex Luthfi made art in dialogue with the 2004 presidential elections, shown in Jakarta in 2004. Yulikodo made paintings evoking economic uncertainties and ongoing corruption as it bears upon children's futures. Entang relished his return to Indonesia and the Yogyakarta environs. He turned to making enormous art (twelve feet high by sixteen feet long) in his large, new studio: gold and white paintings decorated with red-white-blue objects that explore his Indonesian and American self through complex teddy bear images (Teddy Roosevelt is referenced, and a popular coffee table book on Roosevelt and teddy bears is in Entang's library) and yellowed arms (Homer Simpson—the universal everyman and Indonesian citizen—is referenced).[32] Today, each artist seeks to paint "life anew," what Entang has so aptly labeled in his democracy paintings, "the sublime."

Studies of individual Indonesian artists, we hope, will contribute to "exploring new forms of Javanese subjectivity, emerging under quite new conditions," a task that we argued, in an essay honoring Clifford Geertz, is critical for understanding Indonesian culture and society today (B. Good and Good 2005: 103). In his commentary on our paper, Geertz responded that "'exploring new forms of Javanese subjectivity, emerging under ("quite new?" well, anyway, "new") conditions' is clearly the way to go and in doing so the one thing I feel quite sure after all these years is that the Javanese themselves will be superb and willing guides in pursuing such an enterprise. It is hard to get a word out edgewise from the Balinese about what is going on *dalem*, 'inside.' It is, it still is, hard, so far as I can see, to get the Javanese to stop talking about it" (C. Geertz 2005: 119). We are indebted to the three Yogyakarta artists, all Javanese, whom we feature in this chapter, for their willingness to talk—about their psychological and political struggles and about their art. And we thank them for their generous guidance in exploring subjective experience and interpretive politics in post-Suharto Indonesia through the medium of art and the making of "truth in painting."

NOTES

We express our deep gratitude to Entang Wiharso, Christine Cocca, Alex Luthfi, Yulikodo, and all within the Yogyakarta art community who spoke with us and shared not only their art and their lives, but their thoughts on art, politics, and the future of Indonesia. Bambang Widojo provided extraordinary help in locating these artists and assisting with interviews, as did Ninik Supartini, who also transcribed and translated many of our formal interviews.

The images in this chapter are central to our discussions. We greatly appreciate Karen Philippi's new photographs of Entang's *Don't Touch Me* and of Alex Luthfi's *Kado Reformasi*, and her contribution of previously photographed images of Entang's paintings we reproduce here; and Seth Hannah's exceptional assistance in meeting the challenge of preparing digital images from photographs as well as preparing the digital text. We thank as well Margo McCool for her attention to the many details involved in the process from draft manuscript to published work, and Nita Sembrowich for her editorial assistance.

Our academic colleagues and students, in particular Michael M. J. Fischer, Atwood Gaines, Setha Low, Vincent Crapanzano, Sabine Koengeter, Shirley Lindenbaum, Mariella Pandolfi, Janis Jenkins, Tom Csordas, Ken George, Mary Steedly, and participants in our Southeast Asian workshops on media, art, and politics, provided engaging and challenging comments on earlier presentations and manuscript drafts. Our coeditor, Sandra Teresa Hyde made helpful editorial suggestions, as did our anonymous reviewers.

A serendipitous spinoff of Mary-Jo's sabbatical year as a visiting scholar at the Russell Sage Foundation in New York City (2002–03) provided the freedom to explore the city's museums and the influences of contemporary American art on contemporary Indonesian art, and to develop in earnest the scholarship that underlies this new work. I (Mary-Jo) thank the Russell Sage Foundation for this wonderful opportunity.

1. Bu Mega (or Ibu Mega), Megawati Sukarnoputri, leader of the PDI-P was vice president (1999–2001), then president of Indonesia from July 2001 to September 2004, following the impeachment of Gus Dur (Abdurrahman Wahid), who was deemed incompetent by the national assembly.

2. Yulikodo refers to the long conflict between the Indonesian military and the forces of the Free Aceh Movement (GAM), who threatened to establish Aceh as an independent nation, free of Indonesian control. This conflict became particularly intense during the years 2001–04. On August 15, 2005, in part as a result of the devastating tsunami and the influx of international agencies into the province, a peace agreement was signed between the Republic of Indonesia and the Free Aceh Movement, which granted Aceh regional autonomy but in which GAM gave up all claims to independence. At the time of this writing, the peace process has continued to be successful.

3. In 1996, when we spent our first Fulbright semester affiliated with Gadjah Mada University in Yogyakarta, our interest in contemporary Indonesian art was piqued by nationalist and modernist paintings by Affandi and others of his generation. Kenneth George, an anthropologist then at Harvard, deepened our interest through his analyses on the contemporary Bandung art world (George 1997) and the personal journey of A. D. Pirous, a leading Indonesian modern artist who had become renowned for the use of Islamic calligraphy (George and Mamannoor 2002; George 1997).

4. This process recalls our observations of authoritarian Iran under the Shah and in the Islamic revolutionary era, in which the subjectivization of the state was played out through innovations in the practice of Taz'iyeh and other Moharram rituals, legitimizing a distinctive public and private emotional discourse and critical commentaries on these (M. Good and Good 1988).

5. Images of the state as a military machine contrasted with those of narcissistic politicians performing for the electorate; poverty and yearning in the face of monetary crisis contrasted with Grandma Moses–style naïve paintings of election demonstrations and motorcycle brigades (Sutejo and Luthfi 1999).

6. George Marcus and Fred Myers (1995) ask similar questions, as does Robert Wuthnow (2001) and Myers and colleagues in the *American Ethnologist* "Contemporary Art Worlds and Their Productive (In)stabilities" issue (2004). Marcus notes the political engagement of contemporary American artists exhibiting in Power (Indianapolis Museum of Art, September 5–November 3 1991): "None displayed an indifference in their interviews to what their work might mean; with critics, they forcefully discuss and elaborate on what they intend. They fully cooperate in explaining their work in the framework of contemporary theories of social and cultural criticism" (1995: 201–203). We have had similar experiences in our conversations with Indonesian artists. Debates about art and politics make sense of critical moments as noted in Louis Menand's essay, "American Art and the Cold War" (2005).

   Adam Gopnik, recounting conversations with Kirk Varnedoe, formerly chief curator of the Museum of Modern Art, wrote that "he had come to believe that in art history description was all the theory you needed; if you could describe what was there, and what it meant (to the painter, to his time, to you) you did not need a deeper supporting theory. Art was not meaningful because, after you looked at it, someone explained it; art explained itself by being there to look at. He thought that modern art was a part of modern life" (2004: 87).

The linking of art and the artists' exegesis remains central to our ethnographic interpretation and to our theoretical formulations on political subjectivity; both the art and artists' commentaries are central to our ethnographic engagement with modern Indonesian art, a different task than that addressed by Varnedoe.

7. Cigarettes figured prominently in the products portrayed by painters. The Phillip Morris Group, which produces Marlboro, is a supporter of the Indonesian Arts Awards and the Fine Arts Foundation. The relationship between tobacco and art was celebrated dramatically in July 2006 in "The Wedding of Art and Tobacco," a party for three thousand guests, including many leading artists, hosted by Dr. Oei Hong Djien, one of Indonesia's great art collectors. His museum, open for public viewing on request, is funded by Dr. Oei's family's tobacco business (Spanjaard 2004).

8. See H. Geertz (1994) for analysis of the bicultural dimensions of Balinese art of an earlier era.

9. This quote, and those that follow, are our translations from the introduction to the exhibition catalog for the FKY XI 1999.

10. The "three generations" referred to the first generation as forty-five years old and older, the second generation as thirty to forty-four, and the third generation as eighteen to twenty-nine.

11. Yogyakarta artists spoke about artists' roles in the nationalist movement, conveying through painting the independence struggle against colonialism and the emergence of a new nationalist ideology. They also recalled the many LEKRA artists who were imprisoned after the coup that brought Suharto to power and during the repressive periods of the New Order regime. Many were not allowed to paint in the earlier years of imprisonment. And then, like Pramoedya Ananta Toer, Indonesia's most famous novelist who was allowed to write only in the last years of his exile, they too were finally allowed to "make art." Paintings of leading LEKRA artists, such as Hendra Gunawan, are preserved in the private collection of Dr. Oei Hong Djien, in Magelang.

Contemporary artists' concerns about accusations of being "communist" are not insignificant. In a *Jakarta Post* article on a housing and studio complex for art students (Sudiamo 2001), the author noted, "Most of the students are pacifists, as reflected in their works of art. They harbor deep suspicions of the police and military. . . . This village is very much open to the general public for art related activities. The accusations made by security authorities and religious groups that it is the headquarters of the Democratic People's Party (PRD) and communists really do not stand to reason."

12. Theodore Friend (2003) recounts how the "insurgent consciousness" of spring 1998, stirred by the Asian monetary crisis and by student-led popular demonstrations against Suharto's reelection to the presidency, infected "artist groups." Friend

recounts that "a movement arose under the banner of Ruwantan Bumi 1998 (Earth Exorcism 1998). It resembled the cultural fever that accompanied the democracy movement in Beijing in the late 1980s. . . . Yet Ruwantan Bumi 1998 included special Javanese qualities of ritual cleansing and cultural purification. Between early April and early May there were at least 170 performances, Internet-linked, in major cities: music, dance, drama, video, pantomime, installation, art, poetry, prayer, and wayang shadow puppetry. Can we really do the Chinese dragon dance? Dare we ridicule Suharto with a wayang story?" (2003: 332)

13. Kenneth George (1997, 1999, 2004, 2005) argues that Pirous, born in 1932, established his painting style in the immediate post-independence era, contributing to the creation of a national aesthetic and nationalist project. He reacted to the limitations on artistic freedom of the Sukarno era through a commitment to abstract painting; then, while on an art fellowship in the United States (1969–70) and during a visit to the New York Metropolitan Museum of Art, he experienced an "intimate self-recognition" when viewing the collection of Islamic art. He increasingly linked his identity as an Indonesian, a modern artist, and an Acehnese Muslim through a set of paintings that drew on the calligraphic traditions of Islam. Only in the post-Suharto years has Pirous begun to explore the violence in Aceh in explicitly political terms.

14. Our initial conversations with Yulikodo were in 2001; some of these were taped. Follow-up conversations were carried out in January 2004 with our Indonesian research assistant and were taped. The main form of the 2001 conversations is quoted here as it was recorded, transcribed, and translated from Indonesian.

15. Indonesia's famed nationalist author, Pramoedya Ananta Toer, uses the pig image in writing of a Dutch colonial boss in his novel *House of Glass*: "He reminded me of a white-skinned wild pig who couldn't see anything around him except what lay directly in front. He did not care what I thought of him, as long as I was ready to come out with my opinions" (1997: 142).

16. Nationalism, internationalism, government by consent, social justice, and belief in one God are the five pillars of Pancasila, the nationalist Indonesian ideology originally proposed by Sukarno in 1945 as the founding principles of an Indonesian state. Under Suharto's New Order, Pancasila was taught as part of national ideology and history throughout the school system; it came to be regarded by many as "a cudgel of control and conformity . . . with political parties required to incorporate the constitution and Pancasila into their charters" in 1975 (J. G. Taylor 2004: 322, 361–62).

17. We tape-recorded two conversations with Alex Luthfi in January 2004. These were transcribed in Indonesian and translated into English with the assistance of Ninik Supartini. Our initial conversations with Pak Alex were in August 2000.

18. Here Yulikodo refers to his super-realist painting of four horses, which he described in 2001 conversations and again in 2004 as symbolizing corruption and greed in the Suharto regime.

19. On July 27, 1996, the Suharto regime ransacked the Jakarta headquarters of the Indonesian Democratic Party (PDI-P) in order to remove the followers of Megawati Sukarnoputri and install more compliant leadership into the party headquarters, leading to deaths of over one hundred of her supporters and the first widespread antiregime rioting in Jakarta.

20. For a fuller discussion of the history of the term *amuk*, from colonial psychiatry to the present, see B. Good, Subandi, and Good (2001); B. Good and Good (2001); and Good, Subandi, and Good (2007).

21. When telephoning Indonesian friends during this period of the political crisis, responses to a simple question such as "how are things in Yogya?" would often be *"aman saja"* (it is secure here). Discussion of security, often voiced in the language of particular communities or groups "running amok," had entered popular discourse.

22. Unless otherwise noted, materials from our interviews with Entang come from unrecorded January 2003 conversations; recorded formal interviews and informal conversations from January and July 2004 in Yogyakarta; recorded interviews in November and December 2004, in Cambridge; and unrecorded conversations in January 2005.

23. Entang told us this story of his humiliation as well, describing how he broke free from surrealism and found his own style of expressionism.

24. See endnote 20.

25. The New God Series includes works from 1998 to 2000; Melting Souls, those from 1999 to 2001; and Community Storage is a set of works from 2000 to 2001. Of these, only Community Storage was not exhibited as a solo show. It is, however, closely linked to the Hurting Landscapes show, exhibited in Rhode Island where we first met Entang in 2003.

26. See Supangkat and Wisetrotomo (2001: 72) for a description.

27. In Javanese: *Nduwure nganggo klambi kok ngingsore wuda.*

28. See also Supangkat and Wisetrotomo (2001: 49–52) for a nicely translated account.

29. Helena Spanjaard, an art historian who has studied Indonesian modern art for twenty-five years, had a comparable experience to our own when she first saw Entang's NusaAmuk exhibition at the National Gallery in Jakarta in 2001: "The enormous power and energy that filled the galleries overwhelmed me in an almost physical sense" (2002: 13). Her essay on Entang's Hurting Landscape exhibit describes the "use of thick paint" as purposeful in Indonesian painting, to achieve spiritual energy, *tafsu*, and *rokh* (27–28). See also Spanjaard's commentaries on Dr. Oie's collection (2004).

30. Entang says he is very "fond" of Homer Simpson because he is the world's iconic "everyman" with the everyman's common problems—whether he be Indonesian or American.

31. See also Michael Fischer's chapter on American artist (of woodblock prints) and physician, Eric Avery (Fischer 2003).

32. The New York Times (2005), featured a picture of Matt Groening, the creator of The Simpsons, with yellow paint on his hands and wrists just like the coloring used by Entang on his teddy-bear self in his 2003–04 paintings.

REFERENCES

Adelman, Bob. 1999. Roy Lichtenstein's ABC's. Boston, MA: Bullfinch Press.

American Ethnological Society. 2004. In "Contemporary Art Worlds and Their Productive (In)stabilities," American Ethnologist 31 (1).

Anderson, Benedict R. O'G., ed. 2001. Violence and the State in Suharto's Indonesia. Ithaca, NY: Southeast Asia Program Publications, Southeast Asia Program, Cornell University.

Aretxaga, Begoña. 2003. Maddening States. Annual Review of Anthropology 32:393–410.

Carr, David. 2005. Will The Simpsons Ever Age? New York Times, April 24, A22.

Entang Wiharso. 1999. Entang Wiharso. Exhibition catalog. Yogyakarta, Indonesia: Bentang Budaya.

———. 2001. NusaAmuk (Artist Plates and Interviews). Exhibition catalog. Yogyakarta, Indonesia: Antena Projects.

———. 2002. Hurting Landscape: Entang Wiharso. Exhibition catalog. Yogyakarta, Indonesia: Antena Projects.

Festival Kesenian Yogyakarta XIII. 2001. Exhibition catalog. Gedung D Museum Benteng Vredeburg, Yogyakarta, June 7–July 7.

Findlay, Ian. 2001. A Voyage through Chaos. Asian Art News (July–August): 53–57.

Fischer, Joseph, ed. 1990. Modern Indonesian Art: Three Generations of Tradition and Change; 1945–1990. Jakarta and New York: Panitia Pameran KIAS (1990–91) and Festival Indonesia.

Fischer, Michael M. J. 2003. Emergent Forms of Life and the Anthropological Voice. Durham, NC: Duke University Press.

Friend, Theodore. 2003. Indonesian Destinies. Cambridge, MA: The Belknap Press of Harvard University Press.

Geertz, Clifford. 2005. Commentary. In Clifford Geertz by His Colleagues, ed. Richard Shweder and Byron Good, 108–24. Chicago: University of Chicago Press.

Geertz, Hildred. 1994. Images of Power: Balinese Paintings Made for Gregory Bateson and Margaret Mead. Honolulu: University of Hawaii Press.

George, Kenneth. 1997. Some Things That Have happened to the Sun after September 1965: Politics and the interpretation of an Indonesian painting. Comparative Studies in Society and History 39 (4): 599–634.

————. 1999. Signature Work: Bandung, 1994. *Ethnos* 64 (2): 212–31.

————. 2004. Violence, Culture, and the Indonesian Public Sphere: Reworking the Geertzian Legacy. In *Violence: Culture, Performance and Expression*, ed. Neil L. Whitehead, 25–54. Santa Fe, NM: SAR Press.

————. 2005. Picturing Aceh: Violence, Religion, and a Painter's Tale. In *Spirited Politics: Religion and Public Life in Contemporary Southeast Asia*, ed. Andre C. Willford and Kenneth M. George. Ithaca, NY: Southeast Asia Program Publications, Southeast Asia Program, Cornell University.

George, Kenneth M., and A. Y. Mamannoor. 2002. *Pirous: Vision, Faith and a Journey in Indonesian Art*, 1955–2002. Bandung, Indonesia: Yayasan Serambi Pirous.

Good, Byron J., and Mary-Jo DelVecchio Good. 2001. Madness and Violence in Indonesian Politics. *Latitudes* 5 (June): 10–19.

————. 2005. On the "Subject" of Culture: Subjectivity and Cultural Phenomenology in the Work of Clifford Geertz. In *Clifford Geertz by His Colleagues*, ed. Richard Shweder and Byron Good, 98–107. Chicago: University of Chicago Press.

Good, Byron J., and Mary-Jo DelVecchio Good, Jesse Grayman, and Matthew Lakoma. 2006. *Psychosocial Needs Assessment of Communities Affected by the Conflict in the Districts of Pidie, Bireuen, and Aceh Utara*. Jakarta: IOM.

Good, Byron J., Subandi, and Mary-Jo DelVecchio Good. 2001. Le sujet de la maladie mentale: Psychose, folie furieuse et subjectivité en Indonésie. In *La Maladie mentale en mutation: Psychiatrie et société*, ed. Alain Ehrenberg and Anne M. Lovell, 163–95. Paris: éditions Odile Jacob.

————. 2007. The Subject of Mental Illness: Psychosis, Mad Violence, and Subjectivity in Indonesia, in *Subjectivity: Ethnographic Investigations*, ed. João Biehl, Byron Good, and Arthur Kleinman. Berkeley: University of California Press.

Good, Mary-Jo DelVecchio, and Byron J. Good. 1988. Ritual, the State, and the Transformation of Emotional Discourse in Iranian Society. *Culture, Medicine and Psychiatry* 12:43–63.

Gopnik, Adam. 2004. Last of the Metrozoids: A Teacher's Final Lessons. *The New Yorker* (May 10): 82–91.

Kerton, Sudjana. 1996. *Nionalisme Dan Perubahannya: Refleksi Karya Sudjana Kerton/Nationalism and Its Transformations Reflection on Works of Sudjana Kerton*. Jakarta: Gedung Pameran Seni Rupa, Departemen Pendidikan dan Kebudayaan.

Kristeva, Julia. 1982. *Powers of Horror: An Essay on Abjection*. Trans. Leon S. Roudiez. New York: Columbia University Press.

Marcus, George. 1995. The Power of Contemporary Work in an American Art Tradition to Illuminate Its Own Power Relations. In *The Traffic in Culture: Refiguring Art and Anthropology*, ed. George E. Marcus and Fred R. Myers, 201–23. Berkeley: University of California Press.

Marcus, George E., and Fred R. Myers, ed. 1995. *The Traffic in Culture: Refiguring Art and Anthropology.* Berkeley: University of California Press.

Menand, Louis. 2005. American Art and the Cold War. *The New Yorker* (October 17): 174–79.

Philip Morris Group of Companies and the Indonesian Fine Arts Foundation. 2001. *Indonesia Art Awards: 2001.* Exhibition catalog. Jakarta: Philip Morris Group of Companies and the Indonesian Fine Arts Foundation.

Phillips, Lisa. 1999. *The American Century: Art and Culture 1950–2000.* New York: Whitney Museum of American Art, New York, in association with W. W. Norton & Company.

Rosenquist, James. 2003. *A Retrospective.* New York: Guggenheim Museum.

Shweder Richard A., and Byron Good, eds. 2005. *Clifford Geertz by His Colleagues.* Chicago: University of Chicago Press.

Spanjaard, Helena. 2002. The Shouting Universe of Entang Wiharso. In *Hurting Landscape: Entang Wiharso,* by Entang Wiharso, 13–28. Yogyakarta, Indonesia: Antena Projects.

———. 2004. *Exploring Modern Indonesian Art: The Collection of Dr. Oei Hong Djien.* Singapore: SNP International.

Steedly, Mary Margaret. 1999. The State of Culture Theory in the Anthropology of Southeast Asia. *Annual Review of Anthropology* 28:431–54.

Sudiamo, Tarko. 2001. A Glimpse into Yogyakarta's Exclusive Arts Settlement. *Jakarta Post,* July 22.

Supangkat, Jim, and Sarah E. Murray, curators. 1999. *Entang Wiharso.* Exhibition catalog. Yogyakarta, Indonesia: Bentang Budaya.

Supangkat, Jim, and Suwarno Wisetrotomo, curators. 2001. Text in *NusaAmuk (Artist Plates and Interviews),* by Entang Wiharso, 21–93. Yogyakarta, Indonesia: Antena Projects.

Sutejo, Godod, and Alex Luthfi R, curators. 1999. *Three Generations of Yogyakarta Artists (Tiga Generasi Perupa Yogyakarta)/FKY XI 1999.* Exhibition catalog. Yogyakarta, Indonesia: Fine Arts Festival Yogyakarta and Bentara Budaya.

Taylor, Jean Gelman. 2003. *Indonesia: Peoples and Histories.* New Haven, CT: Yale University Press.

Taylor, Nora A., ed. 2000. *Studies in Southeast Asian Art: Essays in Honor of Stanley J. O'Connor.* Ithaca, NY: Southeast Asia Program Publications, Southeast Asia Program, Cornell University.

Toer, Pramoedya Ananta. 1997 [1988]. *House of Glass.* Trans. Max Lane. New York: Penguin Books.

Willford, Andrew C., and George, Kenneth M. 2005 *Spirited Politics: Religion and Public Life in Contemporary Southeast Asia.* Ithaca, NY: Southeast Asia Program Publications, Southeast Asia Program, Cornell University.

Wright, Astri. 2000. Lucia Hartini, Javanese Painter: Against the Grain, Towards Herself. In *Studies in Southeast Asian Art: Essays in Honor of Stanley J. O'Connor*, ed. Nora A Taylor, 93–121. Ithaca, NY: Southeast Asia Program Publications, Southeast Asia Program, Cornell University.

Wuthnow, Robert. 2001. *Creative Spirituality: The Way of the Artist*. Berkeley: University of California Press.

Venezia, Mike. 2001. *Roy Lichtenstein (Getting to Know the World's Greatest Artists)*. New York: Children's Press.

*Fantasy, Conspiracy, and Estrangement among Populist Leaders
in Post–New Order Lombok, Indonesia*

John M. MacDougall

This chapter explores the rise in political and religious vigilance in post–New Order Lombok, Indonesia, and the role that militias played in denying Soleh, a nationalist activist in Lombok, the social horizons (loosely, the nation and its youth) he once relied upon to define his political and, in the end, personal reality. The chapter provides an individual case study in order to examine how social disorder and political violence are experienced by a leading intellectual who has been deeply involved in Indonesian politics on the island of Lombok. It makes clear that resistance is at once a social and psychological experience born in ongoing relations of power that are not simply punctuated by moments of lucidity (sanity) or delusion (illness). Instead, the chapter is an ethnographic example of how political disorder has site-specific social and historical forms while psychopathology has its own psychological forms that can reflect social discord as much as they engage internal conflict.

Soleh was one of Lombok's most outspoken advocates of the populist struggle against state oppression during the New Order. He was also a Balinese noble and recent convert to Islam. More importantly, Soleh appealed to a common national unity, and a concept of justice, capable of leveling primordial divisions and denying the military its control of civic loyalties. Nationalist populism was his passion and, more practically speaking, his unique religious and cultural background left him few other venues to pursue. In short, he was too Muslim to be Balinese and too Balinese to be a good Sasak Muslim. In the post-Suharto era of emergent religious and ethnic collectivism, Soleh's populism rang hollow against the increasingly exclusive communities he once risked life and limb to defend. There is a history to Soleh's situation.

The island of Lombok lies east of Bali and is home to 2.4 million inhabitants. Sometimes called the "land of a thousand mosques," it is overwhelmingly Muslim. Ethnic Sasak Muslims make up 92 percent of the population, with not insignificant minorities of some 60,000 Balinese Hindus and 20,000 Sasak Buddhists, mostly in North Lombok. Historically, western Lombok developed closer ties with Bali while eastern Lombok was economically and ideologically (through Islamic affinities) linked to Buginese Muslim kingdoms in Sulawesi to the north and Sumbawa to the east. For almost 150 years beginning in the mid-eighteenth century, two East Balinese royal houses colonized Lombok until Islamic brotherhoods based in East Lombok revolted against the Balinese colonizers in 1891. Although the Balinese subdued the rebellion, the Muslim brotherhoods invited the Dutch in to assist their movement and, after defeating the Balinese in 1894, ushered in a new period of Dutch-style indirect rule. After the Dutch took over control of Lombok, continuous revolts against the Dutch tax laws plagued European administrators until the Japanese ousted the Dutch when they invaded Lombok and Indonesia in 1941. Over Lombok's long history of conflict, organized resistance against foreign invasion has always begun in East Lombok, where ethnic Sasak identity was equated with Islamic reformism, and ritualism became an index for the political residue of Balinese cultural domination. The conflation of the intimate world of Sasak rites with Balinese colonial symbolism introduced an important local justification for Islamic reformism and antiritualist censure throughout the twentieth century.

The New Order government under President General Suharto took over Indonesian politics and, after the massacres of between five hundred thousand and two million suspected Indonesian communists, began a series of five-year economic development plans. To ensure absolute compliance with his development programs in agriculture, birth control, and migration, Suharto used the military's regional battalions to enforce civic compliance with Suharto's brand of guided progress. Mandatory education in national ideology was carried out at all levels of public and private education. The Department of Information and Military Intelligence (Bakin) monitored all publications and radio and television programming for potentially subversive content. Resistance to Suharto's standards invited arrest, abuse, and sometimes disappearance. Political rights were revoked and public memory acquired a muted, haunting presence in the lives of those who fell victim to Suharto's brand of punishment.

Soleh's dilemma arose after Suharto stepped down in 1998 and the sudden removal of the New Order matrix of state terrorism provided activists such as

Soleh with the opportunity to imagine a return to idealistic politics and the restoration of justice to Indonesia's proletariat. Unfortunately, Lombok's own communal politics did not follow Soleh's romantic dreams of democratic promise. In fact, when the police state lost its monopoly over violence, violence was "democratized" to incorporate new actors with new claims to vigilante dominion over the communities Soleh once mobilized in his demonstrations against the state. To Soleh's dismay a hybrid mixture of community-level vigilance and national conspiracy steadily erased his source of self-worth and activism. Soleh's "master signifier," the State to be resisted or reconstituted as Just Ideal, splintered into factionalized corporate identities. Soleh's former youth activists joined these new groups to become vigilantes, a local and more intimate means of restoring cultural vitality, for the sake of community and not nation. The sudden absence of the social coordinates for his style of romantic resistance forced Soleh to construe his own private war with the maddening effects of the phantomlike military agents he believed were set to destabilize the populist movements and any hope of real reform.[1] During Soleh's increasingly lonely battle against the mysterious efforts of Suharto's cronies, he placed his faith in nationalist leader and PDI-P party head Megawati Sukarnoputri, a figure he believed to be able, through auspicious quietism and nationalist fantasy, to sustain her popular and romantic support for a "once and future" nation.

Soleh's imaginary was not unique to his own vision of nationalist struggle. Elsewhere in Indonesia, the unsettling effects of the economic crisis, intercommunal violence, and political conspiracies had forced many Indonesians to create a style of moral vigilance to conjure some sense of surrogate order in their villages. The material justifications for Suharto's development myth (i.e., cheap rice, affordable schooling, and medicine) had turned out to be a dream on loan and Suharto's oppression merely a justification for his own corrupt rewards. For lack of a police state, new forms of moral vigilance enabled Indonesians, in Soleh's case the ethnic Sasak Muslim youth of Lombok, to repossess the social, political, and personal domains once policed by Suharto's New Order regime. New forms of mass entitlement made theft, a common event among Lombok's long-standing thief heroes, into a betrayal of community. After the election of 1999, Lombok's Muslim leaders began to form anticrime militias to patrol their village roads for criminals and provocateurs. In only a few months' time, these groups were able to fill the gap the police state had left with their own spectacles of murder and internal purification of the thieving Other. While these militias made their rounds, and Lombok youth rallied to support the moral authority of the movement, Soleh felt his populist fantasies slip from his grasp.

One must first possess something in order to lose it. Soleh's fantasies are not pure delusion but are rooted in a decade-long set of social and political transformations, some cordoned by the frames of national resistance, some incidental to Lombok's wayward style of militarized development. Soleh became an activist in the early 1990s when dramatic signs of change and prosperity appeared in Indonesia. The rise of the educated middle class, private business, and access to information via the Internet and private cable companies ushered in a flood of information for millions of Indonesians who had prospered during Suharto's rule. The ban on "lefty" books, the presence of intelligence agents on university campuses, and the state ideology courses mandatory for students and professors alike inspired students and intellectuals to form secret "reading groups." By the early 1990s, increasingly large numbers of idealist activists like Soleh joined the critical branches of Indonesia's Legal Aid Institute and a plethora of theory-inspired NGOs to begin what they called *advokasi* (community-based activism).[2]

There were also political developments afoot. In the late New Order (1993–98), outside of the separatist movements in Aceh, East Timor, and Irian Jaya, the power and economic wealth Suharto amassed while leading one of the world's most corrupt bureaucracies went largely unchallenged. In 1995, one of the nation's largest newspapers conducted one of the nation's first pre-election polls. When asked whom they supported to win the 1997 election, 40 percent of the respondents chose Megawati Sukarnoputri, the daughter of Sukarno, Indonesia's nationalist leader and founding father. On July 27, 1996, Suharto punished Megawati and her political party, PDI-P, for her statistical hubris and ordered a military attack on her party headquarters. Megawati was subsequently disqualified from formal party participation in the 1997 election. In protest, Megawati supporters boycotted the election through a movement called Golput.[3] By not voting, they were in essence voting for Megawati. When they discovered Suharto had won, yet again, they celebrated their loss as a victory. Megawati had, in the course of the election, turned Suharto's style of civic quietism into the catalyst of her nationalist movement. That is, Megawati's absence from party politics was even more powerful than her presence. In a similar act of resistant quietism, millions of otherwise apolitical students, farmers, and village youth rallied to Megawati's cause and refused to vote. By not doing or saying anything, or not voting, they were performing the first political protest of their hitherto politically inactive lives.

In May 1998, less than a year after the 1997 election, Suharto stepped down. Because of the heroic demonstrations of Indonesia's students, a few reformists in the military, and the overpowering pressure of the economic crisis, Indonesians had a chance at a new future. Besides the highs of political reform, however, there were more troubling developments on the horizon. Political rivalries intensified and regionally organized vigilante groups or militias grew throughout Indonesia's villages. During this same period, reformist leaders and authorities alike warned communities to beware of *oknum-oknum gelap*, or dark conspirators, intent on creating chaos in the archipelago. Reportedly funded by conglomerates and the increasingly disenfranchised Indonesian military, these dark agents became more than just bits of conjecture. They were real but not identifiable.

In response to the threat of provocateurs, the dimensions of social and political participation in Indonesia experienced a distinct shift. While during the New Order the tensions of state terrorism were felt between the compliant citizen and the government official, these new dark elements were organized to inflame repressed tensions between communities.[4] The presence of such phantom New Order antagonists combined with the rise of partisan campaigns around the 1999 election delineated new dimensions for civic participation. National resistance to oppression no longer lay in the hands of rebellious students, but was contained within the boundaries of the neighborhoods and of religious or ethnic communities of Indonesians' immediate surroundings.

In this atmosphere of community vigilantism, the sociopolitical horizons of insider and outsider, neighbor and oppressor, shrank (in modernist Islam's case, expanded) to the coordinates of community. With twenty-two million of Indonesia's ninety-million-person workforce left unemployed by the economic crisis, there were plenty of "guardians" eager to protect and be recognized by their endangered communities.[5] This mixture of community vigilance and national politics bore little resemblance to New Order Indonesia, when the only people involved in singing the song of resistance were the misfit activists and lawyers Suharto once termed the "bald devils" (*tuyul-tuyul botak*) of the nation.

SOLEH'S DREAMS: NATIONALIST ACTIVISM

Soleh was one such "bald devil." During the late New Order, Soleh was famous for his successful record in the defense of the oppressed Lombok peasants and, most notably, for his street smarts. Among his heroes were populist nationalists such as Lombok's own nationalist martyr, Saleh Sungkar, and President Sukarno, the famously charismatic founding father of Indonesia. Just prior to the 1999 election, Soleh's loyalties and political fantasies came to revolve largely around Sukarno's daughter, Megawati Sukarnoputri, who was rumored to have inherited her father's charismatic spirit. Meanwhile, Soleh's enemies—the abusive members of the military, Suharto's conglomerates, and the unseen dark elements—were, or so he believed, conspiring to destroy the reformist movement and him.

In 1993, the Suharto-appointed governor of West Nusatenggara, Warsito (1987–98), began using the military to force Lombok's peasants to leave their land to be developed for tourism. In response to these threats, NGOs and a few mavericks from the Legal Aid Institute ran to defend their cause. Among these mavericks was Soleh. Like many of the initial founders of the Legal Aid Institute of Indonesia, his courage against the oppressive measures of the state won less respect from the theory-minded university students than from the preman, or roughhouse youth, of the province.[6] Where NGO activists wrote of the plight of Lombok's poor in articles and internationally funded case studies, Soleh mobilized the same peasants to protect their lands from attacks by the military. Soleh was all about action. Like the famous thieves of Lombok, Soleh's style of fly-by-night advocacy was always habis-habisan (to the bitter end). Soleh had not only been a Golden Gloves boxer in his youth, but in 1994 he also single-handedly organized Lombok's first branch of the notorious Suharto-backed thug club called Pemuda Pancasila.[7]

Even though Soleh's populist ideals quickly soured his relations with the more militant and gang-minded Pemuda Pancasila officials in Jakarta, he had provided the Sasak youth who joined his cause with an identity and a uniform associated with defenders of state authority and nationalist ideals. Soleh was a Marhaenist or, to put it simply, a Sukarno-style populist-nationalist. Credited with several victorious "last stands" against the government, Soleh became a kind of celebrity in Lombok. After the reform movement was well under way in 1999, many reformists even thought he might be elected mayor of the provincial capital of Mataram.

During the demonstrations and reformist movement prior to Suharto's fall in 1998, Soleh and his youth idealists demonstrated against the local parliament. Soleh's popular support in Lombok made him attractive to Megawati Sukarnoputri's party. It was largely through support from populist toughs like Soleh that Indonesia's nationalist party, PDI-P, was able to mobilize such a large national following during the election campaigns. Having lived a life as a renegade lawyer, Soleh found his calling when the PDI-P asked him to be one of their party cadres in Lombok. Throughout the island, Soleh converted the old members of Pemuda Pancasila into Pemuda Banteng, or PDI-P youth bulls. Although he was disappointed when Megawati Sukarnoputri lost the 1999 election to Abdurrahman Wahid, Soleh himself had accomplished the task he had fought so long to achieve. For the first time since the 1950s, Lombok had a broad-based political party organized for the revitalization of the people of Lombok. There were other developments growing in Lombok, however, which would compromise Soleh's romantic vision and far-sighted partisan goals.

THE RISE OF MORAL MILITIAS

After Abdurrahman Wahid was elected president in October of 1999, I eagerly set out to discuss the political implications with the Buda Buddhist leaders in my research area. I found that not only were people ambivalent about Wahid's presidency, but it wasn't even on the table for local discussion. Of much greater importance was the development of *pamswakarsa*, or anticrime militias, in East and Central Lombok. These groups were of particular concern to the Buda leadership because of their swelling membership after the general election in June 1999, their regionalist bases in East and Central Lombok, and their Islamist orientation. What worried the Buda leaders was the uncanny resemblance of the *pamswakarsa* vigilante groups to the political terror waged against them during the killings of suspected communists in 1965, prior to their "evasive" conversion to state Buddhism to avoid being cast as pagan atheists and therefore suspected communists. Even without the traumatic echoes of the communist massacres and intimidation of the past, the term *pamswakarsa* itself had a more contemporary but violent national heritage of its own.

In October 1998, President Habibie and General Wiranto drafted legislation proposing that a paramilitary civilian corps be trained and developed to assist Indonesia's weak police force to maintain order in the archipelago. The groups were to be called *pamswakarsa*(self-reliant security corps).[8] Since the bloody riots of November 1998, when these military-backed *pamswakarsa* were mobilized to "protect" the special parliamentary session in Jakarta from student "anarchists," several groups throughout Indonesia had used the *pamswakarsa* label for their own military-backed killing teams. Organized along ethnic, regional, and religious lines, *pamswakarsa* established armed civilian police patrols in order to "restore order" in their respective regions. *Pamswakarsa* in Jakarta, East Java, and most notably in East Timor fed on the aforementioned atmosphere of neighborhood and regionalist allegiance to run antireformist terror campaigns against "subversives" or historical enemies in their respective regions. *Pamswakarsa* or militias have been responsible for the deaths of thousands of random victims scapegoated for partisan, regionalist, or even internationally inspired tensions. By December 1999, *pamswakarsa* membership in Lombok had swelled to over 220,000 members, four times the number of men who razed East Timor after the referendum in September 1999.

Bujak and Amphibi: Economies of Moral Vigilance

Two of the largest and oldest of Lombok's anticrime militias are Bujak and Amphibi. While the government funded East Timor's militias and the Islamic right sponsored Maluku's jihad militias, Lombok's pamswakarsa relied largely on members' dues to fund their operations and, in return, to provide security against crime in their region. The rise of pamswakarsa in Lombok is particularly unusual simply because Lombok, especially East and Central Lombok, is famous for its accomplished thieves.[9]

The restoration of a "local Real," a community-based sense of dominion, might suggest an explanation of how, in postelection Lombok, young men justified the hunting and killing of the criminals they once held in such high esteem. On the other hand, a deeper inquiry into the ritualized and doctrinal power of moral militarism may help us unpack why the executions of criminal heroes were seen as spectacles of both political and moral power of post–New Order Islam. Regardless of the hermeneutic approach, with Suharto's military taking care not to stir up public disfavor Lombok's youth were allowed to exercise a novel moral and political legitimacy in their late-night patrols of Lombok's streets and in the killing of their former heroes. The moral and political legitimacy I speak of can be found in a twofold resonance evident in both political and religious practices. The first is national and regional while the second is scriptural and ritualized.

The rise in communal vigilantism emerged simultaneously with the explosion of partisan participation that mobilized millions of unemployed young men. Recruiting from vigilante youth groups, each party developed its own party police (satgas partai), largely comprised of young men with experience in martial arts or with a regional reputation for toughness. In addition to Lombok's pamswakarsa, there were also other militant Islamist youth security groups active in all of Indonesia's religious organizations and parties. The family resemblances between the political, regional, religious, and "mock" reformist agendas that youth vigilante groups were recruited to protect imbued Lombok's pamswakarsa with an indirectly nationalist and religious credibility. This resulted in, for lack of a better term, a contextual modernist ethic where a local assault (criminal or interfamilial) on the community could also be interpreted as an ideological assault on the village, the region, the nation, or on Islam.[10]

RITUAL RESONANCE: THE MORAL RECOVERY OF SECURITY

Differences between the ritual ideologies of Lombok's traditional and orthodox ritual practices inform similar junctures between more traditional and bounty-oriented anticrime militias and their more blood-letting Islamic groupings. Where earlier, and not explicitly religious, *pamswakarsa* focused on the recovery of stolen goods (and not the immoral criminal), Islamist militias shifted their focus from the recovery of possessions to the extermination of criminal self. Sasak ritual practices of "spirit theft" and "retrieval" follow a similar economy. Almost all Sasak ritual practice, whether elopement, spirit theft (Sasak: *ketemuq*), or head-shaving rites (Sasak: *ngurisang*), revolve around the weakening effects of a "theft" and the rites of the recovery (Sasak: *tebusan*) of what has been taken. The most pervasive and frequent of these rites is spirit theft/recovery, or *ketemuq/nebusang* (Sasak; *nebusang* means "recovery through payment").[11] A crucial cleavage between traditionalist practices of repayment (Sasak: *tebusang*) and Islamist alienation of immoral spirits in these rites helps us to gain a better sense of how morally reconstituting economies conspire to draw men to take lives for the sake of themselves and their communities.

As early as 1994, the Bujak militia, literally meaning "tracker" (*pemburu jejak*), was organized in Central Lombok as an alternative method for retrieving stolen goods. Organized by two Central Lombok nobles, Bujak served as a traditional bounty-hunter organization. For a fee, Bujak would use its connections among networks of thieves to retrieve the articles stolen from Bujak clients. Bujak was formed largely because it was discovered that the police themselves were often involved in laundering stolen goods. (In 1998, a police station in Janapriya, Central Lombok, was burned down as a result.) Most important to note here is the resonance of Bujak's bounty practices with Sasak anxieties and exchange-based rites regarding weakening effects of "loss" and the empowering recovery of what is lost through repayment.

In late 1997, there was a dramatic increase in crime due to the economic crisis and failed harvests. By early 1998, Bujak's bounty service was in full swing. Not all of Bujak's members were morally upstanding, however. In fact many of them were ex-criminals, hence their access to crime networks throughout the island. Because of their *preman*, or thuggish, reputation and the absence of moral or religious leadership in the organization, in early 1998 another group was formed in the Islamic heart of East Lombok. At the time, Soleh and many of Lombok's NGOs tacitly supported Bujak's efforts to break the chain of criminality through recuperative bounty practices. They were not prepared, however, to address Bujak's new Islamist competitor growing in East Lombok.

The new *pamswakarsa* was called Amphibi (as in "amphibious"). Under the moral leadership of the charismatic Muslim cleric, Tuan Guru Haji Sibaway, Amphibi's ranks swelled to sixty thousand in only three months' time. Tuan Guru Haji Sibaway's immediate success was partly because, in October 1997, the founder and leader of Lombok's largest Islamic organization, Nahdlatul Wathan

(NW), had died. Surviving him were two daughters and a fragmented network of lesser Tuan Guru religious leaders without any clear heir to his once authoritarian control over the organization's religious, economic, and educational institutions.[12] Although Tuan Guru Haji Sibaway lacked the notoriety of NW's founder, he picked a good time to fill the power vacuum of East Lombok's Islamic community. By late 1999, Amphibi's vigilante militias had replaced the educational institutions of NW as the single largest "moral religious" force on the island. Bujak didn't have a chance. The combined effect of Amphibi's modernist-Islamist orientation, its recruitment of *santri*, or orthodox youth, and its disavowal of the thuggish former criminals employed by Bujak won Amphibi a form of religious legitimacy that Bujak could never achieve. At the national level, the formation of Amphibi overshadowed the Bujak-style gangsters and replaced them with the vigilant Islamic moralism growing throughout postelection Indonesia (e.g., Maluku's *jihad* forces, the Kabah Youth movement, and Islamic Party Security).

Amphibi, unlike the more exchange-based bounty service of Bujak, was a modernist *pamswakarsa*.[13] Amphibi did not retrieve goods through healers or a network of thieves, or even rely on recuperative bounty payments for the return of stolen goods. As orthodox families used scriptural alienation of the invasive spirit (as opposed to a recuperative payment) of a *ketemuq* victim, Amphibi's focus rested not in the goods stolen but in the immoral actions of the thief. If a thief was caught, he was killed. While Bujak members relied on a the appeal of recovered goods and monetary rewards for services rendered, Amphibi members were supplied with jackets empowered with Arabic script recited into their jumpers (sweaters) by Tuan Guru Sibaway himself. Their powers came not from the street-smart thuggism of activists and criminals but from the supracommunal and scriptural purity of the Koran. While Bujak demanded a *tebusan*, or bounty offering, from the victim of theft, an Amphibi member had to pay 120,000 rupiah. (roughly half a month's wage) just for the honor of wearing the jacket and joining the night guard.

The incursion of Islamic scripture in both Sasak ritual rites of spirit recovery and the restorative powers of anticrime militias' surveillance techniques highlight a crucial ideological difference in how alternately traditional or orthodox Sasaks recuperate endangered vitality. The moral legitimacy of Amphibi's executions rested in many ways on the long-standing cleavage between impure and "primitive" *bid'ah* ritual practice (as reflected in the ritual resonance between nonorthodox *ketemuq* "payments" and Bujak bounty service) and the orthodox scripturalism employed by reformist and modernist Islamic communities throughout Indonesia.

This analysis reveals that these groups are not merely symptoms of a failed government, postauthoritarian regimes, or the mark of a greater conspiracy.

Instead, we should ask what young militia members feel they gain morally, politically, and religiously when they venture into the night in search of locally intimate but morally alienated targets. In her study of rites of violence in sixteenth-century France, Natalie Davis makes a similar point:

> We may see these crowds as prompted by political and moral traditions which legitimize and even prescribe their violence. We may see urban rioters not as miserable, uprooted, unstable masses, but as men and women who often have some stake in their community; who may be craftsmen or better; and who, even when poor and unskilled, may appear respectable to their everyday neighbors. Finally, we may see violence, however cruel, not as random and limitless, but as aimed at defined targets selected from a repertory of traditional punishments and forms of destruction. (1973: 52–53)

As such, we do not have to rely solely on the theories of dark conspiracies the media often employ to depict a "viral" contagion of military-backed militias throughout Indonesia. The young men of Amphibi were not forsaking their communities to join a rebellious group of thugs and ex-criminals to terrorize the countryside. Instead they were ritually and politically projecting new forms of moral surveillance over previously secular and nationally policed sites of dominion. Many of these youth were formerly members of Soleh's nationalist groups and were equally committed to fighting the injustices of the state. In the absence of a formally authoritarian regime, these men relied on Lombok-based practices of ritualized and Islamist ideologies of recovery, the filling of a void: the production of a "local Real." The structure of state power and its boundaries had shifted and were shifting still from center-periphery dynamics of New Order control to the reassertion of religious values in locally authoritative, and, in this case, frighteningly persuasive ways.

THE MATARAM VIOLENCE

On 17 January 2000, over sixty thousand Sasak Muslim men crowded into Mataram to protest the violence against Muslims in Maluku, Indonesia. For three hours, small, organized groups ran through the streets targeting and burning Christian homes and churches. I was caught in the riots myself, and I stopped by several friends' homes as I tried to work my way safely to the port and, hopefully, find a way out of the mess. In each place I stopped, my Sasak friends remarked at how strong the rioters were. One of my friends ran back from the violence to report, "They run without tiring, those Amphibi. They don't drink, eat, or anything and yet they can run the full length of Mataram without stopping to rest."

With scenarios of national and interethnic conspiracy in my head, I returned to Soleh's home to find out what "really happened."[14] In his statement on the motives behind the riots, we begin to see the dark dimensions of Soleh's design, so secular, partisan, and national. We will see these figures again when the territories of Soleh's resistance are taken from him and the convincing yet uncanny mystique of his conspiracies takes on a different life.[15]

In his interpretative description of the political strategies behind the January riots, Soleh laid out the political demise of the new Indonesia, its forces and weaknesses, with Lombok as its trigger for destruction. Soleh's chronology is drawn to match an apocalyptic military plot to restore power to authoritarian leaders. To Soleh, conspiratorial figures, and not local leaders, used religion to incite Lombok militias to riot. At the end of his statement, Soleh attempted to use the president's status as Muslim cleric as a countertrope to defuse the perception that the riots were an Islamic vendetta against Indonesian Christians for the death of Muslims in Maluku. Instead Soleh composed another narrative where the "seeds of hate against Christianity" were no longer articulated within the historical antagonisms between East and West Lombok or even within the inter-religious tensions at the level of the nation. Rather, Soleh believed these strategies were part of a greater political and decidedly military-based strategy to effect a national "state of emergency." In Soleh's scenario the scripturalist ritual power of Lombok Islam was being used as a regional pawn to topple the decidedly pluralist Islamic leadership of the state under Wahid, while ritualistic campaigns of the pamswakarsa were part of a nationwide military effort to weaken the police and to justify the call for military rule.

Unfortunately, Soleh's statist interpretations of the events in January, however right-minded or sound, did not predict what would happen to him and Lombok over the months following the violence of January 2000. After the riots, Amphibi's attraction to the Sasak populace proved efficacious with or without its conspiratorial dimensions. In only three months' time, Amphibi had extended its members' territorial claims into West Lombok. Although before the riots Amphibi was based in East Lombok, now Amphibi's guard posts could be found in almost every community in Lombok. At long last, Amphibi finally controlled the historical divide between colonial West and Islamic East Lombok.

SOLEH'S FALL

Soleh's hard work on behalf of reformist commoner politicians went unrewarded. At the regional PDI-P Congress in June 2000, Soleh was reduced to local party organizer because, according to those who know him, he refused to take money from local businessmen. Several PDI-P and local parliamentarians approached his youth supporters and told them that, even though he was Muslim, Soleh was still a Balinese whose people had colonized and oppressed the Sasak people. Steadily, fewer people visited Soleh's once-bustling home. Finally, in the local paper, it was reported that Soleh's wife was to sue him for divorce because of his incessant accusations that she was producing pornographic films behind his back. What appeared to me at first to be a case of libelous journalism proved to be more true than not when I finally visited Soleh at his home. I approached his veranda, once a hub of activity, only to find him disheveled and alone. His party, the PDI-P and the voice of the people, the Marhaenist dream, had lost the national election and dismissed him for the strictness of his ideals. In fact, his dream of the role party politics would play in restoring pride and self-reliance in the people of Lombok was, in disturbing but effective circumstances, being carried out by Islamic militias. The political and idealist dimensions of Soleh's life had collapsed. When Megawati herself took his name off the list of party cadres, Soleh began to smell a great conspiracy. Soleh explained his "fall" as follows:

"I asked you to come by today, John, because there is a great conspiracy to destroy my life and everyone close to it. At the PDI-P conference two months ago, opportunistic and greedy members of the party removed me from the party cadre register. I was surprised that Ibu Megawati would listen to such gossip and backstabbing when I started to see the signs. A friend of mine brought over a number of pornographic films and, while watching them, I realized that these films were filmed in my house, my very own home. After watching the films over and over again I studied them in slow motion and realized that the actors were from Lombok. The doors of my bedroom, the walls of my main room inside were all part of the set for a pornographic film [filem porno]. Then I remembered that over the last three months, thousands of pornographic films were being sold and watched in villages throughout Lombok. Everywhere you go in Lombok, there is a VCD player and youth watching these films. I checked around and learned how these bootleg films were being brought in to the island. I remembered the way that the films of the violence in Maluku were distributed and it came to me. Since the violence in January I have made several trips to Sumbawa to help some friends there deal with labor issues. While I was gone, people linked to the military and a pornography cartel must have made the films in my home. If news of this got to Megawati or her aides, I'm sure that Megawati would see this as justifiable evidence for my dismissal.

"I called my wife to see the people in the film. I made her watch them because I was convinced she knew too, that they had gotten to her too. I showed her all the parts of the film where it was obvious that it was our house, her friends and expatriates we knew who were featured in the films. There is also a woman in the film who looks exactly like my wife."

"What did your wife say?" I asked.

"She said I was crazy. After watching the films with her she got angry and said, 'You better be careful, Soleh. Someday you might see yourself in that film.'"

Soleh continued, "The military know that we kept their bloodbath from happening last January. They know how we have tried to strengthen the police force so that they can replace the military. We had them running scared but the military intelligence has always been the best and now they have me beat. You don't believe me, do you, John? Come on, I'll show you the films."

I walked into his now bare house. He had taken apart the doors of the rooms and spread them on his living room floor. Until Soleh started to play the film, I thought that it would be some Indonesian pornography filmed in a house that sort of looked like his. Instead, the film he showed me was a European film with big European actors and actresses set in bars and mock hotel settings. Soleh wasn't to be fooled by these camera tricks. "Look at that wooden bed stand," he yelled and ran over to the disassembled door and, angling it up on the floor, showed that it was the same size and cut as the bed stand in the film. "Look at that doorway, the paint on the wall is the same color." He marched all over the house he had taken apart to prove that, in fact, these films had been made in his home. "Soleh," I asked, "What about the actors and actresses? They are European or American. They are blond and white."

"That is what you think," he said. "Before the filming, Sasak girls are painted and powdered with make-up to look white. After the filming they shower it all off and they are Sasaks again." After watching with occasional moments of amusement when the absurdity of the whole situation grew too much to handle, I asked him what he planned to do. Soleh continued,

This is an international cartel, this group. The military and Jakarta business manipulate immigration to produce these films and smuggle them out for editing and production. They are distributed worldwide. These people are so powerful and have so much money they can buy anyone and anything. They are destroying these women's lives. I can't let that happen. My wife is in these films too and that hurts me the most. They destroyed her to get to me. I can't let that happen. Even if she has turned against me, she is still a victim and must be defended.

What power, what dark force of political imagination or delusion had driven Soleh to see his house disassembled and projected onto the set of an erotic film?

As already mentioned, political analysis of the growth of NGOs in Lombok and Soleh's history as an activist-maverick helps us to understand how his romance of the populist-nationalist "peasantry" provided the foundational dimensions for his personal and political conspiracies, fantasies, rivalries, and victories. When other Indonesians were submitting to the standards and scripted modes of being during the New Order, Soleh and the rest of Indonesia's activist misfits were an amalgam of the New Order's primary enemies: the rebellious tough and the leftist student. Grounded in these ideals and social relations, however, Soleh's strict populism and ethnic-caste background (he was a Balinese noble converted to Islam) denied him an effective role in the youth organizations in which he planned to build his dream work: he was too principled for the arch-nationalist thug rings of Suharto's Pemuda Pancasila (1994); too populist for the "theoretical" NGO activists of Lombok (1993–present); and he was too Balinese for the Islamist pamswakarsa that were effectively erasing his influence over Lombok's village-based activists. Soleh was able to actualize the full visionary potential of his dream in Megawati Sukarnoputri's PDI-P in part because Megawati was to him what she was to so many: the silent screen upon which he, and many others, projected their fantasies of a future nation and better lives. Despite the betrayals of PDI-P, Megawati remained pure in Soleh's mind. Megawati, the embodiment of her father's charisma and revolutionary heroism, remained the moral kernel of Soleh's idea of a supra-ethno-religious nation not because of what she did or said, but rather precisely because she did not say or do anything.

Megawati's silence had already made her the object of international and elite ridicule. To her supporters, her silence reflected her purity.[16] During the party campaign period, when all the other political leaders slandered and criticized their opponents, Megawati would not be sullied by such behavior. She remained mute. When the coalition of Islamic parties chose Abdurrahman Wahid over Megawati, the winner of the popular vote, she did not cry foul. In fact, when the rest of the parties were trading to build coalitions, PDI-P and Megawati refused to ply her political wares. She was politically naïve to most observers, but to her supporters she appeared to be loyal to higher values. While other parties clamored for a more federal and pluralist approach to democratic rule, Megawati continued to appeal to Indonesian unity, despite diversity. Her silent script for national unity was also, in its focus on stabilizing centralization of state power and suprareligious solidarity, the bright mirror image of the dark plan Soleh believed the military were creating to reinstate authoritarian rule.

Soleh also believed that Megawati, his sole hope for a nonparochial style of political praxis, was capable of seeing through the lies and slander of his rivals in Lombok. When Megawati banished him from her party, Soleh's political logic, in the absence of a means for counterattack, imploded. Usually, during such attacks Soleh would mobilize youth from villages to reveal the injustice of his rivals. This time, there were no nonmilitia idealists to be found. The media, his youth followers, and now Megawati had provided him no means for recourse. There were no political, spatial, or institutional forces at hand to breathe life into his dying fantasy. In the relatively obscure setting of a Western-made pornographic film, Soleh saw the design behind his fall.

Why, when he watched the pornographic film, did Soleh see the conspiracy, the condemning moral purity of Megawati staring back at him from the images otherwise choreographed to stimulate his own erotic desire? Perhaps it was Soleh's own fantasy of Megawati's moral force judging him from within the film. Soleh saw his home, the onetime grassroots base for rallying Lombok youth to Megawati's cause, broken down and reassembled (in a porn flick) to fit the gross military plot he believed was designed to incriminate him in Megawati's eyes. When Soleh saw his wife and other Sasak women in the pornographic film, hidden under layers of whitening makeup, he did not feel deceived. Instead, he saw them with Megawati's eyes, that is, with his own fantasy eyes, as victims. Unlike his fantasies, Soleh's conspiracies were populated with the dark forces depicted in the realist tonalities of the media. Soleh's conspiracy theories are among the most insightful I have ever heard. These political frameworks were not equipped, however, at least not yet, to address the total absence of a means for resistance to the peasant-based, modernist, militia-run violence growing around him. The presence of the Islamist militias had dissociated the youth, their idealism, and their communities from him and his cause. The militias had empowered the Sasak youth through methods of violence and moral surveillance intimate to their religious and ritual valuation of masculine vitality, or semangat. The militia's rites of vigilance were sensible and "recuperative" to these youth in ways Soleh's fantasy politics could never be. Megawati's disavowal of his worthiness forced Soleh to create new dimensions for his conspiracies and fantasies to live.

They found a new life in pornographic film. In the simultaneously alluring and repellant images of the film Soleh found the new coordinates for his fantasy resistance. In some ways, these films were repulsive because of the personal betrayals he envisioned in the film. The films were wonderful and pleasurable too, however, because the images he saw in the film restored new intimately estranged subjects for fantasy and conspiracy, new desires to defend new "victims." In the film, he saw the familiar foes of the military and the international conglomerates setting the stage for his demise through the moral degradation of Sasak youth. As importantly, the film was proof that his enemies found him worthy of such an elaborate conspiracy. He was not merely a burned-out nationalist. In the repellant-appealing moment of seeing the Euro-American porn stars "doing their thing," he burrowed beneath piles of body paint and military conspiracy to identify yet another desire-laden object of *advokasi*.

CONCLUSION

A month later, I left Indonesia from Jakarta, only an hour after the Jakarta Stock Exchange was bombed, killing and injuring dozens of bystanders. The same conspiracy theorists, the greatest of all being the president, held forth on the dark forces of the military, conglomerates, and Suharto's cronies eager to see Indonesia fall into chaos. Not one of these conspirators has ever been caught, much less punished. Every day in Indonesia, suspected criminals are killed, sometimes burned alive for crimes as insignificant as stealing a chicken. Suharto and his family, the generals and their mercenaries, continue to travel freely throughout the country they are reportedly trying to destroy. To some, this indicates the symptoms of postauthoritarian rule, the absence of law, and the transitional phase in a democracy. Still, to Soleh, it is a part of a grand narrative of sacrifice and conspiracy in which he, Megawati, and other nationalist leaders continue to play an important and vital part. In Lombok, militias continue to grow. In the absence of law, an authoritarian state structure, or the myth of modern development, young men are delineating new localities, moral practices, and forms of surveillance in ways immediate and recuperative, religious and ritualized, terrifying and, to them at least, sensible.

POSTSCRIPT

In October 2001, approximately one year after I first heard Soleh's conspiracy, I visited him once more. He sat on his veranda and, calm and collected, he explained the militia-related conflicts that had torn apart communities in the areas in and around Mataram. Again, his analysis was insightful, eloquent, and well researched. After he had described the militia conflicts in full, I asked him how it was that he was able to recover from his previous obsession (*obsesi*) with the military plot he believed had been concocted to destroy his life. He explained that he was no longer a single activist self forced to project an equally unitary sense of justice against the state. He was composed of many men, many subjectivities, capable of exacting his sense of incidental justice against equally incidental hegemonies. Why? The state was all the more decentralized now, and even the islandwide militias described above had adopted subvillage- (*dusun; gubug*), village- (*desa*) or subdistrict- (*kecamatan*) level identities. Rather than send monies and dues home to militia headquarters in East Lombok, they chose to engage in local rivalries against more localized, sometimes even village-based, militia rivals. Soleh explained,

> I followed the dark figures I told you about last year. The narcotics sellers and the porn syndicate were related, but not in the way I once thought they were. They just wanted money, not power. Then I remarried. I have calmed down since and started to regroup activists without forcing them to adopt my ideals. In the past I was seen to be a Balinese Muslim and my rivals would tell activists that I could not be a proper Muslim so long as my noble blood bore the legacy of the oppression of Sasak Muslims. I turned the argument against the ethnonationalist Sasak activists and said, "Sure I am Balinese and I still spend my days slaving away for the Sasak people. If you are so righteous, why let a Balinese do all the good work? Join forces with me and see what we can do." The young members of the Sasak People's Movement [Geramakan Masyarakat Sasak, GEMAS], an ethnonationalist Sasak group led by a group of conservative Sasak elders, finally joined my effort when they saw that I was defending people's land while others just spouted off to the media.

Soleh continued to believe that there was once a conspiracy against him, his family, and against his ideals. He may have been right, but little proof of the conspiracy was to be found in pornographic film. More importantly, as the political dimensions of state authoritarianism shifted and fragmented into decentralized forms, intra-Lombok power ties, Soleh's sense of idealism shifted and shattered with it. Instead of resisting the inevitable loss of a nationwide reform movement, he rediscovered small-scale loci for his actions, even his identities, to intervene and effect some positive change for people with no legal means to defend themselves. Still, the question remains, was Soleh's pornographic conspiracy the symptom of a delusional self or a delusional ideal? There is no easy answer to this question, for it is one that haunts us, from time to time, still. Soleh's ability to fragment his idealist self to meet the needs of Lombok's activist communities is a sign, nevertheless, that some symptoms are worth believing when the Real (ideal fantasy or its conspiratorial opposite) is found wanting.

NOTES

1. These movements first became apparent prior to the special parliamentary session of November 1998, when pamswakarsa (civilian security corps, self-reliant security corps, or anticrime militias) were organized to stop "anarchistic" students from disrupting the session. Prior to the special parliamentary session the following

year, in October 1999, the anonymous civilian security aspect of militia security was gone. Instead some twenty-three Islamist militias guaranteed security for the parliamentary session under the joint umbrella of the Unified Islamic Front (Forum Umat Islam Bersata, FUIB).

2. Indonesian terms are either Indonesian or Bahasa Indonesia, or are otherwise noted to be Sasak.

3. In Indonesian, "Golput voters" literally means *golonganamily putih*, or "white group voters." The term itself was a slap in the face of Suharto's party, Golkar (Golongan Karya, "functional group"). Because each of the national parties is identified by color (Golkar is yellow, PDI-P is red, PPP is green) the "white group" did not identify so much with a color as with the lack of one. The Golput followers boycotted the elections largely because Megawati Sukarnoputri had been dismissed from PDI-P and replaced by Suryadi as PDI-P's presidential candidate for the 1997 election.

4. "Dark elements" was an obscure reference to the military's special forces and Suharto's cronies who, according to the media and reformist analysts, were conspiring to pit communities against one another to prove that Indonesians could not live without the military's authoritarian control over security matters.

5. Throughout the New Order, and even much earlier, communities developed "neighborhood watch" systems to protect them from crime. During moments of crisis these groups would gather to defend their neighborhoods or villages from targeted foes or criminals. In 1998 these neighborhood watch groups grew more militant and political in part because the *siskambling* stands (small pavilions erected for the night guard) were often transformed into *posko partai*, or places where the village party organizers would gather and plan campaign strategies. The young toughs of these night guards were recruited to join the party security corps (*satgas partai*) and, under the tutelage of a regional leader, join forces with the anticrime militias (*pamswakarsa*) local to their region or religious community.

6. I distinguish theory-minded activists from roughhouse youth because of the simultaneous emergence of environmental and publication-oriented NGOs with Soleh's style of confrontational mass mobilization during the 1990s. While Soleh organized people in their own communities to stand firm against the military attacking their villages, theory-minded NGOs simply wrote about the peoples' social plight.

7. For a more detailed description of Pemuda Pancasila see Ryter (1998). Pemuda Pancasila often claimed high motives (guarding democracy, populist reform, national unity), but was largely employed to intimidate students, merchants, and the business rivals of the military and Suharto's Golkar cadres in the regions.

8. In November 1998, General Wiranto called for the formation of *ratih* (*rakyat terlatih*, "trained civilians"), or a military-trained corps of civilians to assist the police in controlling riots. These groups were to be called *pamswakarsa* (short for *pangamanan swa karsa*, or self-reliant security corps). *Pamswakarsa* were involved in clashes with

students in the Jakarta riots of November 1998. The *ratih* and *pamswakarsa* of East Timor were later called militias (*milisi*).

9. Aside from criminal theft—almost all Sasak marriage rites begin with the secretive "theft" of the bride-to-be—there are also Lombok-wide *ketemuk/sesapaan* (Sasak) rites regarding spirit encounters revolving around the spiritual "theft" of a Sasak person's vital life force (Sasak: *semangat*). Even the more conventional notion of theft is not so much condoned as it is celebrated in East and Central Lombok. Some villages, such as Kebon Jeruk, treat the corpse of a killed criminal from their village like the body of a hero. As late as January 1998, some of the "young guns" of Lombok's capital city, Mataram, spoke to me admiringly of their thief heroes who were so *wanen* (Sasak; brave, invulnerable) that they were capable of stopping a car full of wealthy tourists with their bare hands. There are even several "lords of thieves" (Sasak: *datu maling*), especially in South Lombok, who are treated as royalty simply because of their skill at theft.

10. For instance, when the Australian military invaded East Timor to fight militias, an organization called United Lords of Lombok (Sasak: Desak Datu) searched cars for Australian tourists as a means of noble retribution for the invasion of Indonesia. In a more complicated case, the Amphibi attacked a small Balinese hamlet in the West Lombok village of Perampauan. When Perampauan's own village-based militia decided to defend the minority Balinese hamlet in the name of village autonomy, thousands of Amphibi attacked the village for defending non-Muslim pagans (Arabic: *kafir*).

11. The *ketemuq/nebusang* ritual is conducted when a person has returned from a journey and, after passing a sacred site or cemetery, becomes feverish, weak, and dizzy. When this happens, it means that a deceased member of their village (Sasak: *bapuk-baluk*) or forest spirit (Sasak: *epen pair*) has taken a part of that person's vital life force (*semangat*). In order to find out which spirit is responsible for the theft of the person's vitality, a hair divination ceremony is held. Hairs on the victim's head are pulled as the names of deceased and the spirits of sacred sites (*epen pair*) are said aloud. When the hair answers with a distinctive "pop" sound, this indicates that the spirit just named is responsible for the spirit theft. Once the spirit responsible for the theft is identified, two different remedies are conducted, depending on the Islamic orthodoxy of the victim or the family. The less orthodox family will go to the cemetery or sacred site of the spirit holding the victim's *semangat* and make an offering or payment in the form of betel quid (Sasak: *sesedah*) and sometimes a meal. The victim chews one of the betel quid and draws a line through the hairs of the divination to signify the return of their *semangat*. Once the payment is made and the victim recovers, other rites might be conducted affirming a relation between the victim and the spirit.

For more orthodox families the making of offerings to unseen spirits is forbidden (Sasak: *bi'dah*). Instead, sections of the Koran are read over the victim in his home to exorcise the unclean spirit (Arabic: *jin*) in order to force it to return to its proper place. This scripturalist intervention interrupts the exchange rites of repayment offering for spirit and transforms it into the establishment of a moral gap between the scripturally purified *roh* or *semangat* of the victim and the immoral desires of the invasive spirit. This crucial cleavage between the "rites of spirit encounter and exchange" of a less orthodox family and "encounter and exorcism" in an orthodox family is especially helpful for exploring the transformation of Lombok anticrime militias from bounty hunters for lost goods into hunters of criminals in the name of Islam.

12. Nahdlatul Wathan (NW) is Lombok's largest Islamic organization. Founded and developed by Tuan Guru Haji Zainudin Abdul Majid in 1932, NW developed an educational *dakwah* (Arabic; missionizing) movement to reform Lombok Islam from a ritualistic tradition to a more scripturalist form (with a focus on actual teachings of the Koran), and to build an educational center. Under the guidance of NW, East Lombok Islam worked closely with Jakarta and New Order–based interests and distanced themselves from the more liberal and tolerant schools of modernist Islam in Java (i.e., Nadhlatul Ulama).

13. Since the end of the nineteenth century in Indonesia, there has been a steady move by Indonesian religious organizations to react to the pressing forces of secularized technologies, colonial modernities, and the disavowal of sacred symbols through the ideologization of religion. Islamic political parties, Koranic purism, and scripturalism have steadily denied sacred symbols their internal currency (as have secular education and the world). The ideologized or puritanical variety of Islamic orthodoxy is what many scholars call modernist Islam. For a more eloquent exploration of this theme, see Geertz (1968).

14. In January 2000, President Wahid had left the country and had demanded the resignation of General Wiranto, then leader of the armed forces under charges for the violence after the 1999 referendum in East Timor. Could Wiranto stage such a massive riot in a backwater like Lombok? The promilitary Islamist Eggy Sudjana's visit to Lombok on the day of the riots, and the recent opening of the Front for the Defense of Islam (Front Pembela Islam, FPI) office, suggested that military-friendly Islamists from the national scene had entered the picture. None of these conspiracies explained, however, why so many men (over sixty thousand) were willing to risk life and limb by looting the city.

15. Soleh's long narrative can be summarized as follows:

1995–96:	Conflicts sprang up around the Islamic party campaign.
1995–96:	Interethnic violence broke out between Dayaks and Madurese in Kalimantan.
1995–96:	The government allowed Christians to build churches in Muslim areas throughout Lombok, planting the seeds of hate against Christianity.

1995–96:	Popular support for Megawati forced Golkar, the government party, to prepare a backup plan in case she won.
1996:	Islamic think tanks groomed their leaders, and Golkar leader, Baramuli, rallied all of eastern Indonesia to secede from Indonesia if Golkar lost the election.
1998:	Attacks were perpetrated against "traditional healers" and "orthodox Muslim" leaders in East Java and were believed to be an effort to pit the followers of Megawati and Gus Dur against one another and divide their reformist coalition against Golkar.
1999:	Muslims began to build a militia fortress against crime and narcotics. This was done to embarrass the government and police. They couldn't do their job so the militias would do it for them. This only made the military look all the more necessary to improve the stability of the nation for proper governance.
1999–2000:	Lombok militias were prepared before the violence of January. CDs of Muslim women being killed in Maluku and fake Christian handbooks calling for the extermination of Muslims in Indonesia were distributed to rally the militias and Muslim communities of the island.
1999–2000:	A conservative group of Sasak nobles in Lombok had worked with shady promilitary Islamists to organize the riots and reassert Islamic Sasak nobilities' claim to their birthright.
2000:	Tuan Guru Sibaway, the religious head of Amphibi, signed a letter of support to provide "security" for the Muslim demonstration before it turned into riots in Lombok.

After his long description, a group of Soleh's underlings came back from their PDI-P Youth bases. He said to them, "Go to our people in the villages and tell them that the riots were an effort to use us to effect a coup d'etat. We have to support *presiden kyai kita*, our cleric president [Abdurrahman Wahid]" to protect the country from disintegration (author's field notes, January 2000).

16. Feik (2001). In this article and others, Megawati's "silence" became a matter for academic debate among Australian Indonesianists. For instance, Dick Feik praised Megawati's silence: "Acting in accordance with particularly Javanese notions of power, she has displayed to her predominantly Javanese constituency all of the qualities required in a leader . . . smoothness of spirit, appearance and behavior, as well as refined manners, asceticism, purity and harmony. Her relative inaction may have increased her popularity, for it has served to set her apart from a government that has performed abysmally" (Feik 2001). In reply, Dr. Damien Kingsbury, senior lecturer in international development at Deakin University, Victoria, warned, "To argue that Megawati Sukarnoputri, Indonesia's likely next

president, should not be assessed by Western or indeed universal standards is to adopt a type of cultural relativism that was used to rationalize Australia's acceptance of president Suharto's three decades of brutal rule and robbery" (Kingsbury 2001).

REFERENCES

Davis, Natalie Z. 1973. The Rites of Violence: Religious Riots in Sixteenth-Century France. *Past and Present* 59 (May): 51–91.

Feik, Dick. 2001. Daunting Role for Megawati to Fill. *South China Morning Post*, 1 June.

Geertz, Clifford. 1968. *Islam Observed*. Chicago: University of Chicago Press.

Kingsbury, Damien. 2001. Beware Megawati, a Puppet of the Elite. *The Age*, 31 May.

Ryter, Loren. 1998. Pemuda Pancasila: The Last Loyalist Free Men of Suharto's Order? *Indonesia* 68 (October): 45–73.

4

HAUNTING GHOSTS

Madness, Gender, and Ensekirite in Haiti in the Democratic Era

Erica Caple James

When you see the state of the country, the state of your own
life, sometimes your whole body hurts. You see that it's only
God who is your consolation. I can't do anything. Sometimes
you have to lie down and do nothing. You resign yourself. . . . A
long time ago we didn't have this stuff—you didn't live in fear
and you could eat. Now you can't. We couldn't have foreseen
that this would happen.

   Guitelle Mezidor, interview, spring 1999

Haiti, the first black republic in the world, achieved its independence from
France in 1804 and entered its postcolonial era in the complex position of
being both a pariah for colonizing and slaveholding nations, as well as a source
of hope for the enslaved and colonized. Since its independence, the nation has
been plagued domestically by political instability, economic stagnation, and
environmental degradation, while suffering political nonrecognition, military
occupation, and economic management and sanctions by the international
community. Two hundred years after its independence, Haiti is infamous for
being the poorest country in the Western Hemisphere. Statistics are often unreliable, but the *World Development Report* 2000/2001 lists Haiti as a "low income"
economy (170th out of 206 economies), with a GNP of only US$460 per
capita, per year. The CIA's *World Factbook* (2006) estimates life expectancy at 54.6
years for women and 51.89 years for men, and cites an HIV/AIDS prevalence
rate of 5.6 percent for the entire population of Haiti.[1]

   The United Nations Development Program's *Human Development Report* 2000
states that 63 percent of the population lack access to safe water, 55 percent lack
access to health services, and 75 percent lack access to basic sanitation. Adult
illiteracy rates are at least 55 percent, but possibly higher. Twenty-eight percent
of children under age five are below normal weight. Infant mortality rates are
ninety-three per one thousand live births. Overall, at least 80 percent of the
population lives in abject poverty (CIA 2006). At the time of this writing
(August 2006), unemployment is estimated at nearly 70 percent.

In many respects Haiti is an archetype for the erratic path that many postcolonial, postdictatorial, and postsocialist nations are traversing toward democracy, human rights, economic justice, and the rule of law. In these "transitional" nations the state is in crisis or is failing and has limited capacity to protect the welfare of its citizens. The international governmental and nongovernmental humanitarian assistance and development apparatus often manages populations, the economy, and the institutions of security in place of the state, creating transnational apparatuses of governmentality (Foucault 1991) that resemble those of former colonial and imperial periods. These institutions of management continue to incorporate biopolitical categorization of populations within their techniques of governance (Foucault 1997; James 2003). Nonetheless, they cannot replace the state's role to protect and promote the welfare of its citizens. In Haiti's case, the government's hands are bound.

The proposed means by which the international community envisions the development of Haiti and Haitians—export-led agricultural production, continued privatization of national industries, expansion of the industrial assembly sector, continued stabilization and structural adjustment efforts, among others—require that the nation and its economy once again open to the nearly unlimited global extraction of labor and resources while it finances these efforts through loans. For the most part, profits will accumulate in the hands of the elite or circulate outside of Haiti, rather than "trickle down" to build state infrastructure and improve the status of the poor majority.

Nonetheless, direct foreign assistance efforts have been suspended for years due to Haiti's ongoing political crises, with emergency funds filtered through international nongovernmental humanitarian assistance and development agencies. Close to half a billion dollars in international aid has been withheld stemming from alleged presidential and parliamentary election irregularities from the May 2000 elections. This suspension continued after an escalation in Haiti's sociopolitical instability[2]: on February 29, 2004, democratically elected President Jean-Bertrand Aristide was ousted from office and forced into exile for the *second* time under highly contested circumstances that had pro-democracy supporters of Haiti within the nation and abroad crying, "It's déjà vu all over again."[3] There is a widespread perception that the international community failed in its obligation to support Haiti's democracy through an eventual transfer of power by constitutional elections. Rather, a virtual coup d'état occurred that former president Aristide and others describe as a "kidnapping" (Chomsky, Farmer, and Goodman 2004) that plunged the nation into another cycle of violence.

Haiti's interim government had little legitimacy and was perceived as a tool of external powers. Fighting between Aristide supporters and those of the opposition proliferated and the ongoing instability in the nation deepened.[4] In February 2006, René Préval, the former president who has been viewed as the twin (*marasa*) of President Aristide, was reelected despite challenges from opponents of Aristide supporters. Préval's inauguration of a cabinet viewed favorably by powers outside Haiti, however, resulted in the international community's commitment of US$750 million to be disbursed between July 2006 and September 2007 (Joachim 2006). While the financial commitment has been made, a question that must be asked is at what cost will this aid be disbursed and who will ultimately benefit?

To some extent these ongoing domestic political and economic conflicts concern the process of representative democracy, social equality, and security, but to another degree they concern the protection of Haitian sovereignty against further international political, economic, and social interventions that come with restrictions. Given its recent period of dictatorship (1957–86), the extreme violence of a de facto regime (1991–94), and its fragile path toward democracy in the "neo-modern" era (James 2004), Haiti—state and nation—may not "recover" economically, politically, or socially on a timetable that will satisfy the international community, and it is clear that external powers will force this process either through direct or indirect action. Hanging in the balance are the needs of Haiti's poor citizens who continue to struggle for political and economic justice, security, the right to participation in government, and development assistance from the international community without shackles. While Haiti's case is particular within the arena of geopolitics, its example is one of relevance to many nations that are attempting "postconflict reconstructions."

In this chapter I discuss some of the ways in which "transitions to democracy" can be perilous and unpredictable at the level of the individual, the community, and ultimately, the nation, through an exploration of a troubling case I encountered in Haiti. I conducted more than twenty-seven months of fieldwork in Port-au-Prince between 1995 and 2000—largely during President Préval's first tenure in office. During this time I followed *viktim*—self-ascribed "victims of organized violence" from the 1991–94 coup years[5]—as they sought healing, justice, and security from a plethora of domestic and international organizations that had disembarked or emerged in order to manage this population. Most of those whom I knew well reside in a *bidonvil* (squatter settlement or shantytown) in Martissant, a heavily populated section of southwest Port-au-Prince that was repeatedly targeted by the coup apparatus between 1991 and 1994. My initial contact with *viktim* occurred when I was invited to provide my services as a practitioner of the Trager Approach, a modality of manual therapy, for a women's clinic established in Martissant by a coalition of Haitian and US-based women's organizations. Among the general population of women clientele, I provided physical therapy to rape survivors who also utilized the clinic's services. From my initial work with these women in the summer of 1996, I developed a multisite ethnographic research project that studied the international, national, and community-level responses to the needs of viktim and their families (James 2003). I continued to work in the bidonvil in Martissant from this period through the end of my fieldwork in early 2000.

Throughout my research, it was abundantly clear that social, political, and economic transitions may not necessarily progress according to the rational technocratic plans of the international community and may appear as a state of paralysis or even chaos, rather than one of progress. In order to unravel what is occurring within Haiti's apparent cycles of instability, it is necessary to make more complex analyses of the uncertain geopolitical and cultural spaces of "postconflict transitions." In transitional nations like Haiti, "cultures of insecurity" are the norm, rather than the exception (Weldes et al. 1999). It is within this space of contradiction, ambiguity, and conflict that I want to examine Haiti's so-called culture of insecurity and the gendered effects of insecurity on the lives of individuals and families in the nation.

ENSEKIRITE

In Haiti, "insecurity"—ensekirite in Haitian Creole—is the actual term that describes the social vulnerability that accompanies the crisis of the Haitian state. Ensekirite refers to the ongoing waves of political and criminal violence that have ebbed and flowed within the nation at critical moments of historical transition in the neomodern era. In common usage it signifies the proliferation of political and criminal violence since the fall of the Duvaliers in 1986.[6] Insecurity reached new heights of materiality or factuality (Scarry 1985) during the three years after the September 30, 1991, coup d'état against democratically elected President Jean-Bertrand Artistide. The coup regime overtly controlled and terrorized the pro-democracy sectors of Haiti—whether in the countryside or in the cities. The egregious "style" of violence (Das and Nandy 1985) deployed against the masses escalated in frequency and extremity that had not been imagined or conceived possible by the residents of these zones. Thousands of individuals were detained, tortured, systematically raped, disappeared, or murdered. Furthermore, the economic embargo imposed by the international community upon Haiti to protest the coup regime's usurpation of power worsened the plight of the citizens whom the sanctions were designed to protect (Gibbons 1999). These combined political and economic excesses resulted in the internal displacement of more than three hundred thousand people and the international flight of forty thousand Haitian refugees who attempted to reach asylum in other Caribbean nations and the United States on rickety, over-burdened boats.

Given the threat of Haitian refugees and the politically unstable nation to US national security, democracy was "restored" in Haiti on October 15, 1994, with the reinstatement of President Aristide by the multinational military and humanitarian intervention of the United States, United Nations, and Organization of American States (OAS). The restoration efforts included plans to restructure the Haitian state and economy, to dismantle and disarm the repressive military, to create a new civilian police force, to repatriate Haitian asylum seekers, and to consolidate the democratic process. Nevertheless, with the ongoing crisis in the state, this effort has been viewed as having very limited success. The disarmament process was voluntary and incomplete and the multinational forces were not mandated to enforce the law (Human Rights Watch and National Coalition for Haitian Refugees 1995). The Haitian National Police are still embattled internally as some members attempt to use the institution to control and direct the flow of contraband and narcotics, while others fight to establish it as a legitimate arm of democracy and justice. Given the state's constraints and preoccupation with domestic and international political positioning, the needs of victims of human rights violations—a subset of the general poor population—are generally left to the assistance of international non-governmental organizations, or to the victims themselves.

In the post-1994 era of "democracy," *ensekirite* refers to the proliferation of political, criminal, and gang violence—and more recently, kidnappings (*Miami Herald* 2006)—that has taken on the egregious style of the coup years. No one is immune. The Haitian elite, the middle-class intellectuals, the clergy, the poor, and their expatriate counterparts are all possible targets in both urban and rural areas. *Ensekirite* is both a material and ghostly presence: acts of violence are visible but complex—they simultaneously display motives of personal vengeance, economic profit, and political threat. The ambiguity of *ensekirite* is that it is difficult to categorize each act and to determine who is the author. This uncertainty adds to the climate of fear. Nonetheless, the visibility of the current state of affairs is only the surface manifestation of gaping wounds from the recent coup years and the thirty years of repressive Duvalier dictatorship between 1957 and 1986.

In the postcoup period there is a pervading sense of incredulity and incomprehension at the scale of the violence and economic uncertainty, which most individuals try their best to forget or push out of consciousness. The ongoing *ensekirite* in the nation makes the resumption of a "normal" life difficult, if not impossible. I have found that beyond its literal signification of political and criminal violence, the term *ensekirite* can be used as a trope for the experience of living at the nexus of multiple uncertainties and forms of violence—political, economic, domestic, gendered, spiritual—and *ensekirite* is mediated through the body.[7] The ambiguity and uncertainty of *ensekirite* is experienced in varying degrees at all levels of society and leaves the entire social system "nervous" (Taussig 1992); however, those who were direct victims of organized violence are now disproportionately affected by the instability that *ensekirite* engenders. *Ensekirite* was and continues to be particularly acute, but also chronic, in Martissant.

ENSEKIRITE IN MARTISSANT

Within the broader boundaries of the nation's capital, Port-au-Prince, Martissant lies just southwest along the Carrefour road that leads westward on the southern peninsula. The majority of my clients and their families resided within thousands of homes in the geographic "block" delineated between the fifth avenue of the Bolosse section of town in the east to Martissant 17 in the west, and from the vast slum that has arisen on the landfill bordering the sea in the north to the highest group of squatter settlements on the southern mountain range. The population of this ethnographic block is difficult to determine, but six to twelve individuals, if not more, inhabit nearly every household, from the sea to the mountains. These homes are cramped one-room, corrugated tin roof houses whose haphazard arrangement lends the zone a mazelike appearance. The lack of proper drainage channels and waste management, combined with the extreme population density in some of these areas, yield pungent and fertile ground for the contamination of water, the proliferation of *Anopheles* mosquitoes, and greater risk for bacterial infections for those residing there. Apart from expansion of the Carrefour road to reduce the traffic jams at an intersection leading into the city, the state has done little to address the public health needs of the residents of these areas.

Indeed, much of Martissant is an enclave that has been neglected by the state since the restoration of democracy in 1994. The liberation of Haiti only temporarily decreased the violent immiseration of its residents. In late 1994, just after the restoration of democracy, Hurricane Gordon killed more than fifty residents of the mountainside *bidonvil*. Its eroded hillsides became avalanches of mud that suffocated entire families who were trapped inside their homes. The road that once connected this neighborhood to a more frequently traveled thoroughfare was washed out during the storm, making this part of the zone even more inaccessible to the civilian police force. In the fall of 1998 two hurricanes, Georges and Mitch, worsened the erosion of the hillsides and destroyed property and households in the area.

In addition to the environmental threats to security, many of my clients spoke of the need for me to leave the area by sunset because armed civilian gangs, known as *kò* (corps) or *zenglendo*, patrolled the zone and enforced a curfew within the enclave.[8] Payment—monetary or sexual—is required for safe passage. While I was able to leave the zone each day, its residents must take their children to and from school, continue to engage in petty trade, work in local construction or other trades, or travel to other places of employment in the city and return by nightfall. While the Haitian National Police made greater efforts to rid the area of organized gangs between 1997 and early 2000, their use of excessive force contributed to the ongoing experience of *ensekirite*; however, the irruptions of the police in the zone were also motivated by the desire to control and direct the criminal activity of some of its residents themselves.

The conditions under which residents of Martissant live are represented by the words of Guitelle, a woman in her middle forties who lived in the neighborhood of the clinic, cited at the opening of this chapter. In my Trager work and formal interview with Guitelle at the clinic,[9] she spoke of her resignation and frustration at not being able to live, in which all she could do is recline and pray for deliverance by God. This feeling of resignation is a form of impotence or "paralysis" that is imposed from the outside, where one can only wait in fear for the forces to change again and permit greater action. The uncertainty generated within this zone of insecurity—in its political, economic, criminal, gendered, and even environmental aspects—was unexpected and physically debilitating for its residents. As Guitelle states: "When you see the state of the country, the state of your own life, sometimes your whole body hurts. . . . A long time ago we didn't have this stuff—you didn't live in fear and you could eat. Now you can't. We couldn't have foreseen that this would happen."

The climate of fear engendered by state-sponsored violence and the fragility of life under a failing state is but one aspect of a broader, collective sense of "ontological insecurity" (Giddens 1984) that characterizes the life of the poor in this nation. In his complex structuration theory Giddens defines "ontological security" as "confidence or trust that the natural and social worlds are as they appear to be, including the basic existential parameters of self and social identity" (1984: 375). The fundamental ground of self and body, social action, and, ultimately, the reproduction of the structure of society is the *sense* of security provided by the routinization of daily life. The reality of *ensekirite* in Haiti, especially among the poor, is that there can be no presumption of stability, security, or trust for the individual or collective group. On the contrary, "ontological insecurity" (1984: 62) is the presumed state of day-to-day life in Haiti and many other countries undertaking political and economic transition, where disruptions and fluctuations in social institutions and practices may be the norm.

To some extent post-traumatic stress disorder (PTSD), the new psychiatric diagnostic category recently exported to Haiti, has been useful in describing the broader environment of *ensekirite* and can assist in defining what for many poor Haitians has been a paradigmatic shift in the mode of "being-in-the-world." But PTSD still fails to capture the sequelae of ongoing uncertainty that is common within Haiti in the postcoup period of "democracy." In my discussions and bodywork with women of Martissant, their suffering corresponded to continual stressors, rather than to a single etiological traumatic event from which there was now a "post"—as is commonly conceived of PTSD (Herman 1997; Basoglu 1992; van der Kolk, McFarlane, and Weisaeth 1996; Marsella et al. 1996; Young 1995).

Furthermore, the conception of trauma or the traumatic memory as residing in the individual sufferer and originating in the past is belied by my experience of everyday life in the *bidonvil*. The ghosts of the past are very present in mundane reality and irrupt into conscious awareness from both within and without the individual. But the "landscape of memory" (Kirmayer 1996) is truly geographical in that the environment in which these people live is a constant reminder of the ontological insecurity of their lives. As in the cross-cultural evaluations of so many forms of suffering, the trauma of *ensekirite* is particular in the Haitian context.

States of *ensekirite* force us to ask the following questions: When ruptures in the fabric of social life are routine, and arise within overall climates of political and economic instability, how does this societal "nervousness" influence the experience of subjectivity and embodiment on both individual and collective levels? Of what use is a concept of post-traumatic stress? When ruptures become routine, what possibility is there for hope or for a sense of security? In what way are poor Haitians able to exercise agency in this environment? For the remainder of this chapter I will elucidate what I call "routines of rupture" and their influence on subjective and intersubjective experience in "democratic" Haiti.

THE GEOGRAPHY OF TRAUMA

In early October 1998, I'd arrived at the clinic somewhat later than I'd intended. Already there were several women waiting to either talk or arrange an appointment to receive a Trager session at a later date. Sylvie, my research assistant, waited patiently for me to finish, then we were going to take another of our walks through the neighborhood that surrounded the clinic. An activist in the community who was helping to organize *viktim*, Sylvie had been both a direct and indirect victim of organized violence after the fall of the Duvaliers in 1986. We had done a lot of work together to interview women and families in the community about their difficult experiences during the coup years. In our lighter moments we had been discussing the ubiquitous issue of black women's hair care and she'd told me of a special plant that would help to strengthen the hair and soothe the scalp. I was excited to learn of anything that might be beneficial to my hair and asked where to find the plants. Sylvie said that we needed to get the herbs in the *rak*—the uninhabited wilds that lay above and west of the *bidonvil*—and we set off on what I'd anticipated would be a mundane journey.

I should have recognized that the hike from the clinic was going to be different from our usual walks when Sylvie led me along a different route to the mountains than I'd become accustomed to—one that avoided the eyes of the market women whom I'd come to know well in my work with them at the clinic. After bypassing the market we descended onto a path—not exactly a road—but the sunken remains of the thoroughfare that had been destroyed by Hurricane Gordon in late 1994. Alongside the path were dilapidated houses that appeared to teeter on small precipices where the road had washed away. Haphazardly placed market stalls had arisen on the once unoccupied road. As usual, the ground was wet from the running water that flowed from the public source and from the soiled water that had been discarded from each home earlier in the day. We had to dance somewhat to land on drier sections of the path, to avoid the pigs that lolled about in the slime, and to skirt the places where the rain had caused trash and garbage to collect in mounds. In the distance I could hear the roosters at the nearby *gagè* (the cockfight arena) as we continued along the well-trodden route.

Sylvie and I reached a point at which another decrepit road turned and rose up the mountain. It was a bit tricky to climb up onto the concrete from the muddy path from which we'd come. Again, the destructive legacy of Gordon and subsequent storms was apparent. This section of road was now an abrupt four feet above the path that we'd been traversing, where once they had been joined along a gradual slope. We proceeded to climb, and both of us commented upon the humidity and heat of the day, wishing that we'd brought some water with us. Another ten minutes of walking up this section of the neighborhood road brought us to a ridge overlooking the *siyon* (*sillon*), an open-walled Pentecostal church to which hundreds of the zone's residents went to fast and pray each week. Under a beautiful ancestral tree, the *siyon* had been a place of asylum—physical and spiritual—for many of the internally displaced people during the repression of the coup years. Sylvie had fled there in 1992 after barely surviving a brutal attack by the military upon her and her husband. Tragically, her husband was murdered in front of her and his body was taken by the soldiers, never to be recovered. Left behind by the torturers, Sylvie fled with her children to the *siyon* before finally escaping the city to her natal home in Jacmel.

We continued through yet another turn of the path that rose and wound around a section of the mountain that was not yet heavily inhabited. Here there were wild grasses and flowers on the edges of the footpath, and a lone wooden shack overlooked the siyon fifty feet below it. Another hundred feet above us an open encampment still remained—a sort of flimsy roof of grasses that was supported by poles—where many of the homeless residents of this zone lived. Sylvie and her children had once stayed there after they returned from Jacmel with the "restoration of democracy" in 1994. It was while residing in this place that one of her daughters had been caught walking alone in the neighborhood and had been gang-raped by a group of youths. As we passed the enclosure, I said to her that I remembered that this was where they used to live "back then." She nodded and did not say more.

As we continued past the open enclosure there was a breeze that rustled the high grasses and I was certainly thankful. But then through the wind we began to hear the plaintive prayers of a man who begged God fervently to give him a job, to help his family, to have mercy on him. He was alone and somehow, under the heat of the late-morning sun and the blueness of the sky, my hearing his prayers made me feel like an intruder in a sacred space. Farther up the path we could also hear a small congregation at prayer. Sylvie informed me that it was another evangelical church that had formed recently, and that there was even another Masonic temple beyond it in the hills. She did not seem disconcerted in any way that they should be there; for me, however, a service in the middle of a weekday morning contradicted my experience of reluctant Sunday worship. Sunday mass had been something for me to endure in my childhood and was remarkable only in that it stood between me and breakfast, and made me faint from hunger in the hot summer. In this place, the words that reached my ears felt true, but they also underscored the reality of fear, poverty, and desperation in the zone. In this environment of *ensekirite*, faith, obedience, and love for God might be all that stood between living a moral life and falling into the "gray zone" of petty crime, lies, and betrayal of others for survival (Levi 1989). Finally, we reached an area where all we could see was a lone house at the end of another long path. Several hundred feet above and behind where we stood were the mansions of a posh residential area that overlooked the city below us. When looking off toward the city in the distance in front of us it was easy to see the large public cemetery downtown in the capital, and the harbor, in which a couple of large ships were docked. I thought to myself that this place was peaceful and beautiful, in contrast to what lay below us.

We'd reached our destination. Just off the path Sylvie pointed out the plants we had spoken of and I recognized them to be fresh rosemary. She explained that what I needed to do was boil the thin leaves and stalks in a pot of water for half an hour or so, strain it, and then use it as a rinse after shampooing once it had cooled. After breaking off a few branches for me and taking some for herself, she pointed to a certain spot by some nearby shrubs. I then realized the true reason for this walk, to show me another site in which the horrors of the past were still manifest.

Sylvie explained to me that this was a place where a young man and his father had been hacked up with machetes and burned to death just a couple of years before in 1996. I was somewhat shaken by this revelation and asked her what had happened. At the time she told me that part of the conflict had been over land and a house whose ownership was disputed. I would not receive the full story—or as much of the truth that was possible to ascertain at the time—until a month later, when I was able to speak with the wife and mother of the deceased, Danielle Marcia, who was forty-two years old at the time of the interview. Sylvie had told me that among the people that she knew in the Martissant zone Danielle was one who continued to have serious emotional and economic difficulties as a result of the attack on her family. The story that followed only emphasized how formidable a task it would be for the new Haitian police force to establish itself as a respected institution in this fragile nation and for there to be true justice, democracy, and healing. It also demonstrated the way in which *ensekirite* discriminates against no one. However, the complexity of the narrative challenged my preconceptions of blame or morality.

Danielle, a mother of seven and wife to Joseph Marcia, is a *madanm sara*, a market woman who makes her living buying and selling goods (*fè konmès*).[10] She had gone on a selling trip to the provinces on the 16th of January in 1996. While she was away, her husband and second oldest son were executed. Sylvie had helped to document the facts of the crime and gave the following introduction of what happened in presenting Danielle to me at the clinic:

> S: Yes. . . . The nineteenth of January 1996 at five o'clock. M. Robert, he called George Marcia and Joseph, they're father and son. He called them as friends and said, "Come on out with me." They were used to going out with him and so they went with him. Danielle Marcia, who is the wife of Joseph, went to the provinces. When she returned, she couldn't find either Joseph or George. She left the house and went to the hospital. She went to the morgue. She went to the police and after four days they went to the slope of the land that's called Mount Carmel and found where they'd cut up Joseph and the entire body of his son George with a machete. And one among them had taken the forearm and tongue of Joseph. They left and left the bodies there.
>
> While we went to go testify what we had found, they set fire to the bodies. The clothes were ruined. There were journalists who'd come to report the case, but they didn't want to identify them. They were afraid that the ones

who'd killed them might threaten them. You know this zone. It's one where they are used to disarming justices of the peace [jij de pe] or police, so . . . anyway, they didn't want to identify them [the perpetrators], that's the job of the justice of the peace to get a warrant for the arrest. The justice of the peace prepared a police report [pwosevèbal] but I don't think Danielle has seen it.

The impunity with which crimes were committed in Haiti during the coup years and the inability to disarm paramilitary groups has hampered the processes of justice. Fear of retribution for attempting to follow the rule of law is very real. The fact that the two Marcia men were lured by an acquaintance to their death suggests that some sort of transgression had occurred for which they were being punished. The issue could be as simple as a dispute over property. Beyond this, however, the taking of the tongue and forearm of her husband marked these murders as much more complicated crimes. While at this time I cannot confirm that the acts were related to those of the secret societies known as sanpwèl or bizango, there are elements of Danielle's testimony that suggest the crime had roots in the judiciary practices that these and other magico-paramilitary organizations have administered throughout Haitian history, but particularly during the Duvalier dictatorship (Larose 1977; Laguerre 1980; Diederich and Burt 1986; Davis 1988; Hurbon 1988).

In continuing her introduction of Danielle, Sylvie revealed yet another instance where tragedy struck the Marcia family:

Six months after that on the sixth of June 1996, at six o'clock in the morning, there were Sylvester, Charles, Anthony, and Eric who were looking for Mathieu Marcia [Danielle's older son], a police officer who served the government. They sent one of them to call him and say that they'd show him the person who'd killed his father and his brother. But it was a plot to kill Mathieu himself. Danielle was going to the market and went down with him. When they arrived at the intersection of St. Bernadette Street, Danielle continued on to the market and Mathieu went with the man who came for him. When they arrived at the appointed place the man told him, there's the one who killed your father. Mathieu went to grab him but the other men shot Mathieu, took his badge, his weapon, and left him on the ground. Like that his mother was left empty-handed. They [the police] invited Danielle to her son's funeral but they did nothing to those responsible.

After this introduction, Danielle told me of the many difficulties she'd had in trying to have the police pursue the case. She'd not found any sympathy or support from the bourgeois staff at the police station who she felt were biased against her as a poor resident of the shantytown.[11] But the local perpetrators continued to persecute her in order to thwart her efforts to find justice. The impunity with which these crimes were committed has left her in fear and despair:

> After, at the same time I had that problem, my house was burned to the ground [by the perpetrators]. . . . You, yourself, you see me, my body is weak [ba] . . . but I don't have money to get a treatment for my head . . . now, my head hurts and it reaches into my back and chest. It's an effort. . . . I don't have anyone except God, I don't have anyone but Jesus. . . . When I get to the point when I can't go on, it's time for me to go. The other [children], when you see the other young man and his big brother—he makes an effort but he's on the street. They're all abandoned. They don't go to school. I left them in the old house. I'm there, I'm struggling, and I do what I can, but I don't have the means to send them to school, I don't have the money to do anything.

At this point in Danielle's narrative I was certain that the pain she described in her head and body was a question of depression and "somatization" (Kleinman and Kleinman 1985: 430). I assumed that through idioms of physical weakness she was expressing her anguish and guilt at being unable to fulfill her role as mother, having abandoned her children to another home, and her inability to make up for the support provided by her deceased husband and sons. One could attribute her angst to a failure to fulfill her expected gender role as mother, but a fuller examination of her narrative in the context of Haitian traditional culture makes an interpretation of her experience and those of her family far more challenging. A brief exploration of local notions of personhood and the self, emotion, and illness is necessary in order to conduct a full exegesis of Danielle's lament.

EMOTIONS, BODY, AND SPIRIT IN THE HAITIAN CULTURAL LEXICON

Throughout my field- and therapeutic work, my client base was most often derived from the poorest residents of Port-au-Prince and the provinces. Most often the language through which the subjective experience of emotion, illness, or suffering was articulated was the epistemology of Haitian Vodou, even though many of these individuals were active practitioners of the many evangelical denominations that are proliferating in Haiti.[12] In general, the person or individual, as conceived within Haitian Vodou, is situated in a nexus of relationships that not only includes the living, but also the ancestors and the divine spirits—the lwa (Brown 1989: 257; 1991). Within each relational web there are reciprocal sets of duties and obligations that maintain balance within the individual, family, and larger community. For those who are ritual practitioners of Vodou, personhood and identity are indelibly tied to the lwa (Dayan 1991: 50):

> Everyone has a personal loa as his protector; he is identified with the Catholic guardian angel. This protector is inherited either on the father's or the mother's side. Every family, the family (fanmi) being a large bilateral group of kin, worships its own spirits. . . . The family is the group within which the spirits have power and exercise authority; they do this mainly by "catching" a member of the group, meaning causing him some kind of affliction. The loas act only within the family. They may manifest themselves in many ways; in dreams, by assuming a human or an animal form . . . and finally in a privileged manner by possessing a member of the family. (Larose 1977: 92)

The social relationships between the lwa, the ancestors, the family, and the individual are multifaceted and to some extent these links can be described as "embodied." However, the concept of the body and suffering that arises within the Haitian context challenges Western conceptions of trauma, and even of chronic pain.

Generally, the embodied "person" in traditional Haiti comprises multiple parts. The gwo bonanj (gros bon ange)—the big guardian angel—is a nonmaterial force, consciousness, or energy that is the "metaphysical double of the physical being" and is able to detach from the body during sleep (Deren 1970: 25–26; Dayan 1991: 51; Métraux 1972: 120, 303; Larose 1977: 92; Brown 1991: 351–52). It is also this part that detaches during the course of possession by the lwa, only to return after the lwa has completed its intended action (Bourguignon 1984: 247). Located in the head (tèt), the gwo bonanj is vulnerable to magical attacks and is especially vulnerable at death, when it may become a "disembodied force wandering here and there" known as a zonbi (Larose 1977: 93).[13] The immaterial zonbi, like the lwa, can possess the individual as a malevolent spirit who seeks a permanent home, until it is dispersed by ceremonial means. But before the ritual dispersal has occurred, it can also be sent by a relative to avenge a wrong or injustice (95). The ti bonanj (petit bon ange) is an energy or presence that is deeper than consciousness, but can enervate the individual in times of stress (Larose 1977: 94; Brown 1989: 265). The kò kadav (corps cadavre) is the material body that is separable from the spiritual essences and subject to decay and dissolution (Dayan 1991: 51; Brown 1989: 265–66). Finally, the nanm is the animating force of the body that disappears after the death of the individual (Brown 1989: 264).

Conceptions of the emotions and their effect on health are also related to the notion of the individual's "head" or tèt—the repository of the gwo bonanj and the seat of the lwa who is its master. When an individual is emotionally distressed, he or she may describe that experience by saying that the "big guardian angel" is upset (Brown 1989: 264). Furthermore, "When an individual is worried, his or her head is said to be 'loaded.' In excitement, the head heats up; when the head cools, the individual becomes calm, also sad" (Bourguignon 1984: 262). "Blood" (san) is the mechanism that regulates heating and cooling in the body. The balance of heat and cold in the body directly affects an individual's susceptibility to illness (Laguerre 1987: 70). The state of equilibrium of heat and cold is determined by the foods that one eats, action on behalf of the individual, or environmental factors (70–71). The relationship between the interior and exterior of the body, the blood, and the emotions is dynamic. Thus, when one considers the impact of local behavioral ecologies on mental health, the bounds of the self must be viewed as extended or permeable.[14]

Subjectivity, in some respects, can be viewed as complex or unbounded, and we are presented with an image of an embodied subject whose social relationships and environment are also constitutive aspects of the person. However, the consequences of the complex self/soul mean that disruptions in the relational webs between the individual, community, ancestors, and the lwa may result in disorder, illness, or other material and spiritual problems, not only for the individual, but also for the extended family.[15] Danielle's narrative began with complaints about individual head and body pain in the aftermath of terrible losses; however, her ongoing suffering extended far beyond her physical person and reveals the ruptures in relational webs amid the ensekirite of Martissant:

> Listen to how people are living—especially the young men. If you're a woman, you can do any sort of old trade [vye konmès], but now the young men are abandoned. . . . I am telling you I don't live. I'm in need of a lot of things. Why am I lacking so many things? Because I've come to a position that I cannot speak of—Sylvie knows the details. But when I see the children in the same condition as I am, sometimes boys or other friends humiliate them. They have some skills that can help them live, but they can't read, and the second one—his mind is cracked. I have to just watch them like that and I can't do anything. . . . They say I am not making an effort to send them to school, and I can't see a way to send them to school. Now life is hard. It's hard. We used to say before we're hungry and that life is hard, but now, life is [really] hard. Whatever little money I have is money for the marketing and then I may not even make a sale. When I really think about this, I get so discouraged. I say, well, if I've only gotten to this point with all my children like this in Port-au-Prince, I'm going back to the provinces. Because when you know how you are slaving away, going up and down [the mountain in order to sell her wares], and they don't even have an education, you want to just stop . . . I don't have to carry on. That's all I can say.

With the loss of her older sons and husband, Danielle and her family lost the financial and emotional support that they relied upon to struggle through the daily travails of life in Haiti. Returning to the provinces, where more than 75 percent of Haiti's population struggle in abject poverty, is seen as a better alternative to the misery her family endures on a daily basis. With the declining economy, petty trade is an uncertain and difficult endeavor. Having lost her home in the wake of the violence perpetrated against her family, having lost her husband and sons, her ongoing despair at being unable to provide for her remaining children in her weakened state is the cross that she bears.

For Danielle's younger sons, the possibilities for living are even more limited. Her older son Pierre, who was seventeen at the time of this interview, has been lost to the realms of madness. Sylvie reiterated Danielle's testimony for me about the aftermath of the ruptures she had faced:

> After they finished slaying Mathieu, shooting Mathieu, slaying his brother and his father, they came to threaten Danielle at her own home. She had to flee and she and her children went to sleep in the wilds of a place they call Gerizim Mountain. She has a son who is so disturbed [pote l' nan tèt] . . . you know that men do not menstruate like women, each month. Now I can say that he's crazy because he walks around incessantly everywhere. But I had him see Dr. Catherine at Doctors of the World, with Danielle and all the rest. They gave a card in order to come back, but they set fire to her house while she wasn't there. They burned down the house and they lost everything completely. Now she's left empty-handed. Danielle doesn't have commerce; she doesn't have family who can help her. The kids who stay with her are the youngest. The one who's slightly older, he's crazy [varye]. That's how she has a double problem.

At the time of the interview, Pierre had disappeared. Danielle had tried to restrain him in the shack, but was unable to prevent him from escaping, removing his clothing, and walking naked in the neighborhood. Despite attempts to find assistance for them at one of the few NGOs that housed "victim assistance" programs, Danielle despaired of being able to make contact with such aid again outside the ensekirite of the zone and resigned herself to her tragic fate.

Sylvie provides an interesting psychobiological interpretation of the way in which individuals respond to trauma according to biological sex. Within the hermeneutics of embodiment and illness in Haiti, menstruation is one means by which the balance of blood, heat, and coolness is maintained in the body. In terms of the sex/gender ideology, menstruation is a powerful time of cleansing what is considered putrid or unnecessary in the blood. Furthermore, the presence of menstrual blood was one agent that prevented some women from being raped during the coup years. Men, who do not have the capacity to regulate their systems in this way, remain *cho*, with "hot blood" that rises to the head (*tèt*). The stagnation of blood in the head can lead to madness, as in Pierre's case. But the difficulty that many men faced in recovering from material, psychological, and physical losses was also related to the gendered division of labor.

In the previous two statements, Sylvie and Danielle mark the differences between how men and women are able to cope with the insecurities of life. At the very least, women may have some form of psychobiological "protection" and can resort to historical forms of commerce in order to survive; however, I didn't understand the full truth of their message until later in the interview. I had asked Danielle a question meant to elicit whether or not she had intrusive memories of these traumatic events. Her answer actually addressed other features of PTSD: "In addition to that, the problem that I have, is that each person has their own way of treating you [*abitid li bay-ou*]. Understand? Each time I think about how people treat me, I had the right to have someone with me. When I meet someone, and he comes in the same form as them, my heart jumps! That, it's become a domination [*dominasyon*] for me." Danielle had spoken of having to resort to *vye konmès* in order to survive. On one level this refers to the trade in crops that slaves were able to produce on small garden plots of land during the period of plantation slavery. On another level, the form of commerce to which she referred was one more elemental.

Within the ideal or historical sex/gender system in Haiti, women have been involved in commerce or small-scale trade. They have sold the produce of their male partner's agricultural activities and have become proficient traders in both rural and urban areas. But women are also recognized as possessing wealth within their own physical bodies. According to Ira Lowenthal, the Haitian Creole aphorism *"Chak fanm fèt ak yon kawo tè—nan mitan janm-ni"* (each woman is born with a *kawo* of land—between her legs) reveals some measure of the resources women are viewed to possess innately: "Female sexuality is here revealed to be a woman's most important *economic* resource, comparable in terms of its value to a relatively large tract of land. . . . The underlying notion here is of a resource that can be made to work to produce wealth, like land or capital, or that can be exchanged for desired goods and services, like money" (1984: 22).

Although the truth of Danielle's situation remained unspoken, she was indicating that she'd needed to employ the survival strategy of "prostitution" in order to survive. It is an activity that still carries stigma in this community despite Lowenthal's statement that sexual exchange is simply another form of alienated labor that can produce wealth. It was partially because of her need to "meet someone" that she abandoned her children to the wreckage of the burnt out home, so that she might receive clients in the darkness of night in a shack that overlooked the *siyon*. Sometimes a client would seem to resemble either her husband or one of her deceased sons. The similarity was physically startling to her and would disturb her to the point where she could no longer eat. With the appearance of a client who resembled a family member, the memories of what had happened would irrupt into her conscious thought; but certainly it must also have been disturbing to engage in sexual relations with someone that resembled one of the deceased. In her testimony Danielle laments the loss of her former life, one in which there was greater social support and in which her family treated her well. Now, within the insecure zone of the *bidonvil* she is isolated and faces humiliation, shame, and disrespect from the neighbors who know of her plight. She has been taunted and teased by them and ridiculed for her fall in social and economic status, much like Primo Levi's description of the physical and emotional persecution of the new arrivals within the Lagers (1989: 36–69).

Danielle's statement has yet another layer: throughout my research, many *viktim* used the term *dominasyon* to describe the inability to stop intrusive memories of their victimization and ruminations or reflections on their suffering. Yet *dominasyon* has another sense of being persecuted or "ridden" by an outside, autonomous agent—somewhat like descriptions of possession by the *lwa* or affliction by the *zonbi* discussed above. Not only do her thoughts and memories intrude, she is also persecuted by other sources of distress. One of the CAPS questions asks if a person fears reexperiencing their victimization or suffers from flashbacks. Danielle answered by describing an experience of having been tormented by her deceased husband Joseph on one occasion during the course of a "dream."[16] Joseph confronted her in this state and she struggled with him: "He charges at me. When he charges at me, I grab and pull him, grab and pull him, and I thrown him to the ground. Then he had time to grab a rock and hit me in the temple and then I'm sick, sick, sick." Upon "waking" Danielle had terrible, chronic headaches, to which she referred early in the interview.

Beyond carrying the stigmata of Joseph's wrath, Danielle was also haunted by her son Mathieu, the police officer, whose apparition would appear to her when she felt she was fully awake. The *zonbi* of her son George would torment her at night. She was "persecuted" by them because she had not been able to fulfill her ritual obligations to them at the time of their deaths. Sylvie began the explanation of how this contact was possible:

S: What can allow that is that they did not have the last prayers for the dead [*dènyè priyè*].

E: That's what I don't yet know about.

S: The last prayers are for the *zonbi* of the person, which means the spirit while you're living. When you die, for it to not remain around [*mache*] in the house, for it to leave. When you don't do the last prayers for the person, the body is buried but the spirit [*nanm*] is still in the house and is persecuting [*pèsekite*] you. It's because of the affair of the last rites that he's persecuting her in the house and making her sick. . . . For the last prayers you have to buy coffee, sugar, like when you have a wake, and you have to prepare food for the dead and pay for a *pè savann* [bush priest] to come say the mass for you in the house. They have a burial ceremony [*nevenn*]. They pray for seven to eleven days, they chant the "Libera" inside and after that the *pè* has another thing to do and then the *zonbi* of the person goes. It doesn't stay in the house.

After death: "A dead person will only harass the living if they neglect him, if they omit to wear mourning, if they fail to withdraw the *loa* from his head and finally if they show themselves dilatory in giving him a worthy burial-place. He shows himself in dreams and explains his disappointment; on those who pay no attention he calls down a 'chastisement'" (Métraux 1972: 258). In the quick succession of murders in the family, and her own persecution by the perpetrators of the crimes, Danielle had been unable to pay for the services of the *pè savann* that could contain and dispel the *zonbi* of the deceased in a timely manner. As Alfred Métraux states, the dead will continue their punishment and quest for justice owed by the family until proper restitution can be made, but Danielle did not have the resources to do so. Sylvie affirmed that the inability to properly bury the dead was the ultimate source of shame and stigma that marked Danielle as belonging to the lowest class of the poor within this desperately poor zone.

In sympathy with Danielle's plight, I had offered to help arrange for the services of the *pè savann*, but I was not able to contact Danielle again. The zone became increasingly dangerous in the weeks after this interview and my own life was threatened, requiring that I leave temporarily. When I finally returned to my work in Martissant in the early spring of 1999, I could not find Danielle again. I do not know if she and her family were able to locate her "mad" son Pierre, or if she still suffers from the frustration and anger of the dead. I do not know if Danielle was able to fulfill the burial ceremonies for Joseph, George, and Mathieu, or if she protects herself from the threat of AIDS and other STDs in her need to "meet men." Somehow, the acquisition of condoms seems to be the least of her worries in the face of these ghostly assaults on her person. In sharing her story with me, Danielle made me understand the traumas of Sylvie and others like her who had suffered during the years of the coup regime, had lost loved ones, had been unable to properly mourn them, and who continued to live with humiliation and shame. Such is the reality of *ensekirite*.

Michael Taussig (1987) calls the intersubjective environment created by the culture of torture and terror "spaces of death." They are "nourished by the intermingling of silence and myth in which the fanatical stress on the mysterious side of the mysterious flourishes by means of rumor woven finely into webs of magical realism" (1987: 8). Martissant is only one zone affected by the haunting legacy of past violences and the ongoing threat of ontological insecurity. In these environments it is difficult, if not impossible, to maintain "a sense of trust in the continuity of the object-world and in the fabric of social activity" (Giddens 1984: 60), much less trust in one's own bodily integrity. For those who've not yet resolved their relationships to family, the dead, the ancestors, and the social community—and the number of the dead and disappeared are in the thousands from 1991 to 1994 alone—there is little space that offers hope for recovery, restitution, and democracy. These sites are truly "gray zones," haunted by the ghosts of the living and the dead and patrolled by those who would continue the magico-paramilitary structures of power. The embodied sense of uncertainty and fear that arises amid these desperate scrambles for power represents the reality of *ensekirite*: the routinization of ontological ruptures in everyday life. That ruptures have become routine can be no better demonstrated by a recent report of the massacre of twenty-two men, women, and children in the Martissant zone in which I used to work—"civilians" caught in the crossfire of the escalating struggle between gangs in the zone—whose security has not been provided by the UN peacekeeping mission (*Le Nouvelliste* 2006), just as it was not during the 1991–94 coup period. The failure of international efforts to provide security in Haiti when the state cannot and to support its fledgling efforts at democracy consistently raises troubling questions about the projects of humanitarian and political development assistance abroad.

As other nations move forward from the horrors of the past and attempt to reconstruct polities that accord with the ideals of democracy, human rights, and the rule of law, the specter of insecurity and the complexities of local power politics may impede a "timely" progression along this path that is recognized as legitimate and transparent by the international community. The perception of "chaos," "paralysis," or "noncompliance" that those outside local spaces hold does not help to quell routinized ruptures in environments of insecurity—especially when external powers fail to provide security or foment its demise, while shadowy forces reap the benefit of the lacuna in order. Should assistance be withheld from nations that struggle with consolidating their democracies— nations that still bear the stigmata of centuries of haunting ghosts? It may be that only through "feeding" these *zonbi* will they be laid to rest. But if the *ensekirite* under President Préval's first tenure is any indication of what the future holds for poor Haitians, it may be a case of "déjà vu all over again."

NOTES

1. These rates vary according to region and other factors: At a May 2002 talk at the Boston-based Management Sciences for Health (MSH), Dr. Georges Dubuche, reproductive health and HIV/AIDS advisor for the MSH/HS-2004 project, presented a rate as high as 13 percent in the Northwest Department (based upon a 1998 estimate).

2. International assistance was initially suspended in the spring of 1997 in protest against alleged irregularities in the April parliamentary elections; the disputed seats were up for reelection in May 2000 in order to resolve the long-standing crisis in the government.

3. The tragic period following Aristide's first removal from office on September 30, 1991, is discussed below.

4. Interestingly, the CIA's *World Factbook* 2006 reports 2005 as the first year of economic growth since 1999, despite manifest reports of increasing inflation and an escalation of violence at all levels.

5. Survivors of political violence in Haiti have embraced and appropriated the category of "victim" as a sociopolitical category of activism.

6. According to anthropologist Michel-Rolph Trouillot (1990) the practice of political violence in Haiti had a somewhat predictable character in earlier historical periods in which there was a clearer distinction between the political and civil realm of battle. The Duvalier dictatorships—"Papa Doc" François Duvalier (1957–71) to Jean-Claude Duvalier (1971–86)—were noted for the blurring of the political and civil domains, the specific targeting of civil society, women, the clergy, and other "innocents" with egregious forms of violence.

7. While it has become common to refer to the term "structural violence" in order to explain the pernicious effects of poverty, I have found that such a term tends to leave unexamined the complexity of situations of vulnerability that simultaneously involve international, national, and local relations of power, economy, politics, race, gender, and other factors. While labeling structural inequalities as "violence" can assist in drawing attention to the everyday misery of the disenfranchised individual, community, or nation, it may do more harm than good by crystallizing violence in a fetishistic manner. Attention to security, vulnerability, uncertainty, and complexity may assist with social analyses, but I also fear that my own approach can limit effective social interventions for change in Haiti and nations like it.

8. *Zenglendo* is a term that has its etymological roots in the Haitian Creole word *zenglen*, referring to shards of broken glass, and *do* which refers to the back. *Zenglen* was also the name given to the secret police force that served under President Faustin Soulouque (Emperor Faustin I) and that became the model for François Duvalier's

terrorist force, the *tonton makout*. During the coup years of 1991–94, the *zenglendo* were "criminals . . . recruited from groups ranging from the marginal social strata found in working-class districts to police officers themselves usually acting at night, in civilian clothes and with official weapons" (Human Rights Watch and National Coalition for Haitian Refugees 1994: 5).

9. I was testing a Haitian Creole version of the Clinician Administered PTSD Scale (CAPS) with my clients at the clinic.

10. *Madanm sara* (or *madansara*) is the word for a weaverbird, known to destroy crops, but it is also a term to describe women who transport and sell merchandise. Market women are also referred to as Madam Sara.

11. It is also possible that her son's murder implicated police involvement in the insecurity of the zone.

12. While none of my clients admitted to serving the spirits, the broad formulation of a sociocentric "self/body" (Becker 1991) that follows was commonly expressed regardless of my clients' stated religious practice.

13. The *gwo bonanj* can also be captured by a sorcerer when a person is alive and is also called the *zonbi*; however in this case, the *gwo bonanj* can be used to force the material person to whom it belongs—literally, the living dead—to labor for the sorcerer.

14. Karen Brown notes that these aspects of identity and body are such that "for the Vodou worshipper, each person is at the core of his or her being, a multiplicity of beings, a polymorphous entity and that it is only at the periphery of life, in areas less important to that person, that he or she adopts clearly definable, and consistent roles or modes of being" (1979: 23).

15. I want to emphasize that relational obligations are sometimes sources of threat to the self, even as they are also sources of blessing and healing. Failure to uphold these obligations can result in illness or misfortune for the person who is directly guilty (Métraux 1972: 256) or for others within the community. See also Boddy (1988), Brown (1991), Antze (1996), and Lambek (1996) for further discussions of how the expression of alternate selves through either spontaneous possession or MPD can be viewed as creative presentations of self in everyday life regardless of the "willed" nature of the occurrence.

16. I hesitate to label the state in which this event occurred a dream in that Danielle emphasized that it occurred when she had just lain down to rest. I am going to call such a state "imaginal"—following the work of Csordas (1994) and Nordstrom (1997). This particular space—somewhere between waking and sleeping, but a space of encounter, vision, and action—is another "reality" in which both illness and healing can occur.

REFERENCES

Antze, Paul. 1996. Telling Stories, Making Selves: Memory and Identity in Multiple Personality Disorder. In *Tense Past: Cultural Essays in Trauma and Memory*, ed. Paul Antze and Michael Lambek, 3–23. New York and London: Routledge.

Basoglu, Metin. 1992. *Torture and its Consequences: Current Treatment Approaches.* Cambridge: Cambridge University Press.

Becker, Anne. 1991. Body Image in Fiji: The Self in the Body and in the Community, PhD diss., Harvard University.

Boddy, Janice. 1988. Spirits and Selves in Northern Sudan: The Cultural Therapeutics of Possession and Trance. *American Ethnologist* 15 (February): 4–27.

Bourguignon, Erika. 1984. Belief and Behaviour in Haitian Folk Healing. In *Mental Health Services: The Cross Cultural Context,* ed. Paul B. Pedersen, Norman Sartorius, Anthony J. Marsella, 243–66. Beverly Hills: Sage Publications.

Brown, Karen McCarthy. 1979. The Center and the Edges: God and Person in Haitian Society. *Journal of the Interdenominational Theological Center* 7 (Fall): 22–39.

———. 1989. Afro-Caribbean Spirituality: A Haitian Case Study. In *Healing and Restoring: Health and Medicine in the World's Religious Traditions,* ed. Lawrence E. Sullivan, 255–85. New York: Macmillan Publishing Company.

———. 1991. *Mama Lola: A Vodou Priestess in Brooklyn.* Berkeley: University of California Press.

Central Intelligence Agency (CIA). 2006. *The World Factbook.* www.cia.gov/cia/publications/factbook/geos/ha.html (accessed August 9, 2006).

Chomsky, Noam, Paul Farmer, and Amy Goodman. 2004. *Getting Haiti Right This Time: The U.S. and the Coup.* Monroe, ME: Common Courage Press.

Csordas, Thomas J. 1994. *The Sacred Self: A Cultural Phenomenology of Charismatic Healing.* Berkeley: University of California Press.

Das, Veena, and Ashis Nandy. 1985. Violence, Victimhood and the Language of Silence. *Contributions to Indian Sociology,* n.s., 19 (1): 177–95.

Davis, Wade. 1988. *Passage of Darkness: The Ethnobiology of the Haitian Zombie.* Chapel Hill: University of North Carolina Press.

Dayan, Joan. 1991. Vodoun, or the Voice of the Gods. *Raritan* 10 (3): 32–57.

Deren, Maya. 1970 [1953]. *Divine Horsemen: The Voodoo Gods of Haiti.* New York: Documentext.

Diederich, Bernard, and Al Burt. 1986. *Papa Doc and the Tonton Macoutes.* Port-au-Prince: éditions Henri Deschamps.

Foucault, Michel. 1991. Governmentality. In *The Foucault Effect: Studies in Governmentality,* ed. Graham Burchell, Colin Gordon, and Peter Miller, 87–104. Chicago: University of Chicago Press.

———. 1997. *Ethics: Subjectivity and Truth; Essential Works of Foucault 1954–1984,* vol. 1. Ed. Paul Rabinow. Trans. Robert Hurley et al. New York: The New Press.

Gibbons, Elizabeth D. 1999. Sanctions in Haiti: Human Rights and Democracy under Assault. The Washington Papers 177. Westport, CT, and London:

Praeger Publishers. Published with the Center for Strategic and International Studies, Washington, DC.

Giddens, Anthony. 1984. *The Constitution of Society: Outline of a Theory of Structuration*. Berkeley and Los Angeles: University of California Press.

Herman, Judith. 1997 [1992]. *Trauma and Recovery*. New York: Basic Books.

Human Rights Watch and National Coalition for Haitian Refugees. 1994. Rape in Haiti: A Weapon of Terror. Vol. 6, no. 8 (July).

————. 1995. Haiti: Human Rights after President Aristide's Return. Vol. 7, no. 11 (October).

Hurbon, Laënnec. 1988. *Le Barbare Imaginaire*. Paris: Les éditions du Cerf.

International Bank for Reconstruction and Development/World Bank. 2001. *World Development Report 2000/20001: Attacking Poverty*. New York: Oxford University Press.

James, Erica. 2003. The Violence of Misery: "Insecurity" in Haiti in the "Democratic" Era. PhD diss., Harvard University.

————. 2004. The Political Economy of "Trauma" in Haiti in the Democratic Era of Insecurity. *Culture, Medicine and Psychiatry* 28:127–49.

Joachim, Dieudonné. 2006. 750 millions de dollars pour Haïti. *Le Nouvelliste*, July 25. www.lenouvelliste.com/articleforprint.php?pubID=1&ArticleID=32322 (accessed July 26, 2006).

Kirmayer, Laurence J. 1996. Landscapes of Memory: Trauma, Narrative, and Dissociation. In *Tense Past: Cultural Essays in Trauma and Memory*, ed. Paul Antze and Michael Lambek, 173–98. New York and London: Routledge.

Kleinman, Arthur, and Joan Kleinman. 1985. Somatization: The Interconnections in Chinese Society among Culture, Depressive Experiences, and the Meanings of Pain. In *Culture and Depression: Studies in the Anthropology and Cross-Cultural Psychiatry of Affect and Disorder*, ed. Arthur Kleinman and Byron Good, 429–90. Berkeley and Los Angeles: University of California Press.

Laguerre, Michel S. 1980. Bizango: A Voodoo Secret Society. In *Secrecy: A Cross-Cultural Perspective*, ed. Stanton K. Tefft, 147–60. New York and London: Human Sciences Press.

————. 1987. *Afro-Caribbean Folk Medicine*. South Hadley, MA: Bergin and Garvey Publisher.

Lambek, Michael. 1996. The Past Imperfect: Remembering as Moral Practice. In *Tense Past: Cultural Essays in Trauma and Memory*, ed. Paul Antze and Michael Lambek, 235–54. New York and London: Routledge.

Larose, Serge. 1977. The Meaning of Africa in Haitian Vodu. In *Symbols and Sentiments: Cross-Cultural Studies in Symbolism*, ed. Ioan Lewis, 85–116. London: Academic Press.

Levi, Primo. 1989 [1986]. *The Drowned and the Saved*. New York: Vintage Books.

Lowenthal, Ira P. 1984. Labor, Sexuality and the Conjugal Contract in Rural Haiti. In *Haiti—Today and Tomorrow—An Interdisciplinary Study*, ed. Charles R. Foster and Albert Valdman, 15–33. Lanham, MD: University Press of America.

Marsella, Anthony J., Matthew J. Friedman, Ellen T. Gerrity, and Raymond M. Scurfield, eds. 1996. *Ethnocultural Aspects of Posttraumatic Stress Disorder: Issues, Research, and Clinical Applications*. Washington, DC: American Psychiatric Association.

Métraux, Alfred. 1972 [1959]. *Voodoo in Haiti*. Trans. Hugo Charteris. New York: Schocken Books.

Nordstrom, Carolyn. 1997. *A Different Kind of War Story*. Philadelphia: University of Pennsylvania Press.

Le Nouvelliste. 2006. Plus de 20 morts, dont des enfants, dans des violences en Haïti. July 12. www.lenouvelliste.com/articleforprint.php?PubID=& ArticleID= 31828 (accessed July 24, 2006).

San Martin, Nancy. 2006. "Les Kidnappings" are Haiti's Latest Misery. *Miami Herald*, August 2. www.miami.com/mld/miamiherald/news/world/haiti/ 15176663.htm?template=contentModules/printstory.jsp (accessed August 2, 2006).

Scarry, Elaine. 1985. *The Body in Pain: The Making and Unmaking of the World*. New York: Oxford University Press.

Taussig, Michael. 1987. *Shamanism, Colonialism and the Wild Man: A Study in Terror and Healing*. Chicago: University of Chicago Press.

———. 1992. *The Nervous System*. New York: Routledge.

Trouillot, Michel-Rolph. 1990. *Haiti—State Against Nation: The Origins and Legacy of Duvalierism*. New York: Monthly Review Press.

United Nations Development Program. 2000. *Human Development Report 2000*. New York: Oxford University Press.

van der Kolk, Bessel A., Alexander C. McFarlane, and Lars Weisaeth, eds. 1996. *Traumatic Stress: The Effects of Overwhelming Experience on Mind, Body, and Society*. New York and London: The Guilford Press.

Weldes, Jutta, Mark Laffey, Hugh Gusterson, and Raymond Duvall. 1999. Introduction to *Cultures of Insecurity: States, Communities, and the Production of Danger*, 1–33. Minneapolis: University of Minnesota Press.

Young, Allan. 1995. *The Harmony of Illusions: Inventing Post-Traumatic Stress Disorder*. Princeton, NJ: Princeton University Press.

5

The Humanitarian Governance
of the Postcommunist Balkan Territories

Mariella Pandolfi

Since the end of the colonial era, many of the territories where anthropologists have worked have been witness to an increasingly visible "humanitarian presence." The massive army of volunteer workers, international experts, local staff, and soldiers associated with humanitarian intervention has had a remarkable impact on local cultural landscapes. Despite the increasing proliferation of these zones of humanitarian and military intervention, anthropologists are only beginning to examine the theoretical and practical consequences of these new forms of intervention. Intervention studies present a perilous but necessary challenge to the anthropological community. They force us to consider both new sites of intervention and new actors, such as humanitarian organizations, international institutions, and specific segments of local elites.[1] This chapter traces these emerging actors within the new "biopolitical" landscape of the postcommunist Balkan territories[2] where humanitarian intervention is marked by a "double bind" of forced Westernization, which imposes a monolithic model of intervention that often does not fully consider local contexts. These reflections evolved over the course of my work and field experiences in Albania, as a consultant for the United Nations Drug Control Programme (UNDCP) both before and after the Kosovo war, and in Kosovo itself after the war, as an expert for the International Organization for Migration (IOM) pilot project that experimented with new forms of trauma intervention.

THE POLITICS OF INTERVENTION
AND THE POLITICS OF THE INTERVENING
ANTHROPOLOGISTS

In order to understand the role that anthropologists stand to play in laying bare the dynamics of humanitarian intervention, it is necessary to reflect on how we can conceive of humanitarian intervention in the context of new global and local landscapes. Intervention most often occurs in areas undergoing rapid transformation. Intervention is a necessarily mobile phenomenon and can be conceived of as the complex deployment of a network of military forces, non-governmental organizations (NGOs), and international institutions including, among others, UN agencies, the International Monetary Fund (IMF), the World Bank, and the Organization for Security and Co-operation in Europe (OSCE).[3] It is difficult to define humanitarian intervention according to specific "goals" or technical means because these are constantly changing in light of shifting local and global circumstances.[4]

For example, the United Nations first approached the subject of humanitarian intervention through the notion of "complex emergencies." This concept was used to denote a phenomenon characterized by a host of causes (including conflict, war, and famine) and requiring a diverse array of responses (such as military, peacekeeping, and relief efforts). This militarized approach to humanitarian intervention will later replace the humanist approach, exemplified by the category "the right of interference." This category emerged out of the European, and particularly French, humanist tradition and became a dominant force in the humanitarian realm in the 1980s. Against the backdrop of a new world order, the international community relied upon this new notion to lay claim to its right to interfere in any area for the purpose of upholding human rights. Most recently, the terminology of humanitarian efforts has shifted again, inventing a new discourse: "the responsibility to protect." This term was instituted in 2005 and was specifically aimed at protecting populations from genocide, ethnic cleansing, and other crimes against humanity. If a government is deemed unwilling or incapable of protecting its own citizens, this doctrine asserts that the international community has the duty to assume the protection of that state's citizens. This final categorization of humanitarian intervention represents the merging of prior militaristic and humanist perspectives, for it unites the benevolent responsibility to intervene in times of suffering with the an unquestionable right to employ force in the protection of global citizens.

Indeed, intervention has been the preferred foreign-policy tool of the post–Cold War order, and over the years it has taken on many guises: "humanitarian" when it seeks to redress the suffering of civilian populations; "military" when it seeks to restore international security and order; and "political" when it seeks to reconstruct states and societies. As a flexible tool that can be applied both to postcommunist societies in "transition" and to societies in the aftermath of war, intervention has become a common foreign-policy solution to the varied crises of our times. Intervention is the standard response of an outside force to the local problems of societies undergoing multiple, simultaneous transitions. It is composed of a set of complex social relations that exist within a particular framework of power and a landscape marked by a distinct temporality and a politics of "emergency."[5] The procedures of intervention are justified in the name of coping with "economic" and "democratic" emergencies. The "emergency" period is an administrative definition that permits the loosening of rules for the allocation and distribution of resources, irrespective of the situation on the ground. Yet these procedures often provoke shifts in power where local populations lose control over the agenda of political reform and the processes that create new social hierarchies (Lafontaine 2002).

Whether speaking of the dissolution of Yugoslavia or regime change in Afghanistan and Iraq, intervention entails the invocation of a particular "state of exception" (Agamben 1998, 2000, 2005), a suspension of previously valid norms and rules arising not only from the collapse of existing social and political structures but from the fact of intervention itself. Intervention presupposes the very exceptions it creates. Speaking in terms of power, is it possible to conceive of this reduction in terms of what Michael Hardt and Antonio Negri (2000) define as "empire"? Examining this issue from the point of view of populations, it might be useful to reflect upon Giorgio Agamben's radical biopolitics of "bare life."[6]

As Mark Duffield underlines, "The insistence that humanitarianism is 'neutral' and separate from politics, means that humanitarians can only grasp human life as bare life. By excluding the political, humanitarianism reproduces the isolation of bare life and hence the basis of sovereignty itself" (2004: 13). While Agamben (1998, 2000) worked in a very different context, his theoretically evocative approach to biopolitics offers important insight into the dynamics of power at work in the new realm of humanitarian intervention (Pandolfi 2000c, 2000b).

This deeply political and inherently mobile field poses many challenges for anthropological fieldwork. It is challenging for anthropologists to work in a field that is so widely covered by the media. Yet anthropological expertise has much to offer to this situation, for anthropologists are particularly adept at calling into question the logics associated with emergencies and "humanitarian catastrophes." Humanitarian intervention clings to international institutions and to certain segments of local elites, weakening the society that it proposes to reconstruct. It works upon fragile territories whose tenuous position renders them porous to the imposition of Western political logic. Anthropological studies demonstrate that humanitarian intervention conceals the link between its actions and the priorities of Western states by relying on a rhetoric of generosity and the claim that its actions are independent of political forces. The links between military and humanitarian intervention have long been obscured, necessitating a critical examination of the strategies driving humanitarian intervention and the risks inherent in invoking the right to interfere. As explained by Astri Suhrke and Douglas Klusmeyer, "In securing a humanitarian space, it was argued, the aid agencies had to observe conventional humanitarian codes that called for neutrality and impartiality. By the end of the decade, however, this view was increasingly challenged. Some academic observers argued that all humanitarian activity had an inherent political element" (2004: 277).

Since the mid-1990s, we have witnessed the exponential and uncritical growth of what I call a "gray zone" between humanitarian intervention, military humanitarianism (Pandolfi 2006), and the humanitarian war.[7] The gray zone is a fluid space that is alternatively political, civil, and military in nature. This varied space confronts us with an ambiguity that undermines humanitarian intervention (Prendergast 1997). The mixing of military and humanitarian aid results in a hybrid dislocation of political space (Pandolfi and Abélès 2002) that is "locally constructed" around a mobile international community, comprised of both civil and military experts. This gray space acts as a third social actor within a universalizing, apolitical utopia, intended to promote and maintain peace and bring aid to the victims of emergencies. This procedure is enacted in a top-down manner that places itself squarely within a space that is neither local nor national. This new space is sustained by a standard universal discourse that progressively eliminates all historical and cultural contextualization. This new zone progressively marginalizes the kind of contextualized accounts produced by anthropologists and promotes prefabricated schemes produced by international human rights lawyers and political scientists. These schemes outline standardized responses to violations of human rights, the exportation of democratic institutions, and the construction of new civil societies. Within this new gray zone, humanitarian actors tend to focus narrowly on their work at the local level. For example, a surgeon engaged in humanitarian medical aid often conceives of his or her situation in terms of surgeries performed or lives saved and rarely reflects on the role that his or her presence may play in the larger humanitarian apparatus. This overvaluation of microlevel practices often eclipses a more critical view of humanitarian intervention's broad effects and engenders the tendency to sympathize with an uncritical view of humanitarian intervention. Anthropologists are well situated for drawing links between this form of individual action and the broad totality of actors and practices that comprise the realm of humanitarian and military intervention (Pandolfi 2000c, 2000b).

Positing humanitarian and military intervention as the object of fieldwork raises two important issues for anthropologists: marginality and the politics of collaboration. Political scientists and international law experts have been investigating the limits and legitimacy of humanitarian intervention since the mid-1990s,[8] yet anthropologists have remained outside the purview of the technical arena of humanitarian operations. Given their limited access to the field, anthropologists have not been able to study the impacts that the international military and civilian presence have had on local society.

Anthropological fieldwork in humanitarian and military zones raises thorny issues that can be summarized under the term "politics of collaboration." Anthropologists may take on a collaborative role in such settings, becoming directly involved in the humanitarian industry as volunteer workers or "experts," or as officers or project directors. If an anthropologist becomes professionalized within the industry it is difficult for him or her to maintain a critical perspective. Anthropologists working in these situations are often pulled in opposing directions. Faced with the very real problems of human suffering it is difficult for anthropologists to refrain from intervening. Yet intervention complicates an anthropologist's ability to maintain a critical and distanced stance.

The temptation, therefore, is to treat the humanitarian industry in a way that is perhaps not dissimilar from how our disciplinary ancestors treated their isolated villages: as remnants of a pure precapitalist solidarity. Yet wars and postwar zones are no place for fabricated utopias, and critical anthropological work on humanitarian intervention must testify to the more difficult truths that remain once the media spotlight has dimmed. There is an urgent need for anthropology to critically address this issue that so radically departs from the discipline's classic, focused engagement with a single locality and its local social group, language, and culture. The humanitarian industry is a primary effect of globalization (Stiglitz 2002) and as such invites the attention of contemporary anthropology (Appadurai 1996a; Agier 2002; Fassin and Vasquez 2005; Abélès 2006).

THE HUMANITARIAN APPARATUS IN THE BALKANS

Broadly speaking, Albania, Kosovo, and Bosnia are part of the Balkan region, which is commonly referred to as Southeastern Europe.[9] These areas are geographically inextricable from Europe, yet they are culturally constructed as Europe's "other." The Balkans have served to absorb a number of the externalized political, ideological, and cultural frustrations experienced by neighboring regions. Europeans have constructed a positive and self-congratulatory image for themselves by creating an image of the Balkans as a repository for contrasting, negative characteristics. In the nineteenth century, this treatment of the Balkans was reinforced by the political theory of "Balkanization" (Todorova 1997). Throughout the twentieth century, Albania remained one of the most "mysterious" and unknown regions of the Balkans and of Europe in general. In 1912 a French journalist argued that we have a better knowledge of the Sahara desert or of Tibet than of Albania. Bismarck viewed Albania as a historical anomaly.

Certainly, the fifty-year period of isolation that Albania experienced under the communist regime prevented it from being permeated by the logic of Western capitalist nations. The end of the Cold War added new geopolitical nuances to the problem of classifying this area. The U.S. Department of State began to favor new categories of classification such as "east-central Europe" and "Southeastern Europe" as substitutes for a more generic "Eastern Europe." The unrest in former Yugoslavia gave way to a new fear that led Albania and Kosovo to be defined as the new crossroads for reshaping postcommunist societies. The international community became increasingly aware of this region following the wars in Bosnia (1992–95) and in Kosovo (1999) and following the collapse of the communist regime in Albania in 1991, which instituted a period of violence and anarchy that reigned until 1997 (Independent Commission for Kosovo 2000; International Commission on the Balkans 2005).

Throughout most of the twentieth century Albania was relegated to the impoverished backwater of a communist Europe. Kosovo, on the other hand, experienced a degree of progressive independence as part of the Yugoslavian Federation envisioned and created by Tito. Following the collapse of the communist regime in the early 1990s, Albania experienced an extended period of instability marked by an upsurge of violent conflicts. Many Albanians sought to escape this instability by fleeing to nearby Italy. Yet the violence in Albania paled in comparison to the gruesome situation that would befall the once-enviable region of Kosovo. While Kosovo profited under the stable and flourishing Yugoslavian Federation, when Tito died Kosovo was slowly transformed into a theater of contradictory violence. Under the new reign of Milosevic, Kosovo became the site of massive ethnic segregation. Kosovo Albanians fled to North America, Switzerland, Germany, and other European countries to escape persecution. The periods of intense violence and intervention that marked Kosovo in the 1990s transformed the geopolitical space of the region. After 1999, Kosovo was witness to interethnic conflicts and violence, ethnic cleansing, the massive exodus of 450,000 Kosovo Albanians to Albania, the fleeing of some 400,000 other people seeking refuge from the conflict, and the massive influx of international organizations, NGOs, military, secret-service agents, and finally a slow return to "normality" characterized by an "international protectorate" and by the election of a "territorial" parliament that has no real autonomy.[10] The "humanitarian" war of 1999 brought Kosovo further away from its historical and cultural roots, and the influx of a massive military presence transformed the region into an area that more closely resembles the war-torn geography of Afghanistan, East Timor, or Iraq.

AN EMERGING LABORATORY OF INTERVENTION

I would like to open my ethnographic remarks with Proudhon's disturbing aphorism: "Whoever claims to be humane is trying to fool you" (Zolo 2002). This aphorism has been at the root of my decision to perform fieldwork in Albania, Kosovo, and Bosnia. This work has forced me to directly confront the experience of conflict, the naturalization of violence, and the rise of humanitarian and military intervention. On the one hand, these sites have been witness to the international community dancing on the stage of international crises and extolling a standardized panoply of ideologies, practices, and projects.[11] On the other hand, working at these sites I have witnessed local communities' efforts to establish equilibrium between the promise of an emancipation independent of the international community and the necessity to conform to that community's norms and expectations. Developing Arjun Appadurai's notions of mobility, deterritorialization, and sovereignty (1996b), we can define these transnational formations as mobile sovereignties. Developed by specific "epistemic communities," these mobile sovereignties seek to link transnational forms of domination to local political practices (Pandolfi 2000c, 2003, 2006).

The presence of the international community has affected nearly all forms of local life in the postcommunist Balkan territories, creating both new laboratories of intervention and increasingly intriguing sites for anthropological study. I am reminded of my first arrival at the Tirana Airport in Albania, in the mid-1990s, and of my trip from the airport to the downtown area. I recall the scene of this first trip as a sketch of images marked by armored tanks, Apache helicopters, weapons, combat clothes, and armor-clad military jeeps. The humanitarian war had not yet begun, but combat dress had already arrived in the area. Those living in the military and humanitarian zones had adopted a kind of "aesthetic of the occupied." This aesthetic could be perceived in the small details and colors of combat dress. Cardigans and body armor were donned in both war zones and humanitarian aid zones. For example, in Pristina, Kosovo, the shopping centers that graced areas where the military lived were brimming with tee shirts, pants, berets, and other sorts of gadgets aimed at a market of combat consumers. There was nothing particularly unique about this scene, for these aesthetics were repeated over and over again, wherever military and humanitarian intervention had settled.

The particular aesthetic of military-humanitarian intervention is found not only in what people wear, but in the places that they frequent. This is most evident in the space of restaurants, bars, and meeting places that make up the "green zone." This cordoned-off area of places to eat and drink evokes images of a world beyond conflict. These areas bear a closer resemblance to American cities than to urban areas typical to the region. These scenes in the Balkans are reminiscent of a similar scene in Iraq, invoked in striking detail by William Langewiesche in his article about Baghdad's green zone (2004). The Baghdad that Langewiesche describes is more characteristic of Minnesota than Mesopotamia. His work brings me back to my days in Tirana in the mid-1990s, or in Kosovo, in Pristina, at the end of that decade. Each of these "gray zones" where migratory sovereignties have nested, has the potential to become a "green zone." These protected, and therefore occupied and militarized, zones are reserved solely for the high rollers in the new social hierarchy: the "nostalgic" political men from the communist era or those linked to the area's powerful clans, the new elite that have been identified as members of a new global civil society, the new politicians, and, sometimes, select cosmopolitan youth (Pollock et al. 2000).

Experts, journalists, and high-ranking international military men create and circulate an internal rhetoric among the international community that resides within these "protected" zones. By examining the cafes, hotels, and other spaces occupied by the international community, we can elaborate a new sociology of power relations. The geography of these occupied spaces in Tirana in the 1990s illustrates the emblematic way that the networks between the international community and the local community are formulated and fostered. The atmosphere inside these meeting places harkens back to scenes from the great films of the 1940s, such as Casablanca, where characters met in shadowy spaces that were heavy with smoke and strange odors. The meetings inspired by such places are a far cry from meetings in the West, which are characterized by a specific goal, a quick meeting, and a full agenda. These are the "showcase" places, where people come to see and to be seen and where the new elite can fashion themselves after Western tastes.

The Hotel Dajti is an ideal place for tracing the various forced stages of postcommunist normalization in Tirana. The Dajti is a fiefdom of Berisha sympathizers (Berisha was the former Albanian president and the head of the Democratic Party and was elected prime minister in 2005) and a symbol of underground resistance against the spaces frequented by Westerners. Westerners stayed primarily at the three "international hotels": the Tirana, the Rogner, and the Sheraton, each built in a different period and all bearing the same message. These international hotels are home to military men, journalists, secret agents, and "experts" from the European community, UN agencies, and international NGOs. The style of these three hotels is emblematic of different stages of the postcommunist transition and reflects different relationships between the international community and the local elite. At the Tirana Hotel, a special unit of the Italian military has taken over the first floor and re-created the hotel space according to their own norms of efficiency and technological modernity. The global media has long taken advantage of the Tirana's strategic position by filming televised reports from its rooftop terrace. The terrace looks out over the square, which embodies in its architecture memories of the fascist Italian occupation and the era of "real socialism." More recently, this square has been the site of massive rallies and protests. Rising above the square, one can make out the minaret of an ancient mosque, which creates a convenient televised reminder for global viewers that Albania is largely a Muslim country. Farther beyond the minaret, one can make out the statue of the hero Skanderbeg and, to its left, an imposing staircase. There is an empty space above the staircase that used to house an enthroned statue of the former dictator. The juxtaposition of mythical men and empty spaces in the square evokes both the promise of invincible heroes, and the threat of the fall from grace. Whether this décor is a testimony, or simply a purely fictive space, it is nonetheless ideal for filming short news clips that portray the phases of "democratization," the risks of entering into the realm of Islamic terrorism, and the generosity that the Albanian people demonstrated in welcoming Kosovo Albanian refugees. Finally, the space was ideal for retransmitting interviews with Western ministers and dignitaries during the war in Kosovo.

When the war in Kosovo was still raging, the urban configuration of Tirana continued to produce and evoke images and film sequences that oddly obscured the images of human suffering that the theater of war and expertise was designed to redress. The two refugee camps outside of Tirana, which denounced the horror and human catastrophes of the events, seemed paradoxically on the periphery of the event itself. The humanitarian theater was concentrated in three areas: military zones; the airport, where the airspace was reserved solely for military planes and helicopters transporting volunteers, experts, military, journalists, and political men; or the downtown area, specifically within the network of Tirana's four main hotels. Whereas the Dajti and Tirana hotels evoked an atmosphere of spies, conspiracy, and markets and exchanges of all sorts, the Rogner represented the hotel of "transition," supporting a more neutral and disengaged atmosphere where one did not exchange secrets but myths of nationhood, both past and present. This was a space for developing new strategies and for creating a link between the international community and the part of the local elite that I refer to as "global civil society." Replete with gardens and sunlight, the hotel promoted an atmosphere of "lunch on the lawn," a marked contrast to the majestic yet dim salons of the Dajti and the Tirana. One can still meet members of the new cosmopolitan elite at the Rogner bar. Their institutes and centers are not far from the hotel, so there is a particular logic to frequenting the hotel. However, it is likely that the Rogner's atmosphere, free from identity politics, also makes it a fashionable place for international conferences and meetings. The Sheraton achieved its fame as a "place to be seen" much later, when the phases of emergencies and the process of democratization following the war in Kosovo had already passed. It has become the hangout for modern political men and the new economic elite. A bit removed from the center of town, the Sheraton is less frequented by the international community who in the past were so central to the character of the Tirana and the Rogner. As local elites rise and mingle with one another and with the international community in the safe spaces of hotel lobbies other hot spots, "humanitarianism" takes on a new transactional guise. Hidden away from the lived context of human suffering, elites of all forms can deal in the moral and financial exchanges of the humanitarian market.[12]

HUMANITARIAN INTERVENTION
AND THE NEW MARKETPLACE

How should we interpret the ambiguous and contradictory strategies of humanitarian intervention? Traditionally, humanitarian intervention is legitimized by (1) human rights violations, (2) episodic food insecurity that risks deteriorating into mass starvation, (3) macroeconomic crises with hyperinflation and declining employment rates, and (4) large movements of populations in flight or forcefully relocated as refugees. The fine line separating humanitarian intervention and military operations collapsed in the beginning of the 1990s.[13] While concern has been voiced about this conflation, it appears that the ethics of humanitarian intervention lies beyond the threshold of suspicion. Jean-Christophe Rufin notes that the temptation to conceive of humanitarian matters as inherently innocent is so ingrained in Western consciousness that it is "increasingly at variance with reality, because today humanitarianism has entered the era of high complexity, which can accommodate neither romantic tendencies nor the desire to 'naturalize' war, which forgets that conflicts are not engendered by some sort of barbarian absurdity born out of some kind of tribalism, or the result of an excess of extremist fury, but always have 'political' origins" (1999b: 20, my translation).

The confluence of human rights discourses,[14] antitotalitarian politics, and humanitarian practices brings into view the problem of an unquestionable right of humanitarian interference. Several aid workers who played key roles in humanitarian intervention operations have recently condemned the local impact of the transnational humanitarian apparatus (Rufin 1999b; Brauman and Mesnard 2000). These critiques are not entirely new, yet their presence indicates the importance of engaging in a critical reassessment of the theory and practice of military-humanitarian intervention. Bertrand Badie (2002) has described the irresistible rise of humanitarianism as a new international marketplace. This "pietàs market," as he deems it, represents an investment of both moral value and financial capital gained from dubious origins. This market produces a strategy of "rushing to the rescue" that is justified by discourses that decontextualize and naturalize both the causes and the effects of wars and armed conflicts. Within this complex apparatus, the risk lies in the possibility of breaking all preexistent forms of social life that might hinder the rescue of the victim. This imperative to rescue is achieved by appealing to a principle of high performance that resembles standard business practices. But these means produce their own logic, which strongly favors efficiency and expertise. This problematic disconnection of the bond between ends and means thus results, on the ground, in a strange set of compromises and constraints in what the media hastily label as a "liberated" Kosovo, Afghanistan, or Iraq.

This situation poses many questions for anthropologists. How can we solve the paradoxical predicament experienced by the agents of humanitarian intervention who are caught between a dependence on donor countries and a humanitarianism that is viewed as a "universal" or apolitical ideology? How can we confront humanitarian interventions' dangerous tendency to shed ethical autonomy and become instead a form of parallel diplomacy that can be co-opted and integrated into the agendas of states? Finally, how can we interrogate humanitarianism's adoption of market-driven sensationalism and its position outside of institutional constraints, a position that leads to an ambiguous form of "new politicization" (Badie 2002)?

The new industry of "pietàs," which came to dominate the international scene in the 1990s, was preceded by an early transformation that came to light in the 1960s. This transformation was engendered by a "profound transformation of the status of victims whereby states were delegitimized . . . the end result being the radically privatized management of today's humanitarianism" (Badie 2002: 241). This transformation, and the race to generosity that it inspired, soon revealed its high costs. Political powers were displaced from their institutional sites by a group of "experts sans frontières" whose growing legitimacy allowed them to engage in a form of crisis management that was increasingly free from institutional control.[15]

These business-style modes of operation were characterized by sensitivity to donors' prerogatives and a form of pietàs-oriented broadcasting that engaged in an endless search for "human-interest stories." These operating strategies often contradict the objectives that had first encouraged intervention. The standard justification for military-humanitarian intervention is an appeal to the temporally limited but immediate need to intervene. In the realm of intervention we frequently hear terms such as "effectiveness," "coherence," "timeliness," and "the opportune moment." Other popular appeals include the technical claim that intervention is only a partial activity, limited to pursuing the application of well-defined goals. Partisans of "empire lite" (Ignatieff 2003a) maintain this pragmatic view of human rights.[16] This pragmatic approach often serves to paint its promoters, among others, into a corner. Supporters of this view are victims of a form of innocent ethnocentrism, which often leads people to unwittingly construct a theoretical system that is based on the liberal notion of negative freedom and a highly coercive doctrine of just war. Their pragmatic operation seeks to generalize human rights, but often ends up legitimizing a banal force that gives rise to a kind of humanitarian fundamentalism (Zolo 2003). Today the paradox of humanitarian and military intervention—or "military humanitarianism"—is nothing short of a war conceived of in "humanitarian" terms. In his perceptive postface to the Italian edition of Michael Ignatieff's *Human Rights as Politics and Idolatry*, Danilo Zolo (2003) stresses that all juridical-ethical universalism "tends to be intolerant, aggressive, and oblivious to the diversity and complexity of the world . . . there is nothing more idolatrous and monotheistic (and naïve) than a war waged in the name of human rights" (Zolo in Ignatieff 2003c: 156, my translation).

CURE, NOURISH, AND SAVE HUMAN BODIES

The zones of humanitarian intervention described above can be conceived of as "laboratories of democratization." The local dynamics at work in these laboratories are quite complex, and these intricate local situations are further complicated by the introduction of a massive international humanitarian presence. In recent years, theoretical reflections about a "just" or "humanitarian" war have been at the forefront of debates both within and outside of academia. These debates have importantly engaged scholars from a vast spectrum of academic disciplines and have led many intellectuals to engage in various forms of political involvement. After a decade of examining military-humanitarian interventions, we have only recently begun to feel the need to engage in deeper theoretical examinations of this phenomenon. Considering the postethical attitude of nonintervention in Rwanda, the reluctant intervention in Bosnia, and the right and obligation to intervene in Kosovo, Afghanistan, and Iraq, it is clear that the trajectory of this phenomenon is in dire need of careful scrutiny.

The humanitarian war in Kosovo offers a key example for establishing the genealogy of a double-sided intervention: on March 24, 1999, NATO intervened in Kosovo with air strikes; on April 11, 1999, the very same NATO opened a new branch of humanitarian relief for Kosovo called Operation Allied Harbour.[17] Indeed, in 1999, following the three-month war in Kosovo and the crises of the postwar period, Albania was witness to an enormous deployment of humanitarian organizations that sought to accommodate 450,000 war refugees.[18] In an effort to maintain efficient operations, these organizations interfered with the ongoing negotiations between local institutions and international diplomats present in Albania. Within twelve days of arriving on the scene, NATO, the International Military Force (AFOR), and other bilateral and multilateral bodies had superseded the roles traditionally played by embassies and the local government.[19] NATO's military logistical infrastructure was deployed with such "efficiency" that it had the entire territory under control within a matter of days, assigning responsibilities and distributing tasks to numerous actors on the ground.

One could gain entry into the pyramid mausoleum built by the dictator Enver Hoxha in the center of Tirana by brandishing the badge of an international organization. The mausoleum was serving as NATO headquarters and was the repository for a panoply of figures and statistics necessary for organizing the deployment of humanitarian services. Resources included maps and a host of reports that indicated the precise number of refugees present in the area (updated every three hours), details on internally displaced people, statistics on epidemic diseases, the quantities of available drugs and where they were needed, the number of showers and toilets needed in a specific location, and the total number of beds that could be built in a given refugee camp. The mausoleum was home to the data that was necessary for deploying a set of extremely persuasive strategies intent on curing, nourishing, and saving "human bodies." The AFOR Web site advertised that it was working in concert with local Albanian institutions and international agencies to swiftly and efficiently respond to emergencies "on the ground."[20] Yet, as those who were present at the time can attest (I was in Albania), the chaos of the first few days was only mitigated when the military arrived to take over the logistical and procedural reigns of intervention.[21]

In June 1999, a few days after the war ended, I was still in Albania. Combat had ended and the limelight of media compassion had been turned off. Hotels were emptied of their swells of journalists, officials, and international aid workers; apartment leases were cancelled. The transnational "army" had rented helicopters and cars to move along to the next site of humanitarian compassion. At the same time, Kosovo Albanians were quickly heading back to their homes in Kosovo.[22] The end of the war and the mass return of Kosovars resulted in the suppression of the "emergency" in Albania. NGOs and international agencies active in Albania closed their local operations and laid off their Albanian employees, leaving behind unused material that had never been cleared by local customs. The emergency had moved elsewhere. The international community and its operations, logistics, and apparatuses were moved to the next site: the new "liberated" territory of Kosovo, which became the priority site of postconflict emergency where all international funds were collected.

Many projects in Kosovo aimed at mitigating the "emergency" of the aftermath of war were funded for only one year. Thus, one year after infiltrating the territory, humanitarian groups found themselves in shortage of funds or provisions. The political power in Serbia had changed, and there were new tensions between KFOR, the UN mission in Kosovo, and the Albanian guerrillas in Macedonia. The "emergency" and its associated projects had once again shifted to new terrain. Ironically, as territories evolve from sites of emergencies to sites of stability, they are deprived of the humanitarian apparatus and the resources that it brings. It would be interesting to trace the flows of experts, international organizations, and military personnel further as they migrated from Kosovo to Afghanistan and then waited in the wings to engage in the "humanitarian" mission in Iraq and Lebanon.

THE TRAUMA OF VICTIMHOOD

A series of categories are applied to territories, and to human beings, as they enter the discursive and operative strategies of humanitarianism. Such categories may be extended to the world system and its potential and real donors, to multilateral and bilateral accords, to ad hoc UN agencies, and to emergency programs whose procedures and budgets are not under the control of more traditional agencies.

Past experiences and individual and collective histories are erased by the new categories in which human beings are cataloged. The categories "victim," "refugee," "trafficked woman," or "trauma case" do not fully relate the experiences of surviving traumatic events. These categories are simply labels intended to activate procedures such as fund-raising, legal and medical protocols, the transport of populations, and, finally, a profit-making business whose pervasive nature is concealed by charitable pietàs (Fassin 2000; Rufin 1999a).

Whether hailing from Bosnia or the Philippines, a person who is classified under one of these international categories is an exportable, irrelevant entity. A trafficked woman enters into repatriation procedures whether she is in Kosovo or in Thailand, and demilitarization is accomplished through similar procedures whether it takes place in Africa or South America. In Kosovo, international organizations and NGOs were extremely active. Documents issued by the United Nations Interim Administration Mission in Kosovo (UNMIK), valid for a few months, were substituted for Yugoslav passports. The World Health Organization took on special powers comparable to a ministry of health. International organizations established priorities and divided the territory according to rationalized criteria of intervention that had been established by donor countries, most of which hailed from the West.

An interesting example of how donor priorities are written into intervention programs can be found in an IOM project, the Psychosocial and Trauma Response in Kosovo.[23] This ambitious project brought together major international experts in trauma, ethnopsychoanalysis, transcultural psychiatry, and medical anthropology. The promotional pamphlet for the project describes its objectives as "responding to the most immediate and urgent needs of the resident and returning population" and "understand[ing] the relevance of the migration/exile/war/occurrences as experiences determining specific forms of psychosocial and mental health suffering." The program established "an alternative training facility for counselors." The role of "counselor" did not previously exist in Kosovo.

Following the waves of returnees in the aftermath of war, I became involved as an expert in this project that distinguished itself from other humanitarian programs by its inventiveness and its aim to develop an alternative approach to the standard "rescue machinery." However, it quickly became clear that all this innovative potential lacked a margin for action in which to experiment and to develop an alternative approach, insofar as the innovative program was implemented in a field of intervention already managed by the humanitarian apparatus and all of its rules. Finally, I can say that this promising initiative became trapped in the requirements and procedures of the donor-led humanitarian system to which it was accountable. In this case, the genuine ambition of the program rendered the paradox even more problematic, leading, concretely, to a lived situation of extreme ambivalence.

In order to attain its goal of training counselors, the project had to accommodate the requirements of its two primary donors: the U.S. Department of State and the International Italian Cooperation, the Italian government's development agency. The first phase of the project was carried out at the time of the emergency, and it reflected two different approaches. The first approach favored the creation of a parallel project (the Archives of Memory), which aimed to preserve the meaning of the war events. Unfortunately, this well-intentioned part of the project linking memory and reconciliation overlooked potential long-term effects of the project, most notably the possibility of recognition and retribution against perpetrators. The second approach insisted that the trained counselors practice in hospitals and other structures in order to substitute for absent Serbian psychiatrists, many of whom had abandoned Kosovo territory or were taking refuge in established safe zones. This inevitably produced confusion among the prospective counselors, who ended up becoming the "traumatized" actors to be remembered in the Archives of Memory.

Moreover, there emerged a slow but inexorable normalization of counselor training courses that would satisfy the criteria developed by the World Health Organization (WHO) as a part of their plan for reestablishing mental health in Kosovo. The U.S. Department of State would disperse funds only according to the WHO guidelines, and soon the Italian donor adopted similar requirements. The category of "emergency" and even the category of "trauma" were no longer considered viable for raising funds because they did not correspond to prevailing donor priorities. Following the priorities of these new guidelines, the project turned to the construction of psychosocial support in minority zones in order to demonstrate its adherence to the WHO criteria.

The project tried to develop an alternative approach by offering training in the theories and practices of contemporary ethnopsychiatry. However, its fluctuating and ambiguous strategy repeatedly tended to produce the opposite effects. Why was this so? I have struggled with this paradox for a long time, and I continue to do so. In this example, good intentions and creativity confronted a machinery that did not allow alternatives, compelling us to reevaluate means and ends and the relationship between them. In the absence of such reevaluation, all we can do is acknowledge the "collateral damage" the humanitarian device incurred. And even worse, trapped in the machinery, we risk producing—by constructing new programs from pieces cut, assembled, repositioned, and recombined from other projects—what humanitarian actors in their unique, cynical vocabulary call "Frankenstein projects."

THE EXPERTISE AND ETHICS OF WITNESSING

The world media's insistence on portraying "distant suffering" has gradually legitimated the category of "intervention" (Boltanski 1993). Media images of human suffering often hide the processes entailed in different types of intervention. This is evident in the media coverage of the crisis in Albania in 1991. Televised images showed thousands of human bodies crowding onto ships that were destined to cross the sea and deposit them in Italy, where they could pursue their Western dreams. In 1999, the world watched as 850,000 Albanians fled Kosovo to seek refuge in Macedonia, Albania, and a few Western countries. These poignant images generated a widespread consensus around the category of intervention, legitimating the presence of humanitarian and military experts and their political, economic, and juridical procedures.

The ethics of witnessing and the logistics and politics of emergencies have developed into a specific form of political agency. "Humanitarian intervention" as a form of political agency has become increasingly independent from national and governmental institutions. It has become an autonomous interlocutor with the international community as experts in humanitarian matters (including food, logistics, drugs, hospitals, weapons, security, institution-building, human rights). Intervention has begun to act as a sort of mobile sovereignty.

Soldiers and humanitarian experts have found common ground in the immediacy of wars and humanitarian catastrophes. The capability or possibility of intervening on the ground, free from political and institutional ties, is welcomed by (1) local governments and communities, (2) the United Nations, (3) governmental institutions of donor countries who support intervention, and (4) independent donors who prefer expertise to entrenched bureaucracies. Since the mid-1990s, the intertwining of these four levels has ensured the tacit acceptance of any kind of intervention. Under the label of "humanitarian intervention," national governments have furthered their own interests while marketing a "human-friendly" form of international politics. Saving the bodies of children, women, the elderly, and the suffering has become part of the standard electoral ticket for many governments seeking to further their claims of efficiency and expediency in the international arena. By looking at the discursive practices that have characterized recent electoral campaigns in countries engaged in military-humanitarian operations, we see that increased spending on humanitarian operations, and the promotion of media images of human suffering, can be more effective in gaining electoral support than promoting other domestic issues such as unemployment or health care.

The progressive legitimization of humanitarian action, and thus of humanitarian "experts," does not stem solely from electoral interest in overdeveloped countries. Under the pressure of the right/duty to intervene (the rallying cry of Bernard Kouchner, founder of Médecins sans Frontières, 1971, and Médecins du Monde, 1980), the United Nations is also increasingly recognizing NGOs as political actors. The heterogenous composition of international NGOs has been swiftly identified in international meetings as a form of "civil society," an ambiguous term that seeks to capture the "mobile" actors that sell expediency and expertise at the expense of less mobile forms of civil society, which though operating exclusively at the local/national level play an important role in democratizing their societies. This obsession to define project managers or NGO experts as "representatives of civil society" has increased tremendously since the mid-1990s. It can be argued that this is the weakest aspect of humanitarian intervention. Indeed, if such actors are recognized and legitimized as political partners in the international arena, this presents the new problem of representation and begs the question of why this new set of actors has escaped democratic control.

This anomaly has had a tremendous impact on local communities in contemporary Eastern and Southeastern Europe. In postcommunist European territories, many tend to respond to the ghost of their recent political past by demonstrating a weak identification with their current state institutions. As a result, new lobbies emerge that consist of individuals whose cultural resources enable them to successfully interact with the international community. Such individuals are likely to start their own NGOs in order to tap into international funding networks. Eventually they become experts at navigating the maze of international funding organizations. Gradually these groups become private-interest or pressure groups that are able to influence or even control the media and local and national politicians. Many of these mobile and local communities have acquired international renown and have emerged as new political actors whose presence in the realm of global politics is legitimated by their presumed "expertise" in local affairs.[24] This expertise allows these individuals and groups to bypass the canonical procedures of democratic legitimization, whether on a local, national, or European scale.

The humanitarian style of imposing oneself on the international scene requires both the ability to generate a media image that spurs transnational generosity and the ability to create a veneer of respectability that is based on technically rational protocols of intervention. An individual actor or group must demonstrate his or her ability to create intervention programs that can be exported from one area of the globe to another, breaking down any "institutional barriers" that could hinder "helping the victims." Organizations and individuals must strike a balance between "performance" and "profitability," maintaining a positive image and an acute entrepreneurial acumen.

The spiral of generosity resulting from these processes comes at a high political and social price. The locus of politics is increasingly removed from more traditional institutional seats of power. The growing legitimacy of new "men without borders" creates management crises that escape institutional control and take on the new guise of entrepreneurship. In their effort to promote a visible image of productivity, these individuals and groups tend to lose sight of the humanitarian impulse that initially propelled them in to this world, favoring instead the priorities of international donors and the whims of a media that thrives on a pietàs aesthetic.

Paradoxically, these processes produce a new politicization of humanitarianism (Badie 2002). As these new men and groups gain independence from institutional frameworks they must conform to the rules of the market and the media of visibility. If we look at the past decade of humanitarian intervention we cannot fail to notice that another new form of politicization calls into question the "privatized" legitimacy of humanitarian action. NGOs, international and bilateral organizations, and UN agencies intervene in numerous conflicts both to alleviate suffering and to proclaim their right as a member of international civil society to participate in all phases of diplomatic negotiation. Here a new chapter of the humanitarian saga begins. Pure and simple "humanism" is no longer the autonomous referent called upon to justify intervention. Instead, humanitarian action is defining itself through its role in parallel diplomacy, defining itself as an actor that is banally implicated in the actions and strategies of nation-states. The logic of political neutrality is fading away in favor of a logic of responsibility that is articulated in the formula of the right/duty to intervene as a full participant in the political affairs of states.

GLOBALIZING LEGITIMACY

In addition to creating new spaces and political logics, modern guises of humanitarian intervention also bring new sets of actors to the fore of local and international politics. The rise of these new actors seems to follow a standard trajectory, irrespective of local specificities. These actors come from English-speaking sectors of local society, and they are frequently youth or established intellectuals who by virtue of their position are already plugged into international networks (the strategy of the Soros foundation is emblematic in this respect).[25] Soon these elite players come to be viewed by the international humanitarian network as the sole social group to have gained international legitimization. This newfound legitimacy comes with the right to full participation in a parallel society composed of representatives of local and national institutions and local "strongmen" who represent the new interlocutors of the international community. Sometimes these strongmen are government officials, members of parliament, ministers, or ambassadors. More often, however, strongmen do not hold institutional positions. In this case, they often feel threatened by English-speaking locals whom they perceive to be an emerging counter-elite. These strongmen attempt to strengthen their position by seeking international legitimization through this newly formed parallel society. In Kosovo, Veton Surroi provides a good example of a man who has followed this social and political trajectory.[26] Surroi's father was a Yugoslav ambassador under Tito. Surroi was a representative at the Rambouillet meeting and is a well-known journalist. He is the director of an independent television station, Koha Vizion, and owns a major newspaper, *Koha Ditore*, which is financed by the international community.

Though not a strongman himself, Surroi has become one of the major local "representatives" to the international community. Anthony Borden, director of the Institute for War and Peace Reporting, described Surroi as "a signal voice for democracy in Kosovo; he played a central role in salvaging the process— signing his name alone to the commitment in principle, a paper that Kosovo Liberation Army (KLA) representatives only finally formally backed several weeks later in Paris. Long considered to be a future key political figure in Kosovo, Veton, 38, has so far kept independent from organized politics and claims to be 'just a journalist'" (Borden 1999). While Surroi has been hailed as an apolitical figure promoting the pure interests of civil society, it is important to note that in the summer of 2004 he founded a political party called the Ora, which holds seven seats in the Assembly of Kosovo.

The international humanitarian realm has enshrined these elite as representatives of a local civil society, as a comprehensible voice of the people. Yet in an effort to maintain their international positions of power, these elite have had to adopt the language, priorities, and practices espoused in humanitarian discourse. The international community turns to these elite to express the opinions of local people, but most have completely lost touch with the experiences and views of civil society. Therefore these select elite act more as a mirror for humanitarian priorities than as a window to the people. This profound, radical, and accelerated transformation of local channels of negotiation is often overlooked. When noticed, it is not interpreted in terms of relations of power and domination, but is viewed as a "natural" and necessary moment in the transition from totalitarianism to liberal democracy. Yet this process is far from linear, and unforeseen "collateral damages" undermining the transition to democracy may emerge in the future.

The key figures described here are charged with managing the postwar process. They rose to prominence through an international circuit of conferences, meetings, and interviews. They monopolize the media's attention, and while claiming to speak for the local people they often merely represent themselves. Their positions as members of a parallel diplomatic corps ensure that they are exempt from all forms of institutional accountability. Surroi has argued that Kosovo would provide an ideal place in the region for the European

Union to experiment with building a stable democracy. Hearing such a proposition, one would like to know whether he is speaking as a reporter, a head of state, a senior member of government, or as the representative of a "western strategic think tank" supported by the OSCE.

Furthermore, who is someone like Surroi speaking for? In the end, what are the media spectacles of postwar democratic stabilization, military-humanitarian intervention, peacemaking and peacekeeping operations all about? Perhaps to answer these questions we must examine the logic and democratic practices of local institutions and assess whether these figures are indeed representative of a larger civil society or whether they are simply members of a newly formed oligarchy without democratic endorsement. Territories subject to military and humanitarian intervention occupy an ambiguous position where foreign armies are responsible for both peacekeeping and humanitarian operations.

Multilateral organizations are responsible for a multiplicity of activities at the institutional, administrative, and managerial levels. Local and international NGOs may play a parallel diplomatic role at the global level (which is legitimated by their status as witnesses and experts), while at the local level they calibrate their performance on the basis of the ever-changing priorities of donors. Zolo notes that the definition of civil society that emerged in the 1980s as "the economic and social space where social actors emerge in opposition to the established regime on the basis of modern citizenship values and institutions is gradually superseded by the notion of global civil society, that is, the complex international agency of social movements and voluntary organizations that often oppose established public institutions" (1997: 154, my translation). It is precisely this transformation that generates the ambiguity experienced by the territories subject to military-humanitarian intervention. How can such a stark contradiction be resolved?

Natural and humanitarian catastrophes are most certainly precipitated by distinct forces, yet the human tragedies resulting from events as diverse as civil wars and tsunamis are approached by the international community in much the same fashion. The procedures of saving bodies are portrayed as separate from the specificities of local contexts and political struggles. People are dying and displaced and international and local actors are left to debate about tents and toilets. This technical approach is often the same in various contexts of emergencies, and as anthropologists we must begin to review the links and disjunctures between these ideologies of humanitarian intervention in cases of natural and human disasters. Anthropologists must remain rooted in the constantly shifting terrain of humanitarian intervention, parsing the new forms of social interaction and relationships of power that circulate within this mobile web of people, politics, and technologies.

The barbed wire that surrounds the "militarized safety zones" in Pristina, Sarajevo, East Timor, Kabul, Baghdad, and soon other unforeseen corners of the globe, can be viewed as the jagged border on a detailed map that portrays the contradictory character typical of laboratories of democracy around the world. In some areas, war has ended ten years ago, or perhaps five. In other areas, war still rages. In the meantime, Web sites keep updating their pages, and conference participants continue to speak about questions of peace and security and the role of NATO, the United Nations, or global civil society. Crises are still being managed, and conflicts resolved, and reports are published under titles that mix genres in a way that both announces and obscures the Orwellian novelty of the military-humanitarian intervention.[27]

NOTES

This chapter provides an overview of the various trajectories that my work on humanitarian intervention has taken in recent years. For more detailed discussions of the questions explored here, please refer to my work cited in the reference list. This research has been funded by grants from the Social Sciences and the Humanities Research Council of Canada and the Fonds Québecois de la Recherche sur la Société et la Culture. I greatly benefited from fruitful interactions with friends and colleagues, including those at Byron Good and Mary-Jo DelVecchio Good's Friday Morning Seminar on Medical Anthropology and Cultural Psychiatry (Harvard University); seminars at EHESS in Paris directed by Marc Augé, Jean-Pierre Dozon, Didier Fassin, and Jean-François Gossiaux; and the conference that I organized in 2003 with Laurence McFalls and Marie-Joëlle Zahar titled "Intervention: Protagonists, Logics and Effects." I am grateful to Marc Abélès, Marie Cuillerai, Vincent Crapanzano, Mikhaël Elbaz, Michael Fischer, Judy Farquhar, Ellen Judd, Deborah Gordon, Vinh-Kim Nguyen, and Francine Saillant for our many rich exchanges. I would like to extend my special thanks to Hannah Gilbert, a doctoral student in medical anthropology at McGill University who reviewed the English text, and to Chowra Makaremi, my doctoral student at the Université de Montréal, for many rich intellectual exchanges. Thanks also to Marie-Claude Haince and Phillip Rousseau, my doctoral students at the Université de Montréal, for their precious assistance.

1. "Intervention" could be defined as a laboratory of a new form of domination overriding all preexisting forms of governance in the name of humanitarian action. This supracolonialism produces a constant erosion of democracy, collective participation, and political negotiation (Pandolfi 2000b, 2000a, 2006). For a critical viewpoint see also Zolo (1997, 1998, 2002, 2004, 2006) and Duffield (2001, 2004, 2005).

2. The concept of Balkanization emerged toward the end of the First World War to refer to the fragility of a territory driven to fragmentation by nationalism. With the advent of decolonization, the term was no longer restricted to Eastern Europe, but was employed as a metaphor for any instance of political and economic disintegration. In the mid-1990s the Balkans began to reemerge as a separate entity

within the restructuring of more classic divisions in central and Eastern Europe (Fischer 2002; Todorova 1997).

3. Acronyms for the military and humanitarian missions are as follows: operation Allied Harbour, NATO's first humanitarian mission to Albania, took place between April and September 1999 and was led by Albania Force (AFOR). Kosovo Force (KFOR) was a NATO-led international force responsible for establishing and maintaining security in Kosovo. The Organization for Security and Co-operation in Europe (OSCE) describes itself as "the largest regional security organization in the world with 55 participating States from Europe, Central Asia and North America." The United Nations High Commissioner for Refugees (UNHCR) describes its core mandate as "the protection of some 20 million uprooted people." All of these agencies work in concert with the International Monetary Fund (IMF), the World Bank, and the International Organization for Migration (IOM).

4. On these changes see Clark (1995).

5. As Zaki Laïdi notes, "As soon as emergency is professionalized, it tends to structure itself as social supply waiting for its demands. And if the demand does not exist, one tends to create it" (1998: 57, my translation).

6. I use the term "biopolitics" in the manner developed by Michel Foucault (see generally 1978, 1994, and 2003) to refer to the ensemble of administrative practices— schooling, policing, caring—that came to be used to administer populations within the rise of the modern state. Giorgio Agamben writes, "According to Foucault, a society's 'threshold of biological modernity' is situated at the point at which the species and the individual as a simple living body become what is at stake in a society's political strategies" (1998: 3). Michael Hardt and Antonio Negri (2000) have further developed this concept to examine how these practices produce regimes of rule in the contemporary world that are radically limited to the management of life in the barest terms, as in concentration or refugee camps or in capitalist production.

7. Veronique de Geoffroy (2000) discusses the unification of two realms of vocabulary, that of military humanitarianism or the civilian military. See also Rieff (2002) and Chomsky (1999).

8. In an interview General Clark, the commander in chief of NATO during the war in Kosovo, stressed that every air strike had to be evaluated beforehand by a staff of international law experts to determine its legitimacy.

9. Today, Bosnia and Albania are independent nation-states. Albania has had this status since November 28, 1912. Bosnia-Herzegovina achieved its independence in 1992, but, since the end of the war (1992–95) and after the Dayton Peace Agreement (November 1995), the Office of the High Representative (OHR) continues to play an important role in Bosnia politics. Kosovo was part of the former Yugoslavia and as of June 1999 is a protectorate of the United Nations Mission in Kosovo (UNMIK), an interim administration under the responsibility of the special representative of secretary general. In 2006, only a few responsibilities "are shared" with

the Provisional Institutions of Self-Government (PISG). The unresolved status of Kosovo and the provisional constitutional frameworks determine a permanent uncertainty in the region. The Independent Commission for Kosovo (2000), and member countries of the Contact Group support the Kosovo "conditional independence." A four-stage transition in the evolution of Kosovo's sovereignty is advocated in the last report of International Commission on the Balkans (2005).

10. One of the ways in which the international community seeks to maintain peace is by creating "national" or "territorial" parliaments. These parliaments remain under the guardianship of the United Nations. In Kosovo two elections have been attempted since the end of the war. Both attempts failed because large numbers of voters living in Serbian enclaves failed to vote. The nature and mandate of these parliaments, especially those that do not correspond to the definition of a sovereign nation as in the case of Kosovo, remain ambiguous and could potentially provide new spaces for the outbreak of violence. This military and civilian guardianship feeds the phenomenon that I refer to as "permanent transition."

11. The international community is represented either by NATO or by ad hoc military expeditions such as AFOR (Albania Force), KFOR (Kosovo Force), IFOR (Implementation Force in Bosnia), SFOR (Stabilization Force in Bosnia), or by international police forces such as the European MAPE. Civil personnel are represented by a wide array of agencies and organizations including the United Nations (UNDP, UNHCR, UNDCP, WFP, WHO, etc.) the IMF, the World Bank, the IOM, state-sponsored aid agencies (such as USAID), OSCE, and the European Union (PHARE, ECHO). NGOs that feature prominently on the scene include such agencies as CARE, Save the Children, Human Rights Watch, and Médecins du Monde. These NGOs operate either parallel to or in cooperation with bilateral or multilateral bodies. The international presence in these regions is massive in terms of the sheer number of territorial settlements (i.e., buildings, facilities, leisure activities, security apparatuses, etc.) and in terms of the quality of intervention.

12. The preceding part of the ethnography originally was published in French (Pandolfi 2006).

13. During the Cold War, humanitarian intervention was not strongly allied with military activity, and it was carried out primarily at a national level. After the fall of the Berlin Wall, humanitarian intervention became increasingly characterized by military intervention, resulting in the type of "gray zones" that characterize contemporary humanitarian intervention.

14. Michael Ignatieff (2003a) reminds us that the televised images of humanitarian catastrophes and wars are serving to break down the borders of moral space previously built up by citizenship, religion, and race. Without these boundaries we must now live up to a new form of common responsibility. This common responsibility, a form of human solidarity, justifies itself with a one-size-fits-all principle: the principle of human rights. Following the work of Danilo Zolo (2006) and

Gayatri Spivak (2004), among others, these rights are often confused with the armed interventions deployed to uphold them.

15. Bernard Kouchner is the former special representative of the UN secretary general in Kosovo, the current French minister of foreign affairs, the co-founder of Médecins sans Frontières, and the founder of Médecins du Monde. According to Kouchner, "Humanitarian activities have become customary" (1991: 313, my translation). Kouchner's statement points to the new forms of globally organized power and expertise discussed here. See Pandolfi (2003).

16. "Empire lite" refers to the new form of imperialism that does not rely on direct territorial acquisition but on the use of indirect forms of empire building such as diplomacy or humanitarianism.

17. NATO's objectives in the conflict in Kosovo were set out in the statement issued at the Extraordinary Meeting of the North Atlantic Council held at NATO on April 12, 1999, and were reaffirmed by heads of state and government in Washington DC, April 23, 1999 (NATO's Web site, www.nato.int/docu/pr/1999/p99–051e .tm; site discontinued).

18. From April to September 1999, AFOR ranks were comprised of soldiers from over nineteen nationalities, including seven thousand NATO soldiers. Albania was flooded with all forms of humanitarian aid. Tons of goods were supplied to the area but following the sudden end of war, the resources were abandoned in the field. These goods provided the material conditions necessary for a burgeoning underground economy marked by theft, corruption, and a large-scale black market. During the Kosovo conflict, 180 international NGOs were present in Albania. One year after the conflict in Kosovo, NATO continued to form the core of the international peacekeeping mission to Kosovo (KFOR) in which some forty-six thousand military personnel from thirty-nine countries were deployed. In addition to these soldiers, twenty thousand civilians were working for UNMIK and international NGOs.

19. These bilateral and multilateral bodies included four groups of observers, two from OSCE and others from the special missions of Western governments.

20. "Allied Harbour was NATO's first Humanitarian operation. Normally, such operations are almost exclusively the domain of civilian organisations, both international and non-governmental, but, in the case of the Kosovo crisis, by a fortnight over 200,000 refugees had arrived from Kosovo and NATO was the only organisation quickly able to meet the expanding need. HQ AMF(L) was deployed within five days and much credit should be given to the nations and NATO HQ in deploying their forces and augmenting them so quickly. The soldiers and staff arrived 'on the run', setting to work within twenty-four hours of arrival, and within a few weeks, working closely with the civilian sector and the Albanian Government, we had the crisis under control. Of course, the crisis did not end there and by 15 June 1999 there were 479,223 refugees in the country. But the provision by NATO of

medical, engineer, transport, security, and staff support prevented Milosevic from destabilizing Albania and proved instrumental in sustaining the refugees and in their eventual return to Kosovo. The soldiers from all twenty-five nations involved in the operation have much to be proud of. What follows is an outline of their achievement" (AFOR 2003).

21. I was a consultant for the UNDCP program (Albania Project) in 1999 and expert for the IOM project in Kosovo in 2000. In those two positions I had the opportunity to encounter the "parallel circle" of the international community. I wish to thank Pino Arlacchi, director of the UNDCP program in Vienna at that time, and Lino Losi, the project manager of the Kosovo IOM project, for their patience in enduring my continuous critical comments.

22. Operation Joint Guardian (part of KFOR), June 11–December 31, 1999. KFOR's Web site described its "mission" as follows: "The mission is seeking to build a secure environment within the Serbian province in which all citizens, irrespective of their ethnic origins, can live in peace and, with international aid, and democracy can begin to grow" (NATO's Web site, www.nato.int/kfor/objectives.htm; site discontinued).

23. The IOM is an international organization whose task is to organize the logistics of the movement of large masses of people. See the organization's Web site, www.iom.int.

24. Such communities have achieved this fame in at least two respects. On the one hand, they identify themselves with international politics while utterly ignoring local politics. On the other hand, they become the privileged referents of the international community and international media (including such TV networks as BBC, CNN, etc.).

25. The Soros Foundations Network describes itself as "autonomous institutions established in particular countries or regions to initiate and support open society activities" (Soros Foundations 2004).

26. Veton Surroi, born 1961 in Pristina, is the publisher of the most important Kosovar daily newspaper, the *KOHA Ditore*. He founded one of the first opposition groups in Kosovo, the local chapter of the Association of a Yugoslav Democratic Initiative (UJDI) in 1989, and founded one of the first independent trade unions in Kosovo in 1989. Surroi was the president of the second-strongest political party in Kosovo (PPK) from 1991 to 1992. He is a leading member of several Kosovo Albanian negotiating groups, including the Rambouillet and Paris Talks (1999). Surroi was the recipient of the International Federation of Journalists (IFJ) annual award for journalism, the National Endowment for Democracy (NED) award, and the Geunzen Award for Freedom of Holland.

27. For example, "Operational Allied Force March–June 1999: NATO intervened in Kosovo to halt a humanitarian catastrophe and restore stability in the strategic region that lies between Alliance and member states" (NATO's Role in Kosovo, NATO's Web site, www.nato.int/kosovo/kosovo.htm).

REFERENCES

Abélès, Marc. 2006. *Politique de la survie*. Paris: Flammarion.

Agamben, Giorgio. 1998 [1995]. *Homo Sacer: Sovereign Power and Bare Life*. Trans. Daniel Heller-Roazen. Stanford, CA: Stanford University Press.

———. 2000 [1995]. *Means without Ends: Notes on Politics*. Trans. Vincenzo Binetti and Cesare Casarino. Minneapolis: University of Minnesota Press.

———. 2005 [2003]. *State of Exception*. Trans. Kevin Attel. Chicago: University of Chicago Press.

Agier, Michel. 2002. *Au bord du monde, les réfugiés*. Paris: Flammarion.

Albania United Nations Force (AFOR). 2003. NATO's Humanitarian Mission to Albania, Operation Allied Harbour. www.afsouth.nato.int/operations/ harbour/default.htm (accessed November 9, 2003).

Appadurai, Arjun. 1996a. *Modernity at Large: Cultural Dimensions of Globalization*. Minneapolis: University of Minnesota Press.

———. 1996b. Sovereignty without Territoriality: Notes for a Postnational Geography. In *The Geography of Identity*, ed. Patricia Yaeger, 40–58. Ann Arbor: University of Michigan Press.

Badie, Bertrand. 2002. *La diplomatie des droits de l'homme: Entre éthique et volonté de puissance*. Paris: Fayard.

Boltanski, Luc. 1993. *La souffrance à distance : Morale humanitaire, médias et politique*. Paris: Métailié.

Borden, Anthony. 1999. Interview: Veton Surroi—Sharing the Risks of Democracy. Institute for War and Peace Reporting. http://iwpr.net/?p=bcr&s=f&o =251904&apc_state=henibcr1999 (accessed November 9, 2003).

Brauman, Rony, and Philippe Mesnard. 2000. Champ humanitaire et champ de force. *Mouvements* 12:8–12.

Chomsky, Noam. 1999. *The Military Humanism: Lessons from Kosovo*. Monroe, ME: Common Courage Press.

Clark, Ann Marie. 1995. Non-Governmental Organizations and Their Influence on International Society. *Journal of International Affairs* 48 (2):509–24.

de Geoffroy, Veronique. 2000. Militaro-humanitaire ou civilo-militaire? *Mouvements* 12:49–54.

Duffield, Mark. 2001. *Global Governance and the New Wars: The Merging of Development and Security*. London and New York: Zed Books.

———. 2004. *Carry on Killing: Global Governance, Humanitarianism and Terror*. Copenhagen: Danish Institute for International Studies.

———. 2005. Getting Savages to Fight Barbarians: Development, Security and the Colonial Present. *Conflict, Security & Development* 5 (2): 1–19.

Fassin, Didier. 2000. Entre politiques du vivant et politiques de la vie: Pour une anthropologie de la santé. *Les notes de recherche no. 1 du CRESP.* Bobigny: Université Paris 13.

Fassin, Didier, and Paula Vasquez. 2005. Humanitarian Exception as the Rule: The Political Theology of 1999 Tragedia in Venezuela. *American Ethnologist* 32 (3): 389–405.

Fischer, Bernd. J. 2002. The Perceptions and Reality in Twentieth-Century Albanian Military Prowess. In *Albanian Identity: Myth and History,* ed. Stephanie Schwandners-Sievers and Bernd J. Fischer, 134–42. Bloomington: Indiana University Press.

Foucault, Michel. 1978 [1976]. *History of Sexuality,* Vol. 1: *An Introduction.* Trans. Robert Hurley. New York: Pantheon.

———. 1994. *Dits et écrits 1954–1988.* Vols. 3 and 4. Paris: Gallimard.

———. 2003 [1997]. *Society Must be Defended: Lectures at the College de France, 1975–76.* Trans. David Macey. Ed. Mauro Bertani and Alessandro Fontana. New York: Picador.

Hardt, Michael, and Antonio Negri. 2000. *Empire.* Cambridge, MA: Harvard University Press.

Ignatieff, Michael. 2003a. *Empire Lite: Nation Building in Bosnia, Kosovo, Afghanistan.* London: Vintage.

———. 2003b. *Human Rights as Politics and Idolatry.* Princeton, NJ: Princeton University Press.

———. 2003c. *Una ragionevole apologia dei diritti umani.* Trans. Sandro d'Alessandro. Milano: Feltrinelli.

Independent Commission for Kosovo. 2000. *The Kosovo Report.* Oxford: Oxford University Press.

International Commission on the Balkans. 2005. *The Balkans in Europe's Future.* Report of the International Commission on the Balkans.

International Organization for Migration (IOM). 2004. Web site of the International Organization for Migration. www.iom.int (accessed December 18, 2004).

Kosovo Force (KFOR). 2004. Web site of the Kosovo Force. www.nato.int/kfor/welcome.html (accessed December 18, 2004; site discontinued).

Kouchner, Bernard. 1991. *Le malheur des autres.* Paris: Odile Jacob.

Lafontaine, Annie. 2002. Réfugié ou "local staff"? Changement de statut et enjeux de pouvoirs au Kosovo d'après-guerre. In "Politiques jeux d'espaces," ed. Mariella Pandolfi and Marc Abélès, special issue, *Anthropologie et Sociétés* 26 (1): 89–106.

Laïdi, Zaki. 1998. L'urgence ou la dévalorisation culturelle de l'avenir. In *Urgence, souffrance, misère: Lutte humanitaire ou politique sociale?* ed. Marc-Henry Soulet, 43–59. Fribourg: Presses Universitaires Fribourg.

Langewiesche, William. 2004. Welcome to the Green Zone: Our Fortified Bubble in Baghdad is a Microcosm of America and of What Has Gone Wrong in Iraq. *The Atlantic Monthly* 294 (4): 60–88.

North Atlantic Treaty Organization (NATO). 2004. Web site of NATO. www.nato.int (accessed December 18, 2004).

Organization for Security and Co-operation in Europe (OSCE). 2004. Web site of the OSCE. www.osce.org (accessed December 18, 2004).

Pandolfi, Mariella. 1991. *Itinerari delle emozioni: Corpo e identità femminile nel Sannio campano.* Milan: Franco Angeli.

———. 2000a. Disappearing Boundaries: Notes on Albania, Kosovo and the Humanitarian Agenda. *Psychosocial Notebook* 1:27–40.

———. 2000b. The Humanitarian Industry and the Supra-Colonialism in the Balkan Territories. Paper presented at the Seminar in Postcoloniality, Subjectivity, and Lived Experience, Friday Morning Seminar on Medical Anthropology and Cultural Psychiatry, Harvard University, Boston, October.

———. 2000c. Une souveraineté mouvante et supracoloniale: L'industrie humanitaire dans les Balkans. *Multitudes* 3:97–105.

———. 2002. "Moral Entrepreneurs," souverainetés mouvantes et barbelés: Le bio-politique dans les Balkans postcommunistes. In "Politiques jeux d'espaces," ed. Mariella Pandolfi and Marc Abélès, special issue, *Anthropologie et Sociétés* 26 (1): 29–50.

———. 2003. Contract of Mutual (In)Difference: Governance and Humanitarian Apparatus in Contemporary Albania and Kosovo. *Indiana Journal of Global Legal Studies* 10 (1): 369–81.

———. 2005. De l'utopie balkanique à l'utopie méditerranéenne: Tracer une frontière. In *à la recherche de la dimension perdue: La Méditerranée,* ed. Piro Misha, 151–86. Tirana: Book and Communication House.

———. 2006. La zone grise des guerres humanitaires. In "War and Peace/La guerre et la paix," ed. Ellen Judd, special issue, *Anthropologica* 48 (1): 43–58.

Pandolfi, Mariella, and Marc Abélès. 2002. Introduction: Politiques jeux d'espaces. In "Politiques jeux d'espaces," ed. Mariella Pandolfi and Marc Abélès, special issue, *Anthropologie et Sociétés* 26 (1): 5–10.

Pandolfi, Mariella, Mary-Jo DelVecchio Good, and Deborah Gordon, eds. 1990. Traversing Boundaries: European and North American Perspectives on Medical and Psychiatric Anthropology. Special Issue, *Culture, Medicine and Psychiatry* 14 (2).

Pollock, Sheldon, Homi K. Bhabha, Carol A. Breckenridge, and Dipesh Chakrabarty. 2000. Cosmopolitanisms. *Public Culture* 12 (3): 577–89.

Prendergast, John. 1997. *Crisis Response: Humanitarian Band-Aids in Sudan and Somalia.* London: Pluto Press.

Rieff, David. 2002. *A Bed for the Night: Humanitarianism in Crisis.* New York: Simon & Schuster.

Rufin, Jean-Christophe. 1999a. Les humanitaires et la guerre du Kosovo. *Le Débat* 106:3–26.

———. 1999b. Pour l'humanitaire: Dépasser le sentiment d'échec. *Le Débat* 105:4–21.

Spivak, Gayatri Chakravorty. 2004. Righting Wrongs. *South Atlantic Quarterly* 103 (2/3): 523–81.

Stiglitz, Joseph E. 2002. *Globalization and its Discontents.* New York: W. W. Norton & Company.

Soros Foundations. 2004. Web site of the Soros Foundations. www.soros.org/about (accessed December 18, 2004).

Suhrke, Astri, and Douglas Klusmeyer. 2004. Between Principles and Politics: Lessons from Iraq for Humanitarian Action. *Journal of Refugee Studies* 17 (3): 273–85.

Todorova, Maria. 1997. *Imagining the Balkans.* Oxford: Oxford University Press.

United Nations High Commissioner for Refugees (UNHCR). 2004. Web site of the UNHCR. www.unhcr.org (accessed December 18, 2004).

Zolo, Danilo. 1997 [1995]. *Cosmopolis: Prospects for World Government.* Trans. David McKie. Cambridge: Polity Press.

———. 1998. *I signori della pace. Una critica del globalismo giuridico.* Roma: Carocci.

———. 2002 [2000]. *Invoking Humanity: War, Law and Global Order.* Trans. Federico Poole and Gordon Poole. London: Continuum.

———. 2003. Fondamentalismo umanitario. In *Una ragionevole apologia dei diritti umani,* by Michael Ignatieff, trans. Sandro d'Alessandro, 147–65. Milano: Feltrinelli.

———. 2004. Globalizzazione. *Una mappa dei problemi.* Roma-Bari: Laterza.

———. 2006. *La giustizia dei vincitori.* Roma-Bari: Laterza.

PART II: SUBJECTIVITY IN
THE BORDERLANDS

Contestations of Borders and Infectious Disease in Southwest China

Sandra Teresa Hyde

In one strike-hard anticrime campaign [*yanda yundong*], we rounded up 120 drug addicts in one night! Where are we going to place all these young people? Does the government think about that? We fine them six hundred yuan [two months' local salary] hold them for the night and release them in the morning. Prostitution is the same. Like a poisonous weed, it keeps growing back. AIDS is just another problem attached to a long list of problems we face as a border region. Illegal car smuggling and border drug smuggling are much more pressing problems for the police than AIDS.

Police informant, Jinghong, June 1996

When this policeman downplays AIDS, he is not ignoring the emergence of the epidemic; rather, he reflects a recurrent discourse around HIV/AIDS that emphasizes policing and surveillance of China's border regions.[1] Borders here provide a liminal space where many transactions occur and where the spread of HIV in Sipsongpanna, an autonomous minority prefecture bordering Laos and Burma, symbolizes what Arjun Appadurai (1996) characterizes as late-twentieth-century cross-border migrations. These mass migrations of peoples, goods, services, and now viruses color a moving transnational canvas. This chapter focuses on the late-socialist Chinese state and untangles the actions of certain actors, such as the policeman quoted above, as the state began to police, control, and prevent the spread of HIV from its minority borderlands into the Han interior. It traces the actions, institutions, and multiple positions and interests government bureaucrats had in defining and transforming what I term "everyday AIDS practices." All over the globe, associations involving diseases get mapped onto certain places and peoples more readily than others. I argue that these state actors spatialize the identity of HIV disease through their own discursive constructions of diseases and borders.

The intellectual terrain of this chapter is wide. I first discuss HIV as a disorder facing the late-socialist state and the value of the concept of the borderlands for understanding the intricacies of the modern China. Second, I give two brief histories, one on the question of sovereignty and the other on the social epidemiology of HIV in southwest China. I then explore four narratives of the everyday AIDS practices of state actors and their political subjectivity. I use the term "practice" in the Bourdieuian sense (Bourdieu 1977, 1990): to discuss everyday AIDS practices means to capture an array of practices, words, and measures of state actors in the prevention of HIV.[2] I conclude with a discussion of the utility of linking borders, diseases, and political subjectivity. I focus here on the practices and subjectivities of state actors that worked in the Yunnan borderlands in the early years of the epidemic (1996–2000), the years prior to the 2001 official acknowledgment that China even had an epidemic.

DISORDERS OF THE LATE-SOCIALIST STATE

Armed with international and local public health intervention and health education prevention strategies, by the mid-1980s China embraced the idea of risk groups for HIV. Similar to many countries around the globe, China defined HIV through epidemiological categories that linked group rather than individual behaviors to HIV. For while the categories of injection drug user, prostitute, migrant, or foreigner are perceived as having higher rates of HIV than the general population; it is not membership in a group but actual individual behaviors such as sharing dirty needles and having unprotected sex that put people at risk. Furthermore, on the prevention front in the late 1990s, the surveillance of "risky bodies" was intensified in the name of prevention. In previous work I focused on how these risky bodies were also ethnic bodies (Hyde 2001, 2002, 2003, 2006). In this chapter, I discuss these broader categories that designate bodies as risky not only in terms of their ethnicity but also in terms of their location. According to central government reports and interviews with officials, it is borderland peoples who shoot drugs, engage in unsafe sex, and travel to Thailand to work (see Gilman 1988; Arnold 1993; Porter 1997). Here, I emphasize that the strategy of defining risky people rather than risky behaviors brings with it a whole edifice of state controlling practices and regulations. This edifice is not without historical precedent. Chinese historians note that on the eve of liberation in 1953, the Sipsongpanna borderland was perceived as a desolate wasteland of malaria and leprosy-infested jungles, full of barbarians (Yin 1986; Wang 1993).

Given these conditions we need to think about the nature of states and how state actors in the post-1979 reforms, often referred to as late-socialism, address the emergence of a socialist civil society (see Jing 1996; Yan 1996; Liu Xin 2000; Zhang Li 2001). Ralph Litzinger (2000), in his work on the Yao minority group in Yunnan, argues that the state is not merely a static or singular structure, but a series of processes whose social intertextures reveal how the state is reproduced through cultural milieu, ethnicity and local history (see also Shue 1988; Mueggler 2001). Nancy Chen (2003), in her work on "qigong fever" in Beijing, points to the late-socialist state's medicalization of certain martial arts and spiritual practices in order to keep tight controls over public order and space. I build on the work of these scholars and other scholars of late-socialism and postcoloniality who have rejected this notion of the unitary state.

Postreform China offers an excellent counterexample to the problem of what political science labels as the demarcation between civil society and the state.[3] China does so precisely because the state ushered in many of the international NGOs that in the mid-1990s began to work on HIV prevention. At the same time, these NGOs were not independent; rather, all were hybrid organizations of the Chinese government in the sense that every foreign NGO had a government counterpart. Having recognized this state–civil society distinction as spurious, we can more clearly address the centrality of the borderlands to the construction of individual AIDS practices and the state's regulation of risky subjects. Provincial government officials are the vanguard; they create new HIV policies, as they are themselves simultaneously subjected to larger regimes of power within postreform China. HIV policies evolve from a state apparatus that unites multiple discourses and techniques of power that are never straightforward and that create different kinds of political subjectivities and contradictions. These include efforts to survey and police the minority borderlands in the name of disease prevention and sovereignty, as well as cultural ideas about minority gender relations. All of this leads back to the problem of fighting an imagined disease with imaginary figures; who is tested for HIV or marked as an HIV-carrying person often has to do with how one is imagined both epidemiologically and geographically, rather than strictly how one behaves. Before proceeding to questions of sovereignty, I want to explore the notion of the borderlands, which is central to my argument.

BORDERLANDS AND BORDERS

As Thongchai Winichakul (1994: 15) so powerfully argues, modern nations arrive through the very act of imposing boundaries around borders, whether those boundaries are geographic or are categories not yet labeled as such in the case of new, previously unrecognized peoples and spaces. Furthermore, according to the imagined-community approach to modern state building, the

Chinese state's definition of its borders and boundaries allows it to exist as one continuous geopolitical space, because as a nation it is historically perceived and rhetorically revered as having been around for thousands of years (Anderson 1992 in Gladney 2002: 1). In another sense, studying the borderlands of a nation-state, one sees just what the central state considers the essential terrain of government control, including biological control over everyday life.

Whereas anthropologists such as Arnold Van Gennup (1960) studied cultural boundaries and their creation as a way to understand social and cultural expression and identity, recent work in anthropology on borders and boundaries moves away from the notion that they simply divide states, peoples, villages, and communities into two distinct entities—what is inside and what is outside, what is sacred and what is profane. Gloria Anzaldúa (1987) instigated a wave of research and writing on women—how mestizas were divided between two borders and the two cultures of Mexico and the United States. What is crucial about her work for my argument is that she instantiates the idea that borders are not just geographic; borders become embodied through the people identified with them. Building on Anzaldúa's work, Daphne Berdahl (1999: 3) argues, in her research in a village on the former border between East and West Germany, that "boundaries are symbols through which states, nations and localities define themselves" and their distinct territory and cultural limits. The idea of the borderlands allows new possibilities for theorizing subjectivity and actions of the state, the relationship between the center and border, and how center and periphery influence each another in a dialectical dance.

Furthermore, as Akhil Gupta and James Ferguson (1992) point out, "the borderlands are just such a place of incommensurable contradictions" (quoted in Berdahl 1999: 6), and rather than dismissing them as insignificant or marginal, they, and I, want to conceptualize the borderlands as the "normal" locale of modernity and the postcolonial subject. A borderlands approach highlights the fluid and multidimensional aspects of identity and the ways these identities in turn are constantly recreated as the notion of the border shifts within larger political, social, and cultural milieus. Individuals and the state negotiate borderlands in specific ways.

The narratives of the individuals I write about are in one sense about the state; these individuals are the embodiment of the Chinese state through their jobs and Communist Party affiliations. As a very real geographic border here dictates much of the discourse on the disordering effects of HIV on this chaotic and lawless territory, China's geopolitical borders with Laos and Burma must not get lost in this argument (Lyttleton and Amarapibal 2002; S. Lee 2003). In the eyes of the central government in Beijing, the illegal trade in cars, drugs, and sex represents the disorders of this border region. If drug use and sex are

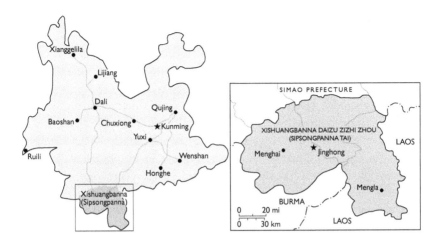

MAP 1.
Yunnan and Sipsongpanna

two of the key routes to HIV, controlling the borderlands must be part of state efforts to limit the spread of these very disorders. As Michel Foucault points out (1977; see also Burcell and Miller 1991), forms of state surveillance and control are never straightforward; they are remade, reinforced, and contested throughout history. Here I draw on the colonial notions of the borderlands as places of barbarian diseases, places that, prior to colonialization by the Chinese, were cesspools of tropical infection and, in the 1990s, were local sites for the spread of the most well-known disease of the twenty-first century.

SIPSONGPANNA AND CONTESTATIONS OF SOVEREIGNTY

The question of borderlands and central state sovereignty is key in contending with the complicated relationship of the central Chinese state to its minority borderlands. Sipsongpanna, a former independent state of the Lan Na kingdom of Thailand, was rechristened Xishuangbanna Dai Nationality Autonomous Prefecture (Xishuangbanna Daizu zizhi zhou) under the Communists in January 1953 (Hsieh 1995: 315; see map 1). Prior to its integration into mainland China, Sipsongpanna had a long history of patronage to Burma and to Ming China. Although many scholars disagree about the strength of Burma and China as the two suzerain states of Xishuangbanna, what they do agree is that after the Communists took over in 1953, the kingdom finally lost any semblance of independent status and became part of China's multiethnic frontier (Sethakul 2000).[4]

Instead of a unified singular Chinese state that transformed and erased the feudal aspects of Tai Buddhist religious practices after 1953, what emerged in the late 1990s was a Tai cultural renaissance that has manifested itself in social practices that capitalize equally on the rising market economy and on what I call an economy of cultural revival. While many Tai citizens of Sipsongpanna complain about the presence of the Han Chinese and their selfish and greedy ways, the Tai themselves have benefited enormously from the rise in economic markets, markets for their religious practices, organizational links to kinship groups in Laos and Thailand, and the resurgence in temple rebuilding and preservation, to name a few of these developments (Borchert 2005).

During previous regimes the religious and cultural habits of the Tai were suspect and suppressed as backward and feudal. Today this shift toward tolerance for ethnic difference occurs in the search for new markets, in this case ethnic tourism. For example, restrictions have been loosened and religious practices encouraged. A burgeoning network of Tai religious organizations throughout Southeast Asia may in the future assist in training young monks, teaching the Tai language, and preserving Buddhist palm leaf scriptures (see Davis 2005). These cultural exchanges often point toward contradictory goals: a Han state intent on raising revenues for tourism, and the Tai minority using tourism to revive and repair aspects of their cultural heritage after the violent suppression of the Cultural Revolution (1966–76).

The prefectural capital city of Jinghong was the capital (formerly Yun-jinghung) of the Tai-Lüe kingdom for over eight hundred years. By the late 1980s it became a tourist destination for Chinese who could afford vacations. Understanding Jinghong's ethnic tourism involves acknowledging its allure as a tropical paradise and exploring its linkage, simultaneously through the rise in sexually transmitted infections (STIs), to a sexual pathology and an urban erotic subculture. The dominant Chinese ethnic group, the Han, believe one of the cultural characteristics of the Tai ethnic group is a high level of sexual promiscuity, and this belief leads the Han to assume the Tai are particularly susceptible to STIs. These cultural prejudices aside, there are real grounds for concern, as Jinghong has a cosmopolitan sex industry that feeds the tourism market. Based on my fieldwork (1996–2000), I found this sexual pathology linked to the notion that beautiful "sex workers" were local Tai minority women. I discovered that 80 to 90 percent of the sex workers were Han Chinese female migrants from neighboring provinces (Hyde 2006). In order to increase their allure, many sex workers wore a modern version of local Tai clothing—a closely cropped long-sleeved top and a sarong. As sexual transmission is now seen as the next wave for the Chinese HIV epidemic, female entertainment workers are viewed as the infectious bridge population to the general population through their male clients (see also Porter 1997; Jeffrey 2002; Gregory 2003; Xia 2004). Therefore, interpretations of sexual risk become highly gendered and accompanied by notions of blame in terms of ethnic identification and territorial social space.

THE SOCIAL EPIDEMIOLOGY OF HIV
ON YUNNAN'S BORDERS

Beginning in the mid-1990s, public health officials in the provincial capital of Yunnan Province stated that the heterosexual transmission of HIV was on the increase in its southern minority border regions, particularly in the Dehong Dai-Jingpo Nationality Autonomous Prefecture in western Yunnan. After compiling three years of epidemiological data in the late 1990s, researchers at the National HIV Prevention and Control Center in Beijing identified eight subtypes of HIV-1 virus, meaning that China had both distinct subtypes of HIV and had absorbed subtypes from neighboring countries in East and Southeast Asia (see Beyrer 1998; Beyrer et al. 2000). According to Chinese HIV experts (Zhang Konglai 2001; Settle 2003), China's epidemic has gone through four distinct phases: (1) from 1985 to 1989 with only sporadic cases; (2) from 1989 to 1994 with cases concentrated in seven counties in Yunnan; (3) from 1994 to 2000 when HIV spread beyond Yunnan; and (4) from August 2001 to the present when every province, municipality, and autonomous region has cases of HIV.

In the mid-1990s, since Dehong Tai Prefecture had high rates of HIV, officials speculated that other regions with a large percentage of Tai minorities would also have high rates of HIV (Zheng Xiwan 1991, 1993, 1995). These officials made the assumption that there could be a cultural link. In these border minority prefectures HIV brings with it a disordering of large proportions, as it also becomes one of the disorders that disrupts the smooth workings of the state in promoting development. By the late 1990s, injection drug users from Yunnan Province made up 78 percent of the total number of people with HIV, and the majority of these were in Dehong (Zhang Xiaobo et al. 2002). As of 2005, the percentage of infections attributed to injection drug use had decreased to 44 percent. The decrease in the numbers of injection drug users is partially due to the increase in iatrogenic infections in the early to late 1990s from unsanitary and deadly practices in rural illegal blood banks in central China. Accounting for over 50 percent of deaths are rural peasants in Henan Province who were infected through giving blood (Ministry of Health et al. 2006: 2).

In Henan Province whole villages had upward of 80 percent infection rates due to entire nuclear families infected by blood-pooling activities of adult blood donors (UNAIDS 2002). Illegal blood banks targeted poor peasants by giving them money in exchange for selling their blood. With frequent extractions of blood, the banks were spinning down the plasma and putting the intermediary cells back with the belief they were preventing anemia and fortifying their donors to repeatedly give blood, thus securing their market. The key here is that these intermediary cells were not put back in the same person donating the plasma and thus were redistributed to several people with the same blood type. This meant that if one pooled donor was HIV positive, all the other donors and often later their wives and newborn children got HIV.

China by global comparison is still considered a low-prevalence country with respect to HIV, with less than a 1 percent prevalence rate (Shen 2004). Joan Kaufman notes that even if China were able to keep rates of new infections at 2 to 3 percent, as has Thailand, tens of thousands of people would require treatment and care (Kaufman 2005). Currently, of the seventy-five thousand people who have already developed AIDS, only 27 percent are receiving antiretroviral treatment (ART) (Ministry of Health et al. 2006: ii). Also, the current distribution of cases is not uniform. After testing close to one hundred thousand individuals from what are defined as "high-risk groups"—injection drug users, those with multiple sexual partners, and migrants—the Yunnan Centers for Disease Control and Prevention report the new rate was up to 1.5 percent. Seven prefectures in Yunnan had the highest prevalence rates, including Ruili County of Dehong Tai Prefecture, and one of the lowest in Sipsongpanna. However, by 2002 the majority of HIV-positive Yunnanese were twenty- to thirty-year-old males, injection drug users, Han Chinese, and unemployed peasants (Zhang Xiaobo 2002: 330).

Risk categories are defined in China, as elsewhere, as epidemiological (such as blood and sexual transmission) and behavioral. Risk groups mark people not by only by their at-risk behaviors but by who they are—homosexuals, heterosexuals, sex workers, migrants, and drug users. HIV is also understood in terms of geographic and political categories. For example, in early 2006, the Chinese Centers for Disease Control and Prevention reissued figures that reduced the count from 850,000 to 640,000 people infected with HIV; however, many Chinese and international AIDS activists contest these figures as far too low (UNAIDS 2002; Ministry of Health et al. 2006: 1). Activists argue that the difference between the official and unofficial estimates resulted from limited reporting in rural and remote areas; widespread fear of HIV and the stigmatization associated with a HIV diagnosis; the relative expense of testing; and the inaccessibility or unavailability of multiple antiretroviral drug therapies (ART). Thus, from central Beijing to the Yunnan periphery bureaucratic action at the local level was often stymied and mired in politics, geography, and notions of blame. It is these notions of blame, politics, and geography that I explore in the following four narratives.

In my fieldwork in Beijing, Menglian, Jinghong, and Kunming, I was able to observe the often shifting and conflicting positions that professionals took in response to local understandings of AIDS. Their positions filtered down into the intimate *guanxi* (personal connections) between professionals and their charges and often were politically motivated and questioned. Because promoting prevention strategies is never easy, China's initial focus on demographic and geographic categories, as opposed to risky behaviors, ensured an edifice of the state controlling practices and regulations over certain groups.

How do individuals who work in the anti-epidemic stations in Menglian and Kunming, and in a high security drug prison outside Jinghong, react in the face of what seems a borderland epidemic? The impact of what state workers say and do is crucial to understanding the decisions that the state makes and how ideas about HIV are created and disseminated through these people's everyday practices.

The individuals I introduce here often occupy multiple positions: their social and professional roles intersect with other institutional roles. One might be a physician, a state-employed health worker, an academic researcher, and a Communist Party member all rolled into one. In the first two narratives, I explore the larger social and cultural context of the forefront of HIV prevention from the point of view of two people in Beijing and Kunming, Dr. Hui and Dr. Jing. These two physicians have diametrically opposed views of AIDS; as such they point toward the contradictory ways that prevention strategies were conceived on the borders of Yunnan.

1. Dr. Hui and an HIV Hotline

I met Dr. Hui, a tall, wiry man with thick glasses, in Thailand in 1995 at an international AIDS conference. We were both delegates with Save the Children–United Kingdom (hereafter referred to as SCF-UK) based in Kunming. Later in Beijing, Dr.Hui invited me to his office in the north of the city. Dr. Hui had a considerable amount of information, education, and communications (collectively known as IEC) material on HIV prevention, and as of August 1996 he operated the only nationwide AIDS hotline staffed with medically trained volunteers. These volunteers worked a four-hour shift every two weeks from four to eight in the evening Monday through Saturday. The funding for the hotline was directly from the Chinese Ministry of Health, although much of the health education material was initially funded by international donor organizations like the World Health Organization and UNAIDS. Dr. Hui explained that most callers just wanted to know where they could get tested for antibodies to HIV. In Beijing, confidential but not anonymous testing was conducted at the anti-epidemic stations for fifty yuan (about six US dollars) per test. The results were returned one week later. As for treatment, Dr. Hui mentioned that clinical drug trials had just begun at Peking Union Medical Center and that those patients enrolled in the trials were given AZT free of charge. Dr. Hui explained, "There is relatively little outreach and information gathering for this hotline, and we do not receive many calls unless there is a program on television or the radio on AIDS." He also kept reiterating, in reference to ethnic groups and their particular subcultures, that "the Tai in Thailand are wild," meaning they engage in too much sex, and "that is why we have so much AIDS in places like Xishuangbanna."

As I wanted to observe the fine workings of the hotline, I simply asked Dr. Hui if that would be possible. He suggested that since I was the expert, I should be the one to answer hotline calls rather than him. I assumed his invitation had more to do with him not wanting to be observed, or rather criticized, than wanting to assist me in my research. I answered two telephone calls on the hotline. The first call was from a young man who was terrified he had contracted HIV from French kissing (my term not his) a foreign male at a gay nightclub in Guangzhou. The second was from a man who had had unprotected sex with a prostitute while traveling south on vacation. The fear in both their voices was palpable; however, I found the first caller compelling, as being a closeted gay male in China was extremely difficult. At the end of the telephone line I could hear the small mild-mannered voice of a young man slowly speaking Mandarin with a clipped Guangdong accent. He explained his recent encounter at a disco: "A foreign male, an exchange student from the USA, kissed me and he used his *shetou* (tongue) and I got some of his *tuoye* (saliva) in me. He didn't only kiss me but he used his teeth and he bit my tongue, and I am so scared. I am too young to get sick and die. My mother is sick and I am worried about leaving her with an ill son."

At first, I suggested that if he thought he caught an STI, he should see a doctor who could treat him. But as his story unfolded, it became apparent that it was a case of mistaken information, indicative of the fact that there was limited access to information about HIV at the time. He was afraid of getting AIDS from kissing an American student on the floor of a Guangzhou disco. I kept saying there are only three ways to transmit HIV and that exchanging saliva and biting someone's tongue posed little risk of transmission. He reported having had a fever, though it had subsided by the time of his hotline call. I began to understand the problems associated with trying to explain one's fears about contracting HIV without admitting to homoerotic activity to a stranger. He was also concerned about getting tested. Dr. Hui pointed me to the telephone number for the anti-epidemic station in Guangzhou, where anyone could be tested for fifty to one hundred yuan, and I told the caller he would receive the results in one week. Again, the young man reiterated, "We didn't have intercourse, we just kissed."

Dr. Hui explained that the majority of calls are made when the hotline numbers are actually advertised in Beijing, Fujian, Hainan, Zhejiang, and Guangzhou newspapers. All these cities and provinces have individual hotlines and materials provided by Dr. Hui, if they have not already developed their own location-specific materials. "Unlike your country," said Dr. Hui, "in China we cannot promote condoms for certain segments of the population, such as prostitutes, who should abstain from having sex; students, who should abstain; farmers, who would be too embarrassed to even read the information; and, migrants, who are too ignorant to read." He also commented on the immorality of prostitution and how it must be stamped out like it was under Mao in the early 1950s. According to representatives at UNAIDS, plenty of money was available for innovative programs, yet Dr. Hui kept reiterating that to prevent HIV, he needed more money. The early IEC brochures he developed in 1996 were questionable depictions of what he deemed both risky bodies and risky behaviors and provided little education other than abstinence.

Dr. Hui represents one attitude in China that HIV is caused by immoral people, a view that parallels those of many Christian groups in the West. Dr. Hui had developed some of the first IEC material on HIV prevention, but at the same time, he did not include information on condom use for fear of offending people. Rumors also circulated that much of his international funding was from the Reverend Sun Myung Moon. One may view this narrative as that of someone struggling with the notions of a changed China, a China no longer under the hold of Maoism and the kind of moralizing that stigmatized, imprisoned, and killed people for not upholding the moral fervor of the state. Dr. Hui was born into the generation of Chinese that came of age after the revolution, in the 1950s, and many of these ideas reflect some of his generation's enthusiasm for the Mao period.

Although the state's everyday AIDS practices are carried out at the local level—for example, the multiple local AIDS hotlines—they are funded by a variety of international donor agencies such as those that supported Dr. Hui's hotline. As William Fisher (1997) contends, one way to assess the work of NGOs is to fathom what they do rather than simply how they are organized. I would add that knowing what NGOs say and what sorts of discourse they encourage also helps in assessing their work. At the same time that Dr. Hui dedicates his life to alleviate suffering of HIV by reducing the numbers of cases through his health-education hotline, he comes down extremely hard on anyone who already has HIV, especially if he or she is a drug addict, a prostitute, a migrant, or someone with multiple sexual partners. Thus, Dr. Hui's individual good will coincides with his personal moral stance that denigrates "immoral" people. Both of his subject positions influence the political will of the state and remake what HIV prevention means according to the central government in Beijing. Through the hotline, Dr. Hui devised his own folk categories for HIV prevention that incorporated the dangers of promoting condoms. Though a government employee working in a national institute with support from the Ministry of Health, he is of a generation whose personal moral views reflect socialist ideas about putting one's country first and one's private desires second.

2. Dr. Jing and Drug-Use Prevention

I first met Dr. Jing, a young psychiatrist, on my first research trip to Menglian County (in the prefecture due west of Sipsongpanna) in 1995 and then on several subsequent occasions in Kunming. Dr Jing worked on the front lines of HIV prevention through a local research institute and with two NGOs that funded the early HIV-prevention programs in Yunnan, the Australian Red Cross and SCF-UK. She also conducted research on drug use and taught psychiatry in Yunnan. Although my interviews and interactions covered many conversations and topics, I focused on her comments on the rise of STIs and HIV and the challenges of prevention.

As in the rest of the world at the time, the HIV epidemic in Yunnan was first seen as a disease of others—foreigners—and then a disease of the internal Other—minorities. More recently, as I argue, it was framed as a question of geography. Dr. Jing said, "Sexual promiscuity may be more prevalent among the Lahu minority than the Tai. AIDS is also a problem of the floating population [people moving from place to place] and perhaps more of an issue for demographers than for epidemiologists. . . . As for those who link AIDS to the Tai, it has more to do with geography and the tourist trade in Xishuangbanna than with cultural ideas." She added, "While both the Tai and Lahu are more sexually open than, say, the Akha or Wa, and they are culturally more open to sexual variations, that does not mean they are conduits for AIDS."

Since the beginning of the millennium, sexual transmission has become an increasing focus of many organizations, including those working on drug use. Dr. Jing argued that people were using heroin more than ever before, and while she agreed in part with the basic premise of harm reduction, she was not sure if the public security bureaus would agree to hand out free needles. "While they give people methadone for free for a period of three months, it is too expensive to give it out for much longer periods. . . . Getting tested for HIV costs one hundred yuan but can be made free for people without means. This means that those who frequent all these clinics are often those with funds, and those without money must face the humiliation of the public hospital.[5] . . .

Drug rehabilitation is a new concept and it will take time to do anything along the lines of exchanging needles like in the United States and Europe." She further explained the difficulties of trying to institute a program of harm reduction like needle exchanges, noting how this difficulty is exacerbated by the complicated authority structures among work units.

Perhaps one of the biggest challenges is the bureaucracy itself. She said, "The relationship of my work unit [danwei] to the Public Health Bureau is only marginal because the provincial level [ting] is under the Ministry of Health [weishengbu] and the high-security drug center [qiangjiedusuo] is part of another ministry. To complicate matters, my work unit is also organizationally related to the provincial public security bureau [gonganting], the bureau for capturing prostitutes, and the army. For example, if my work unit wanted to plan a needle exchange program, we would need the permission from officials in different ministries—Public Health, Public Security, and the People's Liberation Army."

Dr. Jing identified some of the problems associated with health education programs and condom use: "[The] problem with prostitutes and condoms is that the number of condoms women have on them often measures the legal evidence of prostitution. I have been trying to enlighten hotels in Kunming to distribute condoms to customers through informal networks—for instance, sending agents to the Holiday Inn at eight in the evening when most girls start working. Another avenue is an official network, getting health educators to distribute condoms in hotel rooms themselves, but we must convince the managers of the hotels first before we can educate their customers."

In February 2004, the Yunnan Standing Party Committee passed the broad-ranging HIV Prevention and Control Law that required public places such as hotels, inns, guesthouses, and commercial entertainment establishments to provide condoms free of charge, or at the very least for purchase (Zhang Zizhuo 2004). By March 2005, a law was enacted that forced all persons working in these establishments to be forcibly tested for HIV, and if they tested positive their employment was terminated (Zhou 2005). Policies regarding HIV prevention found their way into law and then were made virtually impossible to implement because they compromised both the health and the livelihood of those working in these entertainment establishments.

According to Dr. Jing, early prevention projects in the border minority region of the Dehong Tai-Jingpo Nationality Autonomous Prefecture, in northwestern Yunnan, meant that in the villages with HIV-prevention projects, there had been few new cases. She said, "The biggest problem is finding appropriate materials that will reach out to the non-school-going population, those who don't read or cannot read either Dehong-Tai or Mandarin.[6] I think peer education programs [tongban jiaoyu] are the wave of the future in AIDS prevention."

She discussed the role of the economy in the spread of HIV and STIs: "In places like Xishuangbanna, with development has come the tourism industry, and with tourism has also come the sex industry. Although there is no clear direct connection between development and the sex industry, my colleagues and I do know that certain select places in Yunnan, for example, Ruili, Xishuangbanna, and Menglian, attract people from the border countries who come for sex. With sex tourism also comes prostitution, and some prostitutes buy drugs to keep on working."

In these narratives, Dr. Jing's position is one of a modern scientist; she embraces the latest international drug-prevention techniques of harm reduction rather than incarceration and forced detoxification—the methods currently operative in most of China. Her ideas and interests clearly contrast with those of Dr. Hui; in fact, one could say they are diametrically opposed. Her suggestions for prevention are also on the cutting edge of what was imaginable in Kunming in the late 1990s; her idea to promote condom use in commercial sex followed often widely circulated international discourses, particularly Thailand, with its 100 percent safer-sex condom-use policy in all commercial sex establishments. In fact, Dr. Jing asked me to find her more materials on harm reduction and, while cautious about the identifications of the seven counties in Yunnan with high rates of AIDS, and their location in minority prefectures, she also believed that minority women had a certain predilection to sexual habits that were unlike those of Han women. Dr. Jing belongs to a generation that came of age well after the revolution, and was a small child during the Cultural Revolution. She embraced modernity and science as the hallmarks of international medical development and economic advancement.

In her wonderful description of the difficulties of implementing harm reduction in Yunnan, we see precisely the intricate web of government bureaucracy that makes new ideas and new methods extremely difficult to initiate. Dr. Jing's political position as both a physician and an employee of a state work unit meant she channeled certain contradictory positions in her own mind. Culturally, she thought minority women were more prone to promiscuity; at the same time, she questioned the value of the state's dominant position on minorities and HIV, a view of minority women stemming from preconceived ideas about Tai culture and history. Contemporary Tai culture, according to the Tai themselves, allows for more open alliances between unmarried men and women and for more fluidly defined sexual and gender roles. On the other hand, when translating or interpreting long-held cultural practices by simply mapping them onto current disease categories, we get the distinction that the Tai are prone to HIV because of their cultural beliefs about sexuality and gender.[7]

Although Dr. Jing had a prominent position in the provincial health department and in her research institute, she was somewhat removed from the front line of the epidemic. The agencies involved in on-the-ground decisions about HIV were the anti-epidemic stations (now mini Centers for Disease Control) and the public security bureaus. Each prefecture, county, and city in China is affiliated with a designated anti-epidemic station and public security bureau; these two government offices fulfill the dual purpose of public health: to survey and control bodies through disease prevention and to maintain order and security. In my third and fourth narratives, I explain the second set of prevention processes that evolve around questions of securing the border.

THE FRONTLINE OF DEFENSE: THE ANTI-EPIDEMIC STATION

In the final two narratives, I explore how AIDS was perceived and regulated from within the minority border prefectures themselves. Through their own everyday AIDS practices, we see how government officials, or rather employees of the state, treated minority infections, how they chose to represent themselves versus the Han majority's risk for HIV, and how in turn their own subject positions then marked and actually influenced state policy at the local level. Just how were these border regions, in particular Sipsongpanna Prefecture and Menglian Prefecture, perceived and then targeted in early surveys and later health interventions? In the final two narratives, I introduce the health department structure at the provincial level, because without having a clear understanding of the bureaucracy, the two agencies I discuss, the Menglian Anti-Epidemic Station and the Jinghong Public Security Bureau, appear to be completely disparate institutions when in fact they are linked in the prevention of HIV.

In 1995 the AIDS office of the Yunnan Provincial Department of Health established twelve departments within the provincial anti-epidemic station in Kunming. In 1995 early HIV policy and prevention involved directives discouraging behaviors, namely drug use and multiple sexual partners. The mention of condoms for prevention was considered too sensitive a topic. Dr. Yao, a preventative-medicine specialist, said that difficulties surrounding the use of condoms for HIV prevention reflected the Chinese saying, "One knows what something is but does not understand its purpose." In other words, people can identify that HIV exists but not how it is transmitted or the infectious nature of the disease. Furthermore, the impact of market-oriented policies on health prevention has meant that these local-level health stations must move toward financial independence by generating income rather than relying on the state for full subsidies. Thus, in practice there was no way to assist behavioral change because the local anti-epidemic stations did not have the money or the personnel to carry out their tasks. Dr. Yao further stated, "The other major problem in dealing with AIDS is the paralysis or a constraint placed on structural response by the stations themselves. The idea of building anti-epidemic stations at the local level was a health tactic inherited from the Russians [in the 1950s]. The problem now is that since 1992 we are losing control of the epidemic because individual units under economic reforms are being made financially accountable. They must make money."

For local anti-epidemic stations, the only recourse is to increase activities that generate income: selling vaccines, tests for HIV, and hygiene exams for employees in the food industry. Several informants reported, using the local vernacular, that the anti-epidemic stations "kick their problems to another court" or "merely put out fires"; they have little time and few resources to devote to prevention. In many communities the anti-epidemic stations are simply testing agencies that have been stripped of their capacities as public health educators. They barely keep their heads above water in terms of surviving economically, let alone meeting policy and prevention objectives of the Beijing-based Ministry of Health.

Some anti-epidemic stations, such as the one in Menglian, have some money for testing certain high-risk populations; but their main work is limited to providing health education classes or nurse aides to people who are dying. In a tourist region like Sipsongpanna, these agencies consider it extremely important to maintain an image of a healthy local community. For example, the HIV prevention messages in Jinghong are found only in the back alleys and not on the main streets. Friends I have asked about this reply, "We don't want tourists to disappear." The notion of barbarians and barbarian diseases is revealed not only in historical accounts of northerners' conceptions of southerners' diseases, but also in the everyday speech of northern tourists traveling to Sipsongpanna (Yin 1986). Many Han Chinese tourists speak of their fears of diseases, especially malaria, and would never travel to minority villages on their own, outside of an organized tour. Han tourists were not the only people caught by these fears. Han physicians, originally from the provincial capital, who were working in these autonomous regions reflected on cultural beliefs about the wild and hot climate of the southwest contributing to the spread of HIV. In my final two narratives, I reveal how nonphysicians find themselves in contradictory positions vis-à-vis the institutions they work for and how this in turn reflects their own sense of political subjectivity.

3. Chen and the Menglian Anti-Epidemic Station

Throughout the early 1990s the Yunnan Provincial anti-epidemic stations were criticized for not moving fast enough in developing local HIV-prevention policies. While the criticisms came from those in the Ministry of Health in Beijing, the stations' paralysis can be traced to a reliance on existing channels of expertise. What follows is a discussion of two people who worked on the HIV periphery in a frontline center for prevention; they both regarded the epidemic as an insurmountable problem leading to disorder and thus, they believed, it would become a problem for the border police to solve.

In December 1995, while in Menglian as an adjunct member of the Australian-Yunnan Red Cross survey team, I met Chen, a health worker at what was then known as the Menglian Lahu-Dai-Wa Nationality Autonomous County's Anti-Epidemic Station. During the survey training, she pulled me aside to explain that she had recently been criticized for permitting a Beijing-based television production team to video-tape people with HIV in Menglian. The critique was based not so much on the validity of the coverage as on the notion that Menglian as a result would be marked as a diseased site. Chen noted that many people wanted to believe that AIDS comes from somewhere else. She was extremely diligent and eager in collecting survey information; Chen was up early and motivated the entire survey team to work well into the night. Her participation on the survey soon brought Chen recognition, as she was shortly promoted to a position in the county seat.

Chen and Menglian County's public security officials were most concerned by the recent number of women (about twenty) who were crossing the Burmese border and then moving into northern Thailand to work in the "entertainment industry"—a euphemism for prostitution. The number of HIV cases had apparently risen in Menglian County, and these twenty index cases were seen as a sign of rising rates of migration linked to increasing rates of HIV in Thailand (at the time, Thailand had the highest prevalence in Asia). When I asked what efforts were being made to prevent future infection, it was clear that, apart from Chen's visits to the villages, no systematic prevention information was being given to anybody, least of all to women returning from Thailand.

In Menglian, Chen reported that she knew several women who had worked in Thailand, and she had tried to contact all of them on their return. She was also eager to work on the repatriation of young female prostitutes from Thailand to China. However, one week later, Chen confessed in secret that while she tried to encourage young women to get tested rather than call on the police to arrest them, if they balk, "I bring in the police because these women must get tested to protect their families."[8]

Thus, although Chen was sympathetic to the women and men with HIV in her county, she was concerned about transmission to the degree that she would instruct the police to force women to get tested. She was part of the generation of youth sent down to rural areas such as Menglian during the Cultural Revolution. She saw her political duty arising out of that former Maoist medical regime, which promoted prevention of major epidemics by controlling the individual in the name of the collective. Here a government health worker was, on the one hand, preventing HIV by protecting the individual and, on the other, protecting the community by turning over individuals to the police—actions reflecting the contradictory nature of early practices of prevention in Yunnan.

The contradictions between Chen's ideological position and her sanctioned prevention policies reveal the uneasiness and inconsistency of the HIV discourse in China. Much of the rhetoric about HIV in Yunnan surrounds the protection of the family unit and Chen was merely acknowledging this in her campaign. An early HIV-prevention poster in Yunnan bore the image of a happy family—mother, father, and son—and declared that the happy family knows how to prevent HIV. However, Chen did not just bow to the policy makers in Simao, the county seat; they criticized her invitation to the Beijing film team. Chen's own actions point to the contradictions not only in local HIV policy, but also in how these policies are actually mediated through political subjects who live and work in minority prefectures like Menglian. Chen's own subject position reveals her as an official who felt deeply about people suffering from HIV and who at the same maintained central party-state political convictions that HIV must be controlled at all costs.

4. Lao Yan and the Security Drug Center

My fourth and final narrative is about a policeman who works for the Public Security Bureau in Jinghong. Because HIV was initially associated with drug addicts and trafficking, the public security bureaus mobilized resources to capture and incarcerate HIV-infected individuals. Due to the remarkable efforts of Dr. Samid, SCF-UK's first AIDS advisor, things began to change. Dr. Samid pointed out that since HIV was considered a negative, often polluting disease, one associated with a threat to security due to its appearance in China's most southwestern border, gaining permission to initiate prevention programs required rather difficult political and diplomatic maneuvers. Getting permissions from both the provincial and local Jinghong public security bureaus involved a circuitous route through the military, the military hospital in Jinghong, and finally a drug prison that would become the site of an SCF-UK HIV-intervention program on drug rehabilitation.

In the mid-1990s, most drug addicts were left alone, caught by the police and sent to prison or taken care of by their families; there were no rehabilitation centers. Today, due to careful diplomacy and hard work among several sectors, new options for drug treatment are emerging in Yunnan. One organization, Daytop, modeled on a well-established therapeutic community in upstate New York, began as a harm-reduction project of the Yunnan Institute of Drug Abuse. Chinese drug abuse specialists advocating harm-reduction programs still face uphill battles, but belief in modern science, perseverance, and NGO funding have opened the door to new ways of conceiving drug use as a disease requiring care, rather than a crime requiring incarceration.[9] Previously, SCF-UK became involved because the postreform government reduced state subsidies to the health sector. Thus the state's role in disease prevention, including HIV, was augmented and in many instances taken over by international health NGOs in China. One may argue that transnational NGOs and their development agents prop up the state by injecting their own agendas into China, providing seed money for prevention projects; however, through the power of their organizations they redefine the terrain of everyday AIDS practices (see Pandolfi 2003 and this volume). These seemingly foreign NGOs are not entirely independent of the state bureaucracy; they are hybrid organizations, in part state managed and politically aligned with provincial governments. In fact, in order to register as an NGO, an organization has to have a government counterpart. SCF-UK had the army.

The city of Jinghong sits on the banks of the Lancang River. If one drove across the old bridge over the river, past the army hospital into the hills, past rubber plantations and rock quarries, and up long winding dirt roads peppered with potholes filled with muddy water, one arrived at the high-security drug prison. Vines covered the high red-brick walls, an old Beijing jeep lay in a heap by the side of the road, mangy mongrel dogs barked, and a few inmates and guards squatted in the noonday sun, smoking tobacco from long water pipes. It was here that I first met Lao Yan, a member of the local Tai minority and one of the guards, in his thirties. He welcomed me by showing off his small zoo of bamboo rats (he promised they tasted great), fruit trees, chickens, and dogs. The red-brick buildings at the prison, all in states of disrepair, were organized according to various levels of security: the prison cells where inmates were assigned when they first arrived; the medium-security rooms where inmates shared bunk beds and a courtyard; and finally the unlocked rooms above the prison cells, in which, as a result of the SCF-UK project, female inmates were in rehabilitation.

The high-security section of the prison had four enclosed cells, each surrounded by cyclone-type fencing on all four sides about two stories high. Each cell consisted of a small outer courtyard with an opening large enough to let in the tropical sunlight, and a small room with bunk beds and a window covered by iron grating. Each cell had a water spigot with a small concrete tub in the courtyard and a few stools. About eight inmates lounged around smoking cigarettes while others chopped wood. Xiao Tan, a nineteen-year-old woman, told me, "We are all *yangui* [cigarette addicts]."[10] Above the old prison cells were the newly built rooms funded by SCF-UK. The new low-security wing housed nine young women, including one who had only two days left in her imprisonment. All nine young women appeared to have spent time in the lower section, the enclosed two-story-high cyclone-fence-like cages. Apparently, the previous week three young women had set fire to their wooden bed platforms and burned holes in the mosquito screens, an act the guards regarded as arson. As punishment they were sent back to the high-security cages.

Lao Yan euphemistically said the divisions in types of security among the inmates had to do with their levels of education and their previous occupations. He said that those with more education were easier to control and less likely to become aggressive. Dr. Samid, the SCF-UK HIV advisor, pointed out that where addicts get assigned was based on prejudice and class background. Those of higher social status, despite being addicts, tended to spend less time in the high-security cages, while an old man in his sixties, a former opium smoker, would because of his age and social status never leave the high-security section. According to Lao Yan, 60 percent of the young women addicts had worked as prostitutes to obtain enough money to buy drugs, while the others acquired drugs from friends. He said, "If one works as a successful tour guide, one can fund a habit on one's commissions." Lao Yan reported that most of the inmates ended up back at the center, as recidivism rates were high. Most of the drugs came from Burma near Dehong, not the closer routes through Laos and Thailand. All three of the female inmates I interviewed insisted they used clean needles. Xiao Tan said, "Clean needles are cheap [one yuan each], and are easy to purchase over the counter at local pharmacies, so we wouldn't think of using other peoples' needles; they are so dirty."[11] She continued, "I know about AIDS and am worried about getting it."

On my visits to the center, the guards complained there was never enough money to make repairs, let alone to do HIV testing and counseling with their injection-drug-using charges. Money was so scarce that the resident nurse hadn't received her monthly three hundred yuan salary for two months. Lao Yan said, "We really try to economize. In fact, even Premier Li Peng encouraged us not to buy expensive foreign cars but local jeeps." Later, on reflection, I noted that it was the premier who donated one hundred thousand yuan (over twelve thousand dollars) to build a new brass and gold-glittered gate, a facsimile of a Tai Buddhist temple gate, to mark the entrance to Jinghong's new tourist district, when the only minority technical training school in town had had to close its doors for lack of funds. Lao Yan recounted how the provincial security bureau sent thirty-five middle-level police officers to northern Thailand to review highland tribal police efforts in Thailand's minority tourist belt. The business trip was followed by a trip to Phuket for rest and relaxation, and Lao Yan boasted that the trip cost hundreds of thousands of yuan. Lao Yan's boasting may be related to his coming-of-age years during the Cultural Revolution, which were marked by the scarcity of material goods.

Lao Yan said that in the most recent strike-hard anticrime campaign (*yanda yundong*), which focused on pornography, prostitution, and other illegal businesses, the police had picked up 120 drug addicts in one night. And where were they to put all these people? With the previous *yanda yundong*, the police arrested a total of two thousand drug addicts. Although users are fined six hundred yuan per person (about two months' salary), they are also often held for one night before they are released. The police now concentrate on drugs and the gambling salons and are temporarily ignoring prostitution unless it involves drugs. Lao Yan said, "The police efforts to deal with prostitution amount to literally driving women back to Simao, but we aren't very successful because they come back here a week later. Why would many of the prostitutes who come from Guizhou, Sichuan, and as far away as Guangdong, want to stay in Simao?" He said, "The worst drug addicts work as prostitutes because they need this business to feed their habits." Then he added, "As a border region we have more pressing problems than prostitution and AIDS. Another example is the recent black market in illegal, unregistered cars." Lao Yan explained that smugglers drive cars from Burma to Jinghong to avoid the Chinese government's stiff import taxes, and then they sell these same cars for exorbitant profits on the Chinese side of the border.

Lao Yan revealed his personal views about prostitutes and drug addicts and, through his views, the problems of the Chinese state. There was little money for prevention but then lots of money for tourism; plenty of money for expensive cars, but not for nurses' salaries. Lao Yan showed a mixture of emotions when it came to drugs and HIV prevention, emotions that filtered into everyday practices in his state police job. In not receiving enough money or resources to do his job, he felt maligned by Beijing. He also felt entitled to expensive trips to Thailand for police training.

BORDERLAND DISORDERS AND POLITICAL SUBJECTIVITY

These four narratives—Dr. Hui, Dr. Jing, Chen, and Lao Yan—show that as representatives of the state in Beijing, Kunming, Menglian and Jinghong, and as government health workers, these people are often placed in contradictory positions, positions that reveal multiple political subjectivities. For example, as officials they alternate between personal gain (trips to Phuket, Thailand) and duty to police bodies (forced HIV testing on women who cross the border). As individuals they balance practices that define HIV as a fundamental personal and confidential issue (Chen refusing to disclose the HIV status of women attending our first HIV training) against practices that treat HIV as a border disease requiring forced police intervention (high-security prisons and forced HIV tests for prostitutes). Furthermore, when physicians like Dr. Jing try to map cultural prejudices onto risk variables, the results may reflect their own prejudices more than anything else (see Patton 2002). In addition, these state actors are operating within different historical memories, and thus different generations. Those who are younger were more open to and perhaps better trained for taking into consideration international norms and literatures concerning harm reduction, versus those of an older generation trained under Mao who were more apt to restrict persons with HIV.

In the case of AIDS, the state reacts to the exercise of individual power by trying to craft new sets of boundaries and borders. When geography and politics are wedded in this way, HIV ceases to be a disease without borders and becomes a disease with distinct borders, as if it only seeps through at certain points on a map (see Fischer this volume). Chinese historians argue that even on the eve of liberation in 1953, the Sipsongpanna borderlands were perceived as wastelands of malaria and leprosy-infested jungles full of barbarians (Yin 1986; Wang 1993).[12] These notions of barbarians and barbaric diseases live on in the perceptions of Kunming physicians like Dr. Jing, Menglian health workers like Chen, and Jinghong policemen like Lao Yan. Dr. Hui is concerned with the maintenance of a parochial morality and seeks to control high-risk behaviors between commercial "sex workers" and intravenous drug users. His ways are problematic in the eyes of public health physicians like Dr. Jing. Even Dr. Jing, who is knowledgeable about harm-reduction techniques, maintains that ethnic minorities are more promiscuous than Han women such as herself.

My ethnography of everyday AIDS practices illuminates the internal contradictions of the Chinese state and exposes the differing interests of its bureaucratic actors, who are often devoted to competing goals and feelings. If we understand the state as acting locally (in Menglian), nationally (in Beijing), and internationally (through NGOs), we recognize that HIV policy and action does represent a uniform narrative. HIV policies are often both local and transnational, negotiated by actors who engage in relationships that span the local and the transnational, from the border to the center and back. Chen worked in Menglian in rural Yunnan and catered to Beijing reporters at the heart of party power, to her Simao superiors in more central Yunnan, and to the Australian Red Cross, her international counterpart. Not only do straightforward distinctions between pure civil society and the state become blurred, but so do the distinctions between where power resides and where power resists. Borders and centers constantly highlight the processual and multidimensional characteristics of the Chinese state and reveal how identities are remade as the notion of the borders shifts in and out of prevention projects. NGOs collaborate with state bureaucracies in order to carry out HIV behavioral surveys and prevention in the borderlands, and in turn the state greases the wheels for NGOs to spread international HIV discourses in a postsocialist state, one that not long ago closed off possibilities for international exchange. State and society are integrated at the level of individual everyday AIDS practices, where modes of action are discursively constructed across time, space, and borders. Here, risky bodies and risky practices cast shadows on geography and epidemiology. The habitus of state actors inscribes their political subjectivity, and through their everyday AIDS practices they in turn inscribe the sovereignty of the state onto minority subjects. Political subjectivity for state government bureaucrats means they must balance emotions, personal histories, and moral and political convictions with the goals of the state. In the end, economies of prevention involve more than just biological power over everyday lives; they involve intimate feelings and political and moral ideals that influence government discourses through individuals working on the disorders of late-socialism.

NOTES

My fieldwork between 1996 and 2000 was generously funded by Fulbright-Hays, the Wenner-Gren Foundation, and UC San Francisco's Center for AIDS Prevention Studies. I also received two Foreign Language Area Studies grants, a Regent's Fellowship, and a Lowie Grant from UC Berkeley. An NIMH postdoctoral fellowship at Harvard Medical School made it possible for me to prepare this manuscript. My greatest thanks goes to Mary-Jo DelVecchio Good and Byron Good for their efforts to make sense of my prose and push my ideas forward into a final cohesive essay. I also thank Corina Salis-Gros, Chris Walley, Matthew Kohrman, Sarah Pinto, Angela Davis, June Brady, Nicole Couture, Sarah Friedman, Ann Marie Leshkowich, and Tuulikki Pietila, for their valuable suggestions and critiques on previous drafts. And finally, this chapter, in a somewhat different form, appeared as chapter 2 in my book *Eating Spring Rice: The Cultural Politics of AIDS in Southwest China* (University of California Press, 2007).

1. I follow the UNAIDS May 2006 recommendations on terminology. I use the term "HIV" rather than "HIV/AIDS" (unless specifically referring to AIDS or quoting someone). The acquired immune deficiency syndrome (AIDS) is a disease of the body's immune system caused by the human immunodeficiency virus (HIV). It is

classified as a disease that destroys the body's CD4 cells, an important part of our immune systems, and thus with lower CD4 cell counts the body becomes subject to multiple life-threatening infections and cancers.

2. I use the term "everyday AIDS practices" for two reasons. First, to bring practice theory into an analysis of an epidemic, and this term captures a whole array of practices, thoughts, policies, words, and actions engaged in the process of HIV prevention. Second, to bridge the variety and range of human endeavors that are involved in the social practices and discourses associated with documenting and preventing the evolution of an epidemic. This Foucauldian notion of discursive practice allows me to move away from time-based and spatial analyses of a neat chronology of HIV. I am more interested in what Liu Xin (2000: 24) calls the uncertainty in practice and how practices transform themselves in the very moment when they are actualized.

3. There is a large literature on civil society and the state in China. Due to the length of this chapter, I do not mention them all. China scholars in recent years have debated the power of the socialist state to embrace the emergence of civil society and the degree to which this has succeeded since the post-1979 reforms (Siu 1989; Wasserstrom and Perry 1992; Yang 1994; Jing 1996; Anagnost 1997; Madsen 1998; Lee 1998; Litzinger 2000; Zhang Li 2001; Tsai 2002; Remick 2004).

4. The term "Tai" refers to all peoples speaking the Tai language versus "Thai," which refers to the majority of Tai-speaking peoples in Thailand. In 1951 the Chinese government created the term "Dai" to rename the Tai-speaking ethnic groups inside the People's Republic. "Dai" is often associated with the colonial takeover by the Communist Chinese, and thus the use of the original linguistic term "Tai." The Mandarin term "Dai" in Sipsongpanna Tai sounds like the word "death" and, as scholar Sara Davis (2005) notes, the Tai are not dead yet.

5. A couple of informants mentioned that the recent increases in syphilis in Kunming resulted in the anti-epidemic station holding people with secondary and tertiary syphilis against their will until they completed treatment.

6. The written and spoken Tai language in Sipsongpanna and Dehong is mutually unintelligible, as the two groups, while often linked by Han Chinese, are ethno-linguistically distinct. Taiwanese scholar Hsieh Shih-Chung (1995: 310) argues that the Tai-speaking people in Dehong Dai-Jingpo Nationality Autonomous Prefecture are Chinese Shan because of cultural and linguistic similarities to the Shan people in northern Burma.

7. There has been much made of these distinctions between Han and non-Han in the Yunnan School of Painting. The school often depicts minority women, particularly Tai women, as sexualized nudes (see Lufkin 1990; Gladney 1994; Schein 1997).

8. According to the National People's Congress, in 1989 and 1990 a total of 65,236 people countrywide were arrested for trafficking in women and children (Kristof and Wudunn 1994). According to the Committee for the Protection of Children's Rights and the International Organization for Migration (IOM), both based in

Bangkok, every month there are dozens of women who cross the borders to work in Thai brothels (Feingold 1998).

9. As of 2006, I am working on new research that focuses on the medicalization of drug-use treatment in border communities in Yunnan with funding from the Canadian Social Sciences and Humanities Research Council (SSHRC) and Quebec's Fonds Québécois de la Recherche sur la Société et la Culture (FQRSC).

10. I thank Jay Dautcher for pointing out that *gui* (ghost) is a long-standing metaphor for addiction and a term of dehumanization. Europeans in Chinese history were often referred to as ghosts due to their white skin. Ghosts were people who had died but were not successfully transformed into rightful ancestors by funeral rites; they plagued the living.

11. Outside of the large urban centers, clean needles are not always used in health care facilities despite the Ministry of Health directives.

12. In conversations with local physicians, they often reiterated that diseases such as cerebral malaria and tuberculosis are making a comeback in part due to the lack of medical care in rural areas.

REFERENCES

Anagnost, Ann. 1997. *National Past-Time: Narrative, Representation and Power in Modern China*. Durham, NC: Duke University Press.

Anzaldúa, Gloria. 1987. *Borderlands/La Frontera:The New Mestiza*. San Francisco: Aunt Lute Books.

Appadurai, Arjun. 1996. *Modernity at Large: Cultural Dimensions of Globalization*. Public Words, vol. 1. Minneapolis: University of Minnesota Press.

Arnold, David. 1993. *Colonizing the Body: State Medicine and Epidemic Disease in Nineteenth-Century India*. Berkeley: University of California Press.

Berdahl, Daphne. 1999. *Where the World Ended: Reunification and Identity in the German Borderlands*. Berkeley: University of California Press.

Beyrer, Chris. 1998. *The War in the Blood: Sex, Politics and HIV in Southeast Asia*. London and New York: Zed Books.

Beyrer, Chris, M. H. Razak, K. Lisam, J. Chen et al. 2000. Overland Heroin Trafficking Routes in HIV-I Spread in South and Southeast Asia. *AIDS* 14 (1): 75–83.

Borchert, Thomas. 2005. Of Temples and Tourists: The Effects of Tourist Political Economy on a Minority Buddhist Community in Southwest China. Paper presented at Association for Asian Studies, Chicago, March 21–23.

Bourdieu, Pierre. 1977. *Outline of a Theory of Practice*. Trans. R. Nice. Cambridge: Cambridge University Press.

———. 1990. *The Logic of Practice*. Trans. R. Nice. Stanford, CA: Stanford University Press.

Chen, Nancy. 2003. *Breathing Spaces: Qigong, Psychiatry and Healing in China*. New York: Columbia University Press.

Davis, Sara L. M. 2005. *Song and Silence: Ethnic Revival on China's Southwest Borders*. New York: Columbia University Press.

Feingold, David. 1998. Sex, Drugs and the IMF: Some Implications of Structural Readjustment for the Trade in Heroin, Girls and Women in the Upper Mekong Region. Special issue, *Refuge, Cargo: The Global Traffic in Women and Children*.

Fisher, William. 1997. Doing Good? The Politics and Antipolitics of NGO Practices. *Annual Review of Anthropology* 26:439–64.

Foucault, Michel. 1977. *Discipline and Punish: The Birth of the Prison*. Trans. Alan Sheridan. New York: Vintage Books.

———. 1991. Governmentality. In *The Foucault Effect: Studies in Governmental Rationality*, ed. Graham Burcell, Colin Gordon, and Peter Miller, 87–104. Chicago: University of Chicago Press.

Gilman, Sander L. 1988. *Disease and Representation: Images of Illness from Madness to AIDS*. Ithaca, NY: Cornell University Press.

Gladney, Dru C. 1994. Representing Nationality in China: Refiguring Majority/Minority Identities. *Journal of Asian Studies* 53 (11): 92–123.

———. 2002. Internal Colonialism and the Uyghur Nationality: Chinese Nationalism and Its Subaltern Subjects. In "La Question de l'enchantement en Asie Centrale," *CEMOTI (Cahiers d'études sur la Méditerranée Orientale et le Monde Turco-Iranien)* 35.

Gregory, Steven. 2003. Men in Paradise: Sex Tourism and the Political Economy of Masculinity. In *Race, Nature and the Politics of Difference*, ed. Donald Moore, Jake Kosek, and Anand Padian. Durham, NC: Duke University Press.

Gupta, Akhil, and James Ferguson. 1992. Beyond "Culture": Space, Identity, and the Politics of Difference. *Cultural Anthropology* 7 (1): 6–23.

Hsieh Shih-Chung. 1995. On the Dynamics of Tai/Dai-Lüe Ethnicity: An Ethnohistorical Analysis. In *Cultural Encounters on China's Ethnic Frontiers*, ed. Stevan Harrell, 301–28. Seattle: University of Washington Press.

Hyde, Sandra Teresa. 2001. Sex Tourism Practices on the Periphery: Eroticizing Ethnicity and Pathologizing Sex on the Lancang. In *China Urban: Ethnographies of Contemporary Culture*, ed. Nancy N. Chen , Constance D. Clark, Suzanne Z. Gottschang, and Lyn Jeffery, 143–64. Durham, NC: Duke University Press.

———. 2002. The Cultural Politics of HIV and the Chinese State in Late-Twentieth Century Yunnan. *Tsantsa* (The Review of the Swiss Society of Ethnology) 7: 56–64.

———. 2003. When Riding a Tiger it is Difficult to Dismount: STIs and HIV in Contemporary China. *Yale Journal of Chinese Health* 2 (Autumn):72–82.

————. 2007. *Eating Spring Rice: The Cultural Politics of AIDS in Southwest China*. Berkeley: University of California Press.

Jeffrey, Leslie Ann. 2002. *Sex and Borders: Gender, National Identity, and Prostitution Policy in Thailand*. Vancouver: University of British Columbia Press.

Jing Jun. 1996. *The Temple of My Memories: History, Power, and Morality in a Chinese Village*. Stanford, CA: Stanford University Press.

Kaufman, Joan. 2005. China and AIDS: Epidemic Update and Public Policy Responses. Paper presented at the Rising Peril of HIV/AIDS in China: Sex Workers, Human Rights and the Challenges Facing Public Policy, Luce Lecture Series, Skidmore College, New York, March 24.

Kristof, Nicolas, and Wudunn Sheryl. 1994. *China Wakes—The Struggle for the Soul of a Rising Power*. New York: Times Books.

Lee, Ching Kwan. 1998. *Gender and the South China Miracle: Two Worlds of Factory Women*. Berkeley: University of California Press.

Lee, Stella. 2003. Border Bolsters to Counter Rise in Illegal Sex Workers. *South China Morning Post*, January 25, 4.

Litzinger, Ralph. 2000. *Other Chinas: The Yao and the Politics of National Belonging*. Durham, NC: Duke University Press.

Liu Baoying. 2000. Li Lanqing zai quowuyuan zhaokai de fangzhi aizibing xingbing yantaohui shang qiangdiao geji zhengfu he lingdao yao gaodu zhongshi aizibing fangzhi yu kongzhi gongzuo [At the convening of a meeting of the State Council on the Prevention and Cure of STIs and AIDS, Li Lanqing, urged every level of government and their leaders to attach great importance to working for the prevention and eradication of AIDS]. *Renmin Ribao* [People's Daily] 4 (5).

Liu Xin. 2000. *In One's Own Shadow: An Ethnographic Account of the Condition of Post-Reform Rural China*. Berkeley: University of California Press.

Lufkin, Felicity. 1990. Images of Minorities in the Art of People's Republic of China. MA thesis, University of California, Berkeley.

Lyttleton, Chris, and Amorntip Amarapibal. 2002. Sister Cities and Easy Passage: HIV, Mobility and Economies of Desire in a Thai/Lao Border Zone. *Social Science and Medicine* 54:505–18.

Madsen, Richard. 1998. *China's Catholics: Tragedy and Hope in an Emerging Civil Society*. Berkeley: University of California Press.

Ministry of Health, Joint UN Programme on HIV/AIDS, and World Health Organization. 2006. *2005 Update on the HIV/AIDS Epidemic and Response in China*. Beijing: National Center for AIDS/STD Prevention and Control.

Mueggler, Erik. 2001. *The Age of Wild Ghosts: Memory, Violence, and Place in Southwest China*. Los Angeles, Berkeley: University of California Press.

Pandolfi, Mariella. 2003. Contract of Mutual (In)Difference: Governance and Humanitarian Apparatus in Albania and Kosovo. *Indiana Journal of Global Legal Studies* 10 (1): 369–81.

Patton, Cindy. 2002. *Globalizing AIDS*. Minneapolis: University of Minnesota Press.

Porter, Doug. 1997. A Plague on the Borders: HIV, Development, and Traveling Identities in the Golden Triangle. In *Sites of Desire, Economies of Pleasure: Sexualities in Asia and the Pacific*, ed. L. Manderson and M. Jolly, 212–32. Chicago: University of Chicago Press.

Remick, Elizabeth Justine. 2004. *Building Local States: China the Republican and Post-Mao Eras*. Cambridge, MA: Harvard University Press.

Schein, Louisa. 1997 Gender and Internal Colonialism in China. *Modern China* 23 (1): 69–78.

Sethakul, Ratanaporn. 2000. Community Rights of the Lüü in China, Laos and Thailand. In "Community Right in Thailand and Southeast Asia," special issue, *Tai Culture: International Review of Tai Cultural Studies* 5 (2): 69–103.

Settle, Edward. 2003. *AIDS in China: An Annotated Chronology, 1985–2003*. Monterey, CA: China AIDS Survey.

Shen Jie. 2004. Presentation at the Third Annual Asia Public Policy Workshop, Kennedy School of Government, Harvard University, May 6–9.

Shue, Vivienne. 1988. *The Reach of the State: Sketches of the Chinese Body Politic*. Stanford, CA: Stanford University Press.

Siu, Helen. 1989. *Agents and Victims in South China: Accomplices in Rural Revolution*. New Haven, CT: Yale University Press.

Tsai, Kellee. 2002. *Back-Alley Banking: Private Entrepreneurs in China*. Ithaca, NY: Cornell University Press.

UNAIDS. 2002. *HIV/AIDS: China's Titanic Peril—2001 Update on the HIV/AIDS Situation and Needs Assessment Report*. Beijing: UN Theme Group on HIV/AIDS in China.

Van Gennup, Arnold. 1960. *The Rites of Passage*. Trans. Monika B. Vizedom and Gabrielle L. Caffee. Chicago: University of Chicago Press.

Wang Lianfang. 1993. *Yunnan minzu gongzuo huiyi lu, Yunnan wenshi ziliao xuanze, di sishiwu zhang* [A Memoir and Record of Work among Yunnan's minorities]. Yunnan Cultural History Data Collections, vol. 45. Kunming: Yunnan Renmin Chubanshe.

Wasserstrom, Jeffrey, and Elizabeth Perry. 1992. *Popular Protest and Political Culture in China*. Boulder, CO: Westview Press.

Winichakul, Thongchai. 1994. *Mapping Siam: A History of the Geo-Body of a Nation*. Honolulu: University of Hawaii Press.

Xia Guomei. 2004. *HIV/AIDS in China*. Beijing: Foreign Languages Press.

Yan Yunxiang. 1996. *The Flow of Gifts: Reciprocity and Social Networks in a Chinese Village.* Stanford, CA: Stanford University Press.

Yang, Mayfair Meigui. 1994. *Gifts, Favors and Banquets: The Art of Social Relationships in China.* Ithaca, NY: Cornell University Press.

Yin Shaoting. 1986. Shuo zhang [Speaking of miasma]. *Yunnan difang zhi tongxun* [The Communication Annals of Places in Yunnan] 4:69–74.

Zhang Konglai. 2001. Trends in Sexually Transmitted Diseases and HIV. Paper presented at Health Care East and West: Moving into the 21st Century, MIT, Boston, MA, June 24–29.

Zhang Li. 2001. *Strangers in the City: Reconfirmations of Space, Power, and Social Networks Within China's Floating Population.* Stanford, CA: Stanford University Press.

Zhang Xiaobo et al. 2002. Yunnan sheng 2001 nian HIV/AIDS jiance jieguo fenxi [Analysis of the Surveillance Results of HIV/AIDS in Yunnan in 2001]. *Jibing jiance* [Disease Surveillance] 17 (9): 327–31.

Zhang Zizhuo. 2004. Yunnan AIDS Prevention and Control Law to Take Effect in March. *Yunnan Daily,* February 5. China AIDS Info, www.china-aids.org/english/News/News327.

Zheng Xiwan. 1991. A Preliminary Study on the Behavior of 225 Drug Abusers and the Risk Factors of HIV Infection in Ruili County, Yunnan Province. *Chinese Medical Journal* 12 (1): 12–14.

———. 1993. Cohort Study of HIV Infection among Drug Users in Ruili City and Longchuan County, Yunnan Province, China. *Chinese Journal of Epidemiology* 14 (1): 3–5.

———. 1995. HIV Epidemic in China. *The World Bank HIV in Asia Newsletter: Focus on China,* no. 6.

Zhou Yan. 2005. China Exclusive: Anti-AIDS Campaign Spotlights Sex Workers. Xinhua News Wire, May 4. China AIDS Info, www.china-aids.org/english/news/news416.htm.

OF MAIDS AND PROSTITUTES

Indonesian Female Migrants in the New Asian Hinterlands

Johan Lindquist

Do an Internet search using the keywords "maids" and "Singapore" and a number of employment agencies with names like Maidpower and Noble Maids will appear.[1] Noble Maids, for instance, offers packages from S$488 (Singapore dollars) for an "Indonesian transfer maid." A Christian Indonesian maid will cost you a few hundred dollars more, about the same as a Filipino maid with unlimited replacements within two years. For Indonesian maids there is a free replacement period if she is medically unfit or if you find her unsuitable, but only for the first thirty days. Optional additions to package deals include up to six biannual medical exams for an extra S$210.

Most of these Web sites have pages of photos of primarily Indonesian and Filipino women. Click on the photos to see what prior work experience they have. Susanti, for instance, is a twenty-four-year-old Christian Indonesian woman who has been working as a maid in Singapore for four years. The youngest child she has cared for was 1.6 years old. On the measuring tape in the background you can see that she is about 152 centimeters tall. Soon she will be looking for a new employer.

Find out that all of the women pass through training programs before arrival, most of the Indonesians on the nearby Indonesian islands in the Riau Archipelago. Training is important because, as one site notes, "perhaps, if she is from a remote area, her family would be living in a wood-and-thatch house with a mud floor. Keeping the house spotlessly clean is a futile exercise and they may never have tried." Read the message boards and discuss if Filipinos are preferable to Indonesians. Does it matter that Indonesian maids do not usually speak English? Move on to find out about the dos and don'ts when it comes to dealing with your maid, and finally read about the horror stories—of having a maid, that is, not working as one.

However, there is also, as we might expect, another side to the story. Increasingly women working as maids are portrayed as victims by the mass media in Indonesia, Malaysia, and Singapore.[2] In Indonesia there have even been calls to stop the export of maids, as evidence of widespread abuse mounts. For instance, consider the following headline from the Singapore *Straits Times*: "Abused Maid Speaks: 'My Seven Months of Horror.' She was cut, burned, beaten and bitten. Teenage maid suffered employer's abuse until her badly injured nipple fell out." It appears that not only employers have horror stories to tell.[3]

When you have lost interest in maids, why not choose a less high-tech kind of Web site, "The Batam/Riau Entertainment Update," which offers an intimate guide to the geography of prostitution in the Riau Archipelago, in particular the islands of Batam, Bintan, and Karimun.[4] They all form part of the expanding Growth Triangle, a transnational economic zone that ideally is supposed to bind together Batam, the Malaysian province of Johor, and Singapore. Japanese business guru, Kenichi Ohmae (1990, 1995), among others, takes this discourse at face value and claims that the area is an example of a new "borderless world." But we certainly know better than that. The border between Indonesia and Singapore, as well as Malaysia, has in fact become increasingly regulated since the mid-1990s. This is despite the fact that during the same period there has been a dramatic increase in transnational migration, in general, and female migration, in particular, throughout Asia (Hugo 2002b: 13). In the borderless world, Indonesian labor is supposed to stay in place.

Lonely Planet Indonesia, a popular guidebook for Western tourists, suggests that "there is no reason to stop on Batam for longer than it takes to catch the boat out" (Turner 2000: 602). But many Singaporean men know better than that. With increasing cooperation between Singapore and Batam, ferries take the forty-minute trip every fifteen minutes across the Straits of Malacca. Discos, karaoke bars, and brothel villages offer drugs and sex at bargain prices in a less regulated environment, beyond the reach of the Singaporean state. On the Batam/Riau entertainment Web site, information about hotels, taxis, places of prostitution, and even names of particular women who will perform particular sexual acts are listed. Ways of avoiding scams and getting conned are key themes on the message boards. Questions can be asked. Is Indonesia less commercialized than Thailand? How do you deal with long-term relationships on Batam without getting ripped off? How do you know that they are interested in you and not your money? Comparative examples are drawn from Thailand,

Cambodia, and other countries, all only a short, direct, and inexpensive plane trip away from Singapore's Changi airport.

On the Indonesian side of the border, stories concerning prostitutes are common in the media. On Batam, the local branch of the regional newspaper *Riau Pos*, which was caught up in the hype of borderlessness and changed its name to *Sijori Pos* (short for Singapore-Johor-Riau), took a particular interest in my questions about prostitution when I was conducting fieldwork. "How do you get prostitutes to talk to you?" one journalist asked me, apparently insinuating various forms of transactions. Attempting to humor him, I claimed that all I had to do was buy them iced tea. A few days later I made the section of the newspaper typically devoted to stories of prostitutes, in an article dealing with my research. The title read: "Swedish anthropologist buys prostitutes [*lontong*] iced tea [*teh obeng*]." It featured a cartoon of me walking with a couple of mugs of iced tea while being followed by two prostitutes with their arms forward, as though hypnotized. The journalist's interest in my interest in prostitution obviously did not reach the level of political economy and structural violence that I pushed him to highlight in his article.

In fact, in the Indonesian media, prostitutes are called WTS (*wanita tuna sila*), "women without morals," or in recent years, younger prostitutes, usually in discos or karaoke bars, are identified as ABG (*anak baru gede*), literally "children who have just grown up."[5] In this context, the dividing line between prostitutes and nonprostitutes becomes diffuse. This suggests that these women have a kind of "unruly agency," that they are up to no good and know it. A similar discourse is evident on the Batam/Riau entertainment Web site, where men run the risk of getting conned by women who are just looking for money. In the Singaporean media, this side of the Growth Triangle has also become increasingly publicized, as attention has focused on men who are "secretly taking second wives."[6]

SITUATING GLOBAL CIRCUITS

Saskia Sassen (1991) has noted that particular kinds of places, namely global cities that function as financial hubs, have become increasingly important in the global economy. This leads, she argues, not only to a concentration of financial elites and information technologies, but also to new gendered dynamics of inequality, as low-wage service jobs—which primarily utilize immigrant labor—have expanded. Her main examples are London, New York, and Tokyo, but Hong Kong and Singapore are two more recent candidates in East and Southeast Asia.[7]

Singapore presents a special case since it is also a nation-state where the boundaries of the city converge with those of the state. This means that the state has the ability to regulate the movement of people in and out of the city in ways that are impossible in other global cities. Furthermore, with the emergence of the Growth Triangle, the space between center and periphery is literally compressed. In this context of rapid change, maids and prostitutes are two types of female migrant laborers that have emerged: one in the domestic sphere—regulated but not protected by the Singaporean state—and the other on the opposite side of the border in Indonesia (and earlier in Malaysia), but in an important sense still within the limits of the city.

The increasing mobility of financial capital, ideas, media images, and people are the main "flows" that characterize contemporary processes of globalization.[8] Like Sassen (1998: 82), however, I am primarily interested in tracking the "narratives of eviction" that are silenced in these processes (see also Clifford 1997: 258–59). The experiences and voices of Indonesian female migrants are one example of these types of displaced narratives, constantly lurking in the background of much theorizing concerning globalization.

In this chapter, the Web sites that commodify "maids" and "prostitutes" are juxtaposed with the story of an Indonesian female migrant who first became a maid in Singapore before losing her job and becoming a prostitute on the other side of the border in Indonesia at the height of the Asian economic crisis in 1998 and 1999. My aim in using this account is threefold. First, it brings together and disturbs identities—"prostitutes" and "maids"—that are generally kept separate, instead identifying the "Indonesian female labor migrant" as the figure of interest. Second, this allows me to engage with the "local moral worlds" (Kleinman 1995: 45) of Indonesian female migrants in decidedly multilocal and transnational contexts. I am especially interested in how a particular kind of affect, namely *malu*, meaning approximately "shame" or "embarrassment," is a powerful force in the lives of migrants—binding them to the demands of family, home, and culture while they become engaged with regional and global processes of economic and social change. Third—and this follows from the previous point—this allows me to consider how the experiences of migrants engaged in processes of global change must be analyzed in relation to the cultural contexts from which these migrants emerge.

As Anna Tsing (2000: 330) has pointed out, in much theorizing concerning globalization, "flow is valorized but not the carving of the channel." By this she means that people, objects, and information do not travel randomly, but are rather structured by powerful cultural, economic, and political forces. Rather than taking these channels as given, however, it is important to begin with cultural forms in order to understand the forces that keep migrants on the move. In other words, it is important to open the black box of globalization and interrogate related metaphors such as "channels" and "flows." Within these boxes we find not only regional and local differences, but also the individual's engagement with the burden of culture.[9]

THE GROWTH TRIANGLE

Contemporary Singapore has efficiently been remade from a low-cost export-oriented manufacturing center within the so-called new international division of labor into a global financial hub. By the mid-1980s Singapore had begun to witness slower economic growth for the first time since gaining independence from Malaysia in 1965. Rising labor costs led the PAP (People's Action Party) government, under the leadership of Lee Kuan Yew, to transform Singapore into a "total business hub" (see Perry, Kong, and Yeoh 1997: 113; Rodan 1997: 156–66). While Singapore earlier had thrived on its small size—lacking rural areas that demanded resources and slowed the pace of development—the new economy required an international hinterland with inexpensive labor. The Singapore Economic Development Board pushed multinational companies to keep their main offices in Singapore, but to move their factories to offshore locations throughout Asia, primarily China, Indonesia, Malaysia, and Vietnam. Through this process, Singapore was slowly transformed from an economy based on manufacturing to a center for multinational corporations in the region.

During this same period a communitarian political discourse of "Asian values" has famously been developed in Singapore, primarily in opposition to liberal "Western values." Aihwa Ong (1999: 201) has used the word "caring" to describe the Singaporean style of governmentality. She writes that "the cultural idiom of Asian values is invoked for its familiar 'traditional' appeal to articulate discourses and categories that regulate society while culturally authenticating policies that produce the social conditions desired by global business" (202). C. J. Wan-Ling Wee (1996: 508) has further noted that this discourse has a dual purpose: "the first is to maintain discipline and efficiency in the area of economic production; and the second is to constantly keep Singapore in place in the larger Asian setting—tiny Singapore needs Asia, if not vice versa."

This vision of the New Asia—framed in primarily economic terms—posits a particular relationship between the regional center, Singapore, and the more diffuse periphery.[10] The Web sites that I have discussed, however, suggest that the new transnational imaginary that is developing has moved beyond this official rhetoric and that there are a series of alternative forms of "comparative advantages" to be found in the new Asian hinterlands. Filipinos or Indonesians? Thais or Indonesians? Which do you prefer? The choice is yours.

The transformation of Singapore has resulted in profound changes on Batam, which in the late 1960s was a little known island with only three thousand fishermen and coconut farmers. By 2005, there were perhaps seven hundred thousand inhabitants, though no one really knows exactly how many migrants have been lured there by rumors of the booming economy. Throughout this period of change, the Indonesian government has commonly presented Batam as a competitor to Singapore—the new Houston or Rotterdam of Southeast Asia—the "locomotive" of Indonesian national development. In reality, however, the island has a distinct frontier-town atmosphere: it is a place that has changed too quickly. Golf courses, marinas, and gated communities coexist with factories, squatter communities, karaoke bars, and brothels, while large parts of the island remain covered by jungle. Along with the industrial estates that offer facilities for multinational corporations, a major prostitution industry has emerged, one that is well described in—and indeed implicated with—the Batam/Riau entertainment Web site. Batam is, as one of my Singaporean informants put it, "like Fantasy Island." Working-class Singaporean men, increasingly marginalized in the new economy, can lead a lifestyle of conspicuous consumption, with sex and drugs available at bargain prices, outside of the gaze and grasp of the Singaporean state. While Indonesian women in Singapore labor for the growing middle class, on the other side of the border they cater to the desires of Singaporean men left behind in the process of economic restructuring and the promises of the nation building.

As I have already noted, the understanding of the Growth Triangle as a postnational arena fails to acknowledge that the free flow of people and capital in one direction has been matched by the increasing regulation of Indonesians moving in the other direction.[11] In fact, the period since the 1990s has witnessed new techniques of border control that regulate the flow of people across the border dividing Indonesia from Malaysia and Singapore. In other words, while certain forms of movement are considered crucial to its success, other types of human mobility appear as a threat to the official model of the Growth Triangle. In this context, it is not the cosmopolitans moving comfortably in international space who are of interest, but rather the Indonesian migrants and Singaporean working-class tourists who move within and between nation-states.

This movement is structured not only in national, but also in gendered terms. The Growth Triangle has comprised a number of transformations, creating a demand for increasing quantities of female labor that are localized in a variety of contexts. First, the use of young women in offshore factories has become part of a corporate cultural form that is recognizable around the world.[12] Batamindo Industrial Park, for instance, the flagship of economic development on Batam, employs sixty-five thousand workers, 85 percent of them women between the ages of eighteen and twenty-four. Second, the Growth Triangle has generated a massive market for female prostitution, catering to both Singaporean tourists and Indonesian migrants.[13] Third, the transformation of Singapore into a global city and the expansion of the middle class in Malaysia have together increased the demand for low-paid Indonesian maids in Malaysian and Singaporean households, as middle-class women have increasingly entered the work force.[14] In this context, Indonesian men are often relegated to the margins, working illegally on plantations in Malaysia, on construction sites in Singapore, or wherever they can find jobs on Batam. On Batam, in particular, this turns gender roles on their heads, as women are able to survive more efficiently in both the formal and informal economies.

FROM MAID TO PROSTITUTE

I first met Putri in June 1998 in a dingy hotel area, which was also a center for prostitution and migrants moving in and out of Batam, either to other parts of Indonesia or across the border to Malaysia and Singapore. I had begun spending time there as I found that it was an interesting place to meet people on the move. Putri did not really fit in with many of the other women who waited for clients near the front desks or on the porches of the long row of hotels. Her clothing, style, and demeanor immediately made it evident that she had not been there for long, and when I asked her it turned out that she had only been there for only a month. She had previously worked as a maid in Singapore, but her employer had decided to get rid of her and she had been sent to Batam. I was interested in her story, but it took a month or so before I asked her to tell me what had happened. I explained that I was researching the effects that processes of globalization were having on people in the region and that I felt as though her story was one that should be told. She agreed.

This was at the height of the Indonesian economic crisis. As the krismon, or krisis moneter, worsened in 1998 throughout Indonesia, eventually leading to kristal, or krisis total, and the fall of President Suharto, an increasing number of migrants arrived on Batam, most apparently lured by rumors of an expansive labor market; others hoped to enter Singapore, but mainly Malaysia, in search of higher wages. During the same period, Malaysia and Singapore, fearing a flood of refugees, were closing their borders, making it difficult for individuals carrying Indonesian passports to cross legally. There were frequent raids against illegal migrants in both countries, and in mid-1998 Malaysia initiated Operation Go Away, which aimed at deporting a substantial number of the perhaps one million Indonesians working in Malaysia. Most of these migrants were sent to port towns throughout the Riau Archipelago, and many eventually turned up on Batam, unwilling to return home with nothing. It was in this specific time and place that Putri arrived on Batam.

Putri was born in a small village on the predominantly Muslim island of Lombok in 1970, part of a Balinese Hindu family. Her father died when she was still a child, and since her mother could not afford to care for her, she began working as a maid (*pembantu*) after just a few years of elementary school. The family she worked for raised her in exchange for her services, and, as she put it, "all I could do was wait for someone who would marry me." By the time she was eighteen years old a Balinese man was chosen as her husband and "though I didn't like him, I said nothing. I didn't dare say anything." After a few years, she had her first child, but by the time she was pregnant again she discovered that her husband had a mistress who was also pregnant. "It broke my heart [*sakit hati*]," she said. "Never giving me any money for the household or showing any interest in me or the children was one thing, but this I could not take."

When a *tai kong*, a "labor recruiter," came from to her village one day looking for women who wanted to travel to Singapore to work as maids, Putri and a couple of her friends quickly decided to go together. "Rather than stay in the village and watch my husband remarry, I decided to leave and make some money for my children." She had seen and heard how people had come back from Malaysia and Singapore and built large houses and hoped to do the same. The *tai kong* promised her that she would also be able to make a lot of money and that passports, visas, and transportation would be covered.[15] Since the 1990s, Lombok has rapidly become one of the main sending areas in Indonesia for female domestic servants to Malaysia, Singapore, and, increasingly, to Saudi Arabia. Historically based primarily on an agricultural economy, within a decade transnational migration has become the dominant labor market on Lombok and continues to expand.[16]

Along with twelve other women, Putri left Lombok with the *tai kong* for the island of Bintan in the Riau Archipelago, where for six weeks they were "trained" to cook "Singaporean" food and use electric kitchen equipment. The *tai kong* who had brought them from Lombok was paid about US$50 for each woman when he turned them over to the agent who ran the employment agency and training center. For the first four months in Singapore, the women were told, their salaries would be withheld in order to pay for the costs of their trip and training. After that they would be receive US$150 per month.[17]

Upon arrival in Singapore it turned out that Putri would not just be cooking, as she had been told, but also cleaning, washing, and taking care of a young child and her elderly grandmother in a Chinese Singaporean household. Living in an upscale residential area in Singapore, Putri began work at 5:30 A.M. and was not permitted to sleep until ten or eleven at night. She slept on a mat in the living room and was strictly forbidden to use the telephone.[18]

After four months, when she was supposed to receive her first salary, Putri sent a letter to her mother telling her that she would be sending a money order. Her boss agreed to do this for her but would not let her come along to the bank, even though she tried to insist. A couple of months later, however, a letter arrived from her mother claiming that she had not received the money. When Putri confronted her boss about this he claimed that he did not know what was wrong, but he was unwilling to make any further inquiries.[19] Distressed, Putri began phoning the other women in Singapore who had come from Indonesia with her and tried calling her village on Lombok. When her boss discovered her using the phone he called the agent who was in charge of the maid company and terminated her contract. One day, after seven months in Singapore, Putri's agent from the employment agency arrived to pick her up. She was taken back to Batam without having been paid her salary.[20]

Putri's agent told her that she would have to "train" again on Batam before she could return to Singapore. After a month and a half of working and cleaning in different houses on Batam, Putri was paid a little more than 100,000 rupiah, about US$10 at the time, but knowing that no money had arrived in her village she felt malu, "ashamed" or "embarrassed." Her agent still could not give her a clear answer about when she would be going back to Singapore and, feeling trapped because she was working all the time, Putri decided to leave the employment agent, who had her passport and identity card, and try her chances elsewhere: "It drove me crazy to wait day after day knowing that I wasn't making any money and that my mother and children were waiting for it. Finally I couldn't take it anymore."

After receiving her first salary Putri fled one night together with another woman who had also been waiting to go to Singapore, eventually ending up in the hotel area where I first met her. She thought about looking for work in one of the factories, but when she heard how difficult it was find work, and that they only hired women under the age of twenty-four, she knew that it was no use.

During this period of regional economic crisis the Singapore dollar remained relatively stable, while the Indonesian rupiah fell to as low as one-sixth of its previous value in relation to the Singapore dollar. One effect of this was that while foreign direct investment slowed considerably, prostitution became one of the only expanding industries on Batam and neighboring islands. My rough estimate was that in mid-1998 fifteen thousand women were working as prostitutes out of a total population of one million women and men on Batam and neighboring islands. The number of Singaporeans crossing the border increased substantially and, to the best of my knowledge, the Batam/Riau entertainment Web site was created in the wake of these changes.

It did not take long before the man working at the front desk asked if Putri wanted a client. Within a few days, she decided to accept his offer and work as a prostitute. Putri told me, "of course I felt *malu* at first, but it was nothing compared to the *malu* and responsibility that I felt towards my children. It didn't take long before I got used to it." Like many other migrants I met, she claimed that she refused to return home without a *modal*, a substantial amount of money that would allow her to build a house and open a small shop, not remaining dependent on anyone else.

Merantau, which most directly translates as "migration," was earlier primarily a male activity in Indonesia, but in recent decades women have increasingly entered the *rantau*, the "space of migration." *Merantau* must be understood in relation to a broad range of cultural meanings. Mochtar Naim (1976: 149–50), for instance, defines it as "leaving one's cultural territory voluntarily, whether for a short or long time, with the aim of earning a living or seeking further knowledge or experience, normally with the intention of returning home." While earlier *merantau* was bound to particular cultures, it has become nationalized as a cultural form, as increasing numbers of Indonesians move into wage labor.[21]

The relationship between *merantau* and *malu* is a common theme in this context. *Malu* is a key emotional trope for migrants on Batam and arises in a wide variety of contexts (Lindquist 2004). Most notably, it is connected with anxieties concerning economic failure, thereby making evident the major irony of *merantau* and most forms of economic migration: it demands monetary success that is difficult to attain. One is *malu* to return home without having anything to show for the time one has spent, abroad, in the *rantau*. As another woman I met, who had been deported from Malaysia without receiving her salary, told me, "People will ask, 'for years you have been gone. Where have you been? Where did you work? What do you have to show for it?'"

It was clear from the beginning that it would be difficult for Putri to make enough money, since she rarely found clients. The economic crisis had led to a rapid increase in the number of women working as prostitutes, and competition intensified. Initially, she would go to the discos around the main town of Nagoya, but she claimed that this made her *pusing* (literally, "dizzy"). She refused to "dress like a prostitute," preferring instead to wait in the hotel lobby for potential clients.

I first met Putri a few months before my main round of fieldwork ended. When I saw her six months later on a return trip, she had stopped working as a prostitute and was helping out at a small food stall across the street. She was pregnant and involved in a relationship with the man—a former client— whom she believed to be the father of the child. He had been thrown out of Malaysia during Operation Go Away and was planning to return as soon as it was safe to go back. Putri told me, "He is a good man and I trust him. When he goes back to Malaysia and makes some money we are going to be married." However, when I asked her if she was planning on returning home she looked away and didn't answer.

Rudolf Mrázek (1994: 10–11) has written in the context of West Sumatra that the "*rantau* is a place in which Minangkabau culture's loose elements or excessive tension may be released. But *rantau* is meaningless without 'the heartland.' It has always been acceptable for an adult man in Minangkabau to go to *rantau* at a certain point in his life. But it was, and is, very bad for the *perantau* (the man going to the *rantau*) to become 'destitute in *rantau*,' *melarat di rantau*, to be lost in *rantau*, forgotten by those staying home."

The *rantau* thus appears as a space of freedom and risk, but also, it should be added, of responsibility toward those left behind. In contemporary Indonesia, the moral economy of *merantau* demands economic success.[22] But referring to economic success is not enough. It retains a model of analysis that is too general. Questions remain that cannot be answered from a general perspective. Why do women go when they are called? What does this do to Indonesian men, women, and families? Putri carries burdens and scars, and it is not clear if any form of success would lessen that pain. Soon she will have a new family and she may well become, as in Mrázek's quote above, "destitute in *rantau*."

THINKING THROUGH MERANTAU

A number of scholars have pointed out that most research on transnational migration has focused on two extremes, the "individual" or the "nation"; and to this might be added the "global" (see, for example, Yeoh and Huang 2000; Hugo 2002a; Yeoh, Graham, and Boyle 2002). Such scholars suggest that paying attention to the "family" or the "household" is one way of bridging this dichotomy. The choices and experiences of many transnational female migrants should, they argue, be understood in the context of family networks. Indeed, if we pay attention to Putri's story, it is clear that it is primarily the responsibility and *malu* that she feels toward her children and family—rather than, for instance, any desire for personal fulfillment—that led her to migrate. And, indeed, it is the same form of affect that keeps her from returning home.

During Suharto's New Order regime, there was been a shift in the structure of the Indonesian family "from the emotionally extended to the emotionally nucleated family" (Hugo 2002a: 15). This change "[saw] primary loyalties swing toward one's spouse and children" (15) and should be understood in relation to dramatic declines in divorce in Indonesian during that period of time. In particular, the 1974 Marriage Law made divorce increasingly difficult in legal terms. The fall of official divorce rates, however, hides the fact that there has been an increase in de facto separations. In this changing structure, many households have missing family members, often either the husband or the wife (Jones 2002: 222–24).[23]

Just as importantly, in the same time period there has been an explicit attempt to promote the middle-class nuclear family as the building block of the nation, which is evident in ideals produced through the mass media (Sears 1996). From this perspective, the contemporary Indonesian family should be understood in relation to the nation, and knowledge about how the family should work is to be found among enlightened nationalists, rather than within the household itself (Siegel 1998: 87). It is thus important to ask, as does James Ferguson (1999: chap. 5) in a Foucauldian spirit, not what the "family" fails to do, but what it actually *does*. Concerning the Zambian Copperbelt, Ferguson (1999: 205) claims that the constant reference to "the fiction of the modern family" effectively obscures more basic political struggles between men and women and between generations.

The same is true in Indonesia. The links between the demands of *merantau* and *malu* that emerge when Putri fails to make money that she can send home highlight the tensions between the responsibility that migrants feel toward family members that are left behind and the social and economic forces that keep them on the move. Putri's story, and the cases of many other women I met on Batam, suggest that when the husband leaves and there is a situation of de facto divorce it is often the woman who bears the primary responsibility for supporting the children as well as her parents. It is therefore not surprising that areas such as Lombok and West Java, which have among the highest divorce rates in Indonesia,[24] also have among the highest rates of female transnational migration in the country. The emergence of new labor markets and changing cultural forms that are increasingly offering women the opportunity to migrate therefore generate new kinds of possibilities and problems.

CIRCUITS OF DEBT AND SERVITUDE

Putri's move from working as a maid in Singapore to prostitution on Batam was certainly unusual, but by no means unique. I met a half dozen women like her who had previously worked in either Malaysia or Singapore. Their stories are important, not because they represent a norm, but because they allow us to consider forms of labor and experience together that are generally kept separate, both in economic and moral terms. While maids are often represented in Indonesian media and public discourse as "victims" and prostitutes as "women without morals," the former belonging to the "formal" sector and the latter in the "informal," in fact, both groups are generally recognized as the migrant workers who are "most widely exploited and most vulnerable to abuse and violence" (Stasilius and Bakan 1997: 32).[25] This suggests that it is crucial to reconceptualize and revalorize transnational labor mobility and situate these processes at the center of discussions of economic globalization and the transformation of what the Singaporean government calls the "New Asia."

Maids are among the few Indonesians who are given work visas in Singapore, and this is increasingly the case in Malaysia as well. They are therefore, more often than not, "legal" migrants. Putri's story suggests, however, as do other stories and countless media accounts, that in the context of the domestic sphere, maids in fact tend to be *more* isolated and subject to abuse than men working illegally on, for instance, construction sites. In a historical tradition of servitude, in the homes of the new, primarily Chinese, Singaporean middle class, Indonesian women become located outside of kinship networks as "moral outsiders," thus making them vulnerable to various forms of abuse (Ong 2006: 206–207).

Singaporean state legislation is complicit in this process as foreign domestic servants are offered limited legal protection since they are not covered by the Employment Act (see Yeoh and Huang 1998: 588–89; Human Rights Watch 2005: 24). Work hours and wages are not regulated, women do not have the right to leave the place of work, and there are no guaranteed off days. There are generally salary deductions for between six and ten months to pay off the debt to an employment agency.[26] Furthermore, despite frequent cases of maids falling to their deaths either through accidents or suicides while washing highrise apartment windows, limited legislation has been created to protect their safety.[27] In fact, the Indonesian Department of Manpower imposed a ban on the export of maids to Singapore during the last three months of 1998, in protest against the doubling of fees taken out of Indonesian maids' salaries. The economic crisis had increased competition among agents, and many of them were lowering costs for employers while taking that money out of maids' salaries.[28]

During the economic crisis, as the Indonesian rupiah was collapsing and formal investments had ground to a halt, the informal prostitution industry was booming on Batam. Putri's move from domestic service to prostitution makes evident the position and potential exchangeability of female labor in the shadows of globalization—a move, however, that is by no means automatic, but must be considered in relation to the choices (albeit limited) made by individuals.

One of the customers writing to the Web site for Noble Maids to complain about the greediness of maids notes a historical shift: "For the last 20 years or so when Singaporeans, Malaysians and Thais are no longer interested in working as domestics, my maids have come from the Philippines, Sri Lanka or Indonesia."[29] Taking a step farther back in history, historians remind us that at the end of the nineteenth century Singapore was a coolie town and a center of prostitution in Southeast Asia (see Warren 1986, 1993; Trocki 1990). Most of the women were Chinese or Japanese, a situation that many people have difficulty imagining today. In fact, elderly fishermen on Batam and neighboring islands in Indonesia told me stories of visiting prostitutes in Singapore during the 1950s and early '60s when few were to be found in Riau. Clearly a lot has happened since then.

A lot has changed in Indonesia as well. The days have passed when women stayed at home and the men ideally went on *merantau* to gain experiences before returning to the village to marry.[30] In contemporary Indonesia, women travel to places like Batam or go abroad to Malaysia, Saudi Arabia, and Singapore. The way they get there varies, but it is clear that the movement of women to work as maids and as prostitutes is a lucrative business for the networks that recruit them and that these networks are often similar in form.

My aim in recounting Putri's story is not to reveal "the truth" concerning the experiences of Indonesian female migrants in the Growth Triangle, nor is it to present a kind of "downward spiral" story of the effects of the economic crisis. It is rather to suggest that we bring together different cultural and economic processes. This merging permits us to think about these disparate processes in relation to human experience and local moral worlds—worlds that are increasingly translocal. Putri's story describes a circuit of debt and servitude that leads from a small village in Indonesia, to the Singaporean global city, and on to Batam. This specific circuit, which comes into being through Putri's mobility, brings together practices of servitude in both Indonesia and Singapore, a changing regional economy that demands large numbers of unskilled women and the most intimate forms of experience and emotional debt.

What is most striking when we turn to stories such as Putri's is that there are powerful and contradictory forms of affect at work. In her case at least, the tension between the demands of migration, of sending back money to her children, and the *malu* that she experiences when she cannot do this is one that forces her to make choices in a context of intense constraints. Putri is—needless to say—far from being a "woman without morals," but is rather intensely engaged in a moral economy in which economic success is a necessity. It is precisely this engagement, and the affect associated with it, that is missing from many accounts of globalization as well as from media accounts and Web sites that commodify Indonesian women who are involved in economies that are increasingly transnational, but insidiously violent. And though this is where I end, it is actually from this point that we should begin.

NOTES

Thanks are due to Victor Alneng, Sandra Hyde, Byron Good, and Mary-Jo DelVecchio Good for comments on an earlier version of this chapter.

1. See www.noblemaids.com and www.maidpower.com (both accessed April 10, 2002). There are more than six hundred employment agencies in Singapore that recruit domestic servants.

2. Indonesian transnational female migrants have been represented in Indonesian media and academic discourse primarily as passive victims (Ford 2004).

3. *Straits Times*, March 20, 2002. During the year 2000, I counted at least one hundred articles dealing with maids in the *Straits Times*, Singapore's largest and most influential newspaper. Most dealt with issues of abuse. See also *Jakarta Post*, August 24, 2000, and Hugo (2002b: 168–72).

4. See http://batam-nightlife.hypermart.net (accessed April 15, 2002; site discontinued).

5. See, for instance, the issue of the weekly magazine *Gatra* from October 3, 1998, which included the articles "Sindikat Dagang ABG" or "Syndicate for Trafficking of ABG."

6. See, for instance, *Straits Times*, July 7, 1991.

7. Shanghai should perhaps be added to this list.

8. See Appadurai (1996) for a seminal perspective.

9. This is a response to the work of, among others, Manuel Castells (1996: 475), who argues that "capital and labor increasingly tend to exist in different spaces and times." A similar dichotomy emerges in David Harvey's equally celebrated version of the postmodern condition (1990), in which "ethnography is allowed out of the prison but only to wander around homeless and irrelevant" (Burawoy 2000: 2). Without extended ethnographic fieldwork, however, these perspectives are inevitably restricted to analyzing the "space of flows," while "everyday life" remains beyond reach.

10. See Wee (2002: 22) for a note on the use of the term "New Asia" by the Singaporean government.

11. It is important to remember that borders are created not to stop movement but rather to regulate it.

12. See Ong (1991) and Mills (2003) for two review articles.

13. For studies of prostitution and economic development in Thailand and the Philippines, see Bishop and Robinson (1998) and Law (2000).

14. See Chin (1998) and Yeoh, Huang, and Gonzalez (1999). In 1995 there were 20,000 Indonesian and 100,000 foreign maids in Singapore, one for every eight households in the city (Yeoh, Huang, and Gonzalez 1999: 117). By 2005 there were 150,000 foreign maids in the country, including 60,000 Indonesians (Human Rights Watch 2005).

15. For a discussion of these middlemen, see Hugo (2002b).

16. See, for instance, the report on human trafficking in Indonesia funded by the US Agency for International Development (USAID) (Rosenberg 2003).

17. In comparison, workers in the government category "cleaners and laborers," the occupational group with the lowest gross wages in Singapore, on average made US$827 per month in 2000 (Singapore government wage statistics, www.gov .sg/mom/manpower/manrs/wages/ows_highlight.pdf, accessed November 19, 2001; site discontinued).

18. As the recent report by Human Rights Watch (2005: 66–68) shows, these are within the normal working hours for domestic servants in Singapore. In fact, a widely available handbook on hiring and dealing with foreign maids in Singapore suggests that employers should expect their maid to work these long hours (Chew 2004: 68–69).

19. For a similar case and a discussion of employers' control of wages, see Human Rights Watch (2005: 50–51).

20. Indonesian maids who have problems in Singapore are frequently sent by agents to Batam since it is cheaper than paying for their return ticket home. This is often explicitly stated in contracts.

21. *Merantau* has traditionally been associated with the matrilineal Minangkabau of West Sumatra (Kato 1982), but has recently become widely used among most ethnic groups in Indonesia (Ali 1996; Waterson 1997: 230–31) as more and more people have been transformed into migrants in search of wage labor (Gardiner and Gardiner-Oey 1990).

22. "Moral economy" is a term borrowed from E. P. Thompson (1971), who suggests that there are moral principles that organize productive activities. These become particularly clear in times of crisis, in Thompson's case food riots in eighteenth-century England, in this case the Asian economic crisis. Thompson did not mean for the term to be generalized, but like others (e.g., Kohler 1999), I believe the term is helpful in understanding other social and historical contexts.

23. It is worth noting that the World Bank, around 2000, supported a "widows project" in several provinces in Indonesia, which aimed to support women as heads of households. In East Flores and Lombok, for instance, there are many households where the husband has migrated to Malaysia and has never returned. In both these places the shorthand *Jamal*, meaning *janda Malaysia* or "Malaysian widow," is universally known and used.

24. See Jones (1994) for a discussion of divorce in Indonesia.

25. To a certain degree the discourse on prostitution is changing in Indonesia; countertrafficking campaigns funded by international organizations such as USAID describe prostitutes as victims of sexual exploitation.

26. Off days must be negotiated in the contract between the employer and the maid, usually through the employment agent, who can hardly be expected to consider

the interests of the workers. See Yeoh and Huang (1998) and Human Rights Watch (2005: 62–65). Concerning salaries, see Human Rights Watch (2005: 53). There is, in fact, no legal cap on salary deductions (54).

27. Between 1999 and 2005, 122 Indonesian maids either jumped or fell to their deaths in Singapore (Human Rights Watch 2005: 38). See also *Straits Times*, January 19, 2000. More recently, in 2005, a number of intiatives by Singapore's Ministry of Manpower have been introduced to protect the "quality" of domestic workers (see Human Rights Watch 2005: 29–31).

28. *Straits Times*, October 12, 1998. These deductions from salaries to cover lower prices continues to be prevalent (Human Rights Watch 2005: 34–38).

29. See www.noblemaids.com (accessed April 10, 2002).

30. See Muhamad Radjab's autobiography (1995), which describes the gendered dynamics of *merantau* in West Sumatra during the 1920s.

REFERENCES

Ali, Mariam Mohamed. 1996. Ethnic Hinterlands: Contested Spaces between Nations and Ethnicities in the Lives of Baweanese Labor Migrants. PhD diss., Harvard University.

Appadurai, Arjun. 1996. *Modernity at Large: Cultural Dimensions of Globalization*. Minneapolis: University of Minnesota Press.

Bishop, Ryan, and Lillian S. Robinson. 1998. *Night Market: Sexual Cultures and the Thai Economic Miracle*. New York: Routledge.

Burawoy, Michael. 2000. Introduction: Reaching for the Global. In *Global Ethnography: Forces, Connections, and Imaginations in a Postmodern World*, ed. Michael Burawoy et al. Berkeley: University of California Press.

Castells, Manuel. 1996. *The Information Age: Economy, Society and Culture*. Vol. 1 of *The Rise of the Network Society*. Oxford: Blackwell.

Chew Kim Whatt. 2004. *Foreign Maids: The Complete Handbook for Employers and Maid Agencies*. Singapore: SNP Editions.

Chin, Christine B. N. 1998. *In Service and Servitude: Foreign Female Domestic Workers and the Malaysian "Modernity" Project*. New York: Columbia University Press.

Clifford, James. 1997. *Routes: Travel and Translation in the Late Twentieth Century*. Cambridge, MA: Harvard University Press.

Ferguson, James. 1999. *Expectations of Modernity: Myths and Meanings of Urban Life on the Zambian Copperbelt*. Berkeley: University of California Press.

Ford, Michele. 2004. Beyond the *Femina* Fantasy: Female Industrial and Overseas Workers in Indonesian Discourses of Women's Work. *Review of Indonesian and Malaysian Affairs* 37 (2): 83–113.

Gardiner, Peter, and Mayling Gardiner-Oey. 1990. Indonesia. In *International Handbook on Internal Migration*, ed. Charles B. Nam, William J. Serrow, and Daniel F. Sly. New York: Greenwood Press.

Harvey, David. 1990. *The Condition of Postmodernity: An Enquiry into the Origins of Cultural Change*. Oxford: Blackwell.

Hugo, Graeme. 2002a. Effects of International Migration on the Family in Indonesia. *Asian and Pacific Migration Journal* 11 (1): 13–46.

————. 2002b. Women's International Labour Migration. In *Women in Indonesia: Gender, Equity and Development*, ed. Kathryn Robinson and Sharon Bessell. Singapore: Institute of Southeast Asian Studies.

Human Rights Watch. 2005. Maid to Order: Ending Abuses against Migrant Domestic Workers in Singapore. Vol. 17, no. 10 (December).

Jones, Gavin W. 1994. *Marriage and Divorce in Islamic South-East Asia*. Kuala Lumpur: Oxford University Press.

————. 2002. The Changing Indonesian Household. In *Women in Indonesia: Gender, Equity and Development*, ed. Kathryn Robinson and Sharon Bessell. Singapore: Institute of Southeast Asian Studies.

Kato, Tsuyoshi. 1982. *Matriliny and Migration: Evolving Minangkabau Traditions in Indonesia*. Ithaca, NY: Cornell University Press.

Kleinman, Arthur. 1995. *Writing at the Margin: Discourse between Anthropology and Medicine*. Berkeley: University of California Press.

Kohler, Robert A. 1999. Moral Economy, Material Culture, and Community in Drosophila Genetics. In *The Science Studies Reader*, ed. Mario Biagioli. New York: Routledge.

Law, Lisa. 2000. *Sex Work in Southeast Asia: The Place of Desire in a Time of AIDS*. New York: Routledge.

Lindquist, Johan. 2004. Veils and Ecstasy: Negotiating Shame in the Indonesian Borderlands. *Ethnos* 69 (4): 487–508.

Mills, Mary Beth. 2003. Gender and Inequality in the Global Labor Force, *Annual Review of Anthropology* 32:41–62.

Mrázek, Rudolf. 1994. *Sjahrir: Politics and Exile in Southeast Asia*. Ithaca, NY: Cornell Southeast Asia Program.

Naim, Mochtar. 1976. Voluntary Migration in Indonesia. In *Internal Migration: The New World and the Old World*, ed. Daniel Kubát and Anthony H. Richmond. Sage Studies in International Sociology 4. Beverly Hills: Sage Publications.

Ohmae, Kenichi. 1990. *The Borderless World: Power and Strategy in the Interlinked Economy*. New York: Harper Business.

————. 1995. *The End of the Nation State: The Rise of Regional Economies*. New York: Free Press.

Ong, Aihwa. 1991. The Gender and Labor Politics of Postmodernity. *Annual Review of Anthropology* 20:279–309.

———. 1999. *Flexible Citizenship: The Cultural Logics of Transnationality.* Durham, NC: Duke University Press.

———. 2006. *Neoliberalism as Exception: Mutations in Citizenship and Sovereignty.* Durham, NC: Duke University Press.

Perry, Martin, Lily Kong, and Brenda S. A. Yeoh. 1997. *Singapore: A Developmental City State.* New York: John Wiley and Sons.

Radjab, Muhamad. 1995. Semasa Kecil di *Kampung* [Village Childhood]. In *Telling Lives, Telling Histories: Autobiography and Historical Imagination in Modern Indonesia,* ed. and trans. Susan Rodgers. Berkeley: University of California Press.

Rodan, Garry. 1997. Singapore: Economic Diversification and Social Divisions. In *The Political Economy of South-East Asia,* ed. Garry Rodan, Kevin Hewison, and Richard Robison. Melbourne: Oxford University Press.

Rodgers, Susan. 1995. Imagining Modern Indonesia via Autobiography. In *Telling Lives, Telling Histories: Autobiography and Historical Imagination in Modern Indonesia,* ed. and trans. Susan Rodgers. Berkeley: University of California Press.

Rosenberg, Ruth, ed. 2003. *Trafficking of Women and Children in Indonesia.* Jakarta: International Catholic Migration Commission (ICMC) and American Center for International Labor Solidarity (ACILS).

Sassen, Saskia. 1991. *The Global City: New York, London, Tokyo.* Princeton, NJ: Princeton University Press.

———. 1998. *Globalization and Its Discontents: Essays on the New Mobility of People and Money.* New York: Free Press.

Sears, Laurie, ed., 1996. *Fantasizing the Feminine in Indonesia.* Durham, NC: Duke University Press.

Siegel, James. 1998. *A New Criminal Type in Jakarta: Counter-Revolution Today.* Durham, NC: Duke University Press.

Stasilius, D. K., and A. B. Bakan. 1997. Regulation and Resistance: Strategies of Migrant Domestic Workers in Canada and Internationally. *Asian and Pacific Migration Journal* 6 (1): 31–57.

Thompson, E. P. 1971. The Moral Economy of the English Crowd. *Past and Present* 50:76–136.

Trocki, Carl. 1990. *Opium and Empire.* Ithaca, NY: Cornell University Press.

Tsing, Anna. 2000. The Global Situation. *Cultural Anthropology* 15 (3): 327–60.

Turner, Peter. 2000. *Lonely Planet Indonesia.* Hawthorn, AUS: Lonely Planet Publications.

Warren, James. 1986. *Rickshaw Coolie: A People's History of Singapore (1880–1940).* Singapore: Oxford University Press.

———. 1993. *Ah Ku and Karayuki-san: Prostitution in Singapore, 1870–1940*. Singapore: Oxford University Press.

Waterson, Roxana. 1997. *The Living House: An Anthropology of Architecture in South-East Asia*. Singapore: Thames and Hudson.

Wee, C. J. Wan-Ling. 1996. Staging the New Asia: Singapore's Dick Lee, Pop Music, and a Counter-modernity. *Public Culture* 8 (3): 489–510.

———. 2002. Introduction: Local Cultures, Economic Development, and Southeast Asia. In *Local Cultures and the "New Asia": The State, Culture and Capitalism in Southeast Asia*, ed. C. J. Wan-Ling Wee. Singapore: Institute for Southeast Asian Studies.

Yeoh, Brenda S. A., Elspeth Graham, and Paul J. Boyle. 2002. Migrations and Family Relations in the Asia Pacific Region. *Asian and Pacific Migration Journal* 11 (1): 13–46.

Yeoh, Brenda S. A., and Shirlena Huang. 1998. Negotiating Public Space: Strategies and Styles of Migrant Female Domestic Workers in Singapore. *Urban Studies* 35 (3): 583–602.

———. 2000. "Home" and "Away": Foreign Domestic Workers and Negotiations of Diasporic Identity in Singapore. *Women's Studies International Forum* 23 (4): 413–29.

Yeoh, Brenda S. A., Shirlena Huang, and Joaquin Gonzalez III. 1999. Migrant Female Domestic Workers: Debating the Economic, Social and Political Impacts in Singapore. *International Migration Review* 33: 114–36.

8 AMBIVALENT INQUIRY

Dilemmas of AIDS in the Republic of Congo

David Eaton

The emergence of AIDS has posed profound dilemmas of individual and collective diagnosis in societies of francophone central Africa, as elsewhere. The problems brought by the epidemic have been complicated by the social disruption, insecurity, and violence associated with difficult political transitions in the region over the past two decades.

Field research in the Republic of Congo (hereafter "Congo") revealed to me some of the contradictions these situations engendered in the years leading to the country's devastating civil war of 1997. The volubility of modern medicine about the epidemic in the country during this time, especially in its capital, Brazzaville, contrasted with seeming silences about AIDS in other spheres of public life. By looking more closely at these apparent silences, though, we can discern understandings of social relations, the body, and affliction that animate experience, construct knowledge, and define choice in relation to HIV and AIDS. These practices of interpretation reflect not only modern conjunctures but also longer-term histories in this region of Africa.

In what follows, I consider how these understandings of AIDS have provided many Congolese with languages of life and hope through which they can pragmatically navigate the treacherous terrain in which the epidemic is taking place. I also describe, however, how these ways of knowing AIDS have complicated the acceptance of the epidemic as a real and present threat, undermined the ostensible roles of foreign actors in anti-AIDS programs, and problematized the place of HIV antibody testing as a resource for affected individuals and communities.

I conclude with reflections on the ambivalent potentials of speech about illness, with special reference to the contexts of therapy and to the clinical disclosure of diagnoses of HIV and AIDS.

UNSTABLE STATES

I begin by setting these issues in the context of Congo's difficult national circumstances during the 1990s (see also Eaton 2001, 2006). Indeed, a set of cumulatively disastrous political and economic trends posed similar problems for AIDS awareness and response as the decade unfolded in most countries across equatorial Africa, including not only Congo but also the former Zaire (now the Democratic Republic of Congo), Cameroon, and the Central African Republic. Deepening fiscal crises and political unrest in each of these states, occurring within austere post–Cold War international aid environments, meant that their capacities to respond to the epidemic were limited, and HIV seroprevalences continued to rise as the decade began.[1]

In Congo in particular, response to AIDS was conditioned by social change that began in the wake of *perestroika* and intensified with the collapse of the Soviet Union. After more than two decades of socialist government ended in 1991, the advent of multiparty democracy brought contested elections and accompanying civil convulsions. Factional warfare erupted in Brazzaville in June 1993, paralyzing the country, and soon left hundreds dead and thousands more dispossessed. State salaries remained unpaid for months, and conditions throughout the country—transport networks, factories, state services—continued to disintegrate. The national environment was increasingly that of crisis, and shifting political alliances and conflicts in the reconfigured political landscape cast into doubt existing principles of social cohesion.

Congo had distinguished itself early in the epidemic through its willingness to engage AIDS openly in cooperation with the international medical community. It was the first African country to publish full national statistics in 1986. The government under President Denis Sassou-Nguesso launched extensive radio and television campaigns, together with early and effective blood screening, in coordination with the World Health Organization's African regional headquarters then located in Brazzaville. Further outspoken leadership on AIDS was provided by President Lissouba in the early 1990s. By the middle of that decade, however, the continuing crises had brought the deterioration of public services, infrastructure, and security. Many formal programs had been curtailed or indeed never undertaken. State-sponsored condom sales—never high—were dropping, and HIV test results remained largely unreported to those tested.

AIDS thus came to threaten social life throughout the country and the region at a time when other bases of solidarity and shared purpose were being undermined by political and economic unrest. Questions of diagnosis, therapy, and response were embedded within these larger systems of political discourse and historical consciousness. "*Le pays est malade* [the nation is ill]," said some. Others asked, "Is this country cursed?"

In what follows, I explore how understandings of social relations, of human embodiment, and of affliction specific to this region of equatorial Africa were deeply involved in shaping comprehension of the epidemic. These understandings reflected modes of exchange predominant in Congolese life, and implied and grew from shared idioms, narratives, and senses of the social body. They were adapted to explain the emergence of AIDS and to manage the knowledge stimulated by its appearances as more and more individuals began to suffer physically from its effects. These understandings can be seen in the silences and avoidances so evident in public discourse around AIDS; in the suspicions and accusations that flourished in arenas from local to international; and in the logics of divination and diagnosis that influenced and constrained HIV testing, disclosure, and clinical treatment.

UNSPEAKABLE AFFLICTION

In Congo as in neighboring Cameroon and Zaire during this time, AIDS itself was often described to me in terms of absolute negativity. In these accounts it was evoked as a disease overwhelming humankind, without cure, uniquely catastrophic, which would obliterate the individual and stigmatize the family. Indeed many with whom I spoke doubted the existence of the disease or denied it entirely—"*Ça n'existe pas!*" Others flinched at the sound of the word SIDA (AIDS), dangerous in itself. Deceased musicians who had sung about AIDS were said to have died for their hubris.

Thus it seemed there was constant cultural labor to conceal, to privatize, to deny, to "prevent" AIDS—to keep it from developing as an element of thought and social experience. One man described the psychological shield that he hoped would help protect him against AIDS: he was careful not to think about it. There was a fabric of silences, secrets, and ruptures in knowledge; doctors did not tell their patients, husbands did not tell their wives. "I took the paper from the doctor and tore it up," one friend told me. "I realized . . . it is not necessary to speak this word [AIDS] itself."

References to the epidemic were often absent in public discourse that employed otherwise sophisticated languages of biomedicine. Although tuberculosis is among the most common causes of death for HIV-positive persons in this region, as in many parts of the world, detailed published accounts of the rising incidence of tuberculosis appeared without any mention of HIV or AIDS. One Congolese journal article, for example, described such an epidemic that had "emptied" the town of Mossendjo as its inhabitants fled in fear (*Aujourd'hui* 1993a). The hospital was "submerged," the article stated, and patients arrived "with the disease at an advanced and incurable stage, spitting blood and demonstrating a cruel loss of weight." Although this occurred in the town in Congo with the highest recorded levels of HIV among pregnant women in 1990—almost 12 percent (Congo 1994)—there was no mention of AIDS in the entire account. Instead, the article said the priority was to educate the population about tuberculosis and to face the task of vaccination. The most disturbing problem, it went on to say, was that the local population, "still backwards," attributed the disease to sorcery and possession (*Aujourd'hui* 1993a).

To a Western visitor, this apparent "absence of AIDS" could be striking in other domains as well. Obituaries and homages to eminent men felled by the syndrome made no mention of it (Eaton 2004). Healers in Brazzaville advertised treatments for wasting, prolonged diarrhea, *herpes zoster* (shingles)—all without naming AIDS itself. A North American physician commented to me on the strangeness of this silence about the syndrome itself, in contrast with the evident ubiquity of its effects. "People are spending their time mourning," he observed. "And the deaths are coming to younger and younger people. [Yet when] you ask someone: 'What did your brother-in-law die of?' The answer comes: 'toxoplasmosis.' Toxoplasmosis! They can tell you that he died of toxoplasmosis! You ask—how old was he? 'Thirty-two.' Well, you say, what does that mean about what happened to him? And they will say at this point, perhaps, that he probably died of 'that disease.'"

ACCEPTING THE EXISTENCE OF AIDS

Epidemics of tuberculosis, treatments for shingles, diagnoses of toxoplasmosis—each of these biomedically sophisticated discourses reveals not simply silence or an absence of AIDS, but rather the delicacy of the social pragmatics of discussion of the disease. Indeed, AIDS as a biomedical diagnosis—both individually and collectively, and as one diagnosis among many possible—posed distinctive social problems that could not be easily resolved.

Most crucially, for many of the people I spoke with in my fieldwork, acknowledging the existence of AIDS implied admitting the possibility—usually unverifiable—of their own infection. Without access to antibody testing, they could only infer they might be infected should they become ill or should their infant die. This enormous implication complicated all discussion and changed the stakes of identity: accepting the existence of AIDS meant entering a state of uncertainty as to one's own fate. Further, most sexually active adults found themselves unable to know or accurately judge whether they or their partners were infected. They were forced to risk their lives and the lives of their partners if they wanted to have children.[2]

In this context, fundamental changes in sexual life that could reduce risk often came only subsequent to emotionally charged shifts in interpretive perspective, experienced as crises of realization. For the individual, this might be sparked by a traumatic event, such as witnessing the death of a family member or the suffering of a friend or a lover in an advanced stage of the disease.[3] After oscillations between denial and alarm, changes might be negotiated over time with oneself, with lovers, and with friends and relatives. A man, for example, might begin to use condoms with lovers outside his primary relationship; he might cut back on his drinking with friends in bars; he might take more care in his choice of partners or cut back on the numbers of such partners; he might turn more fully to the practices of a church or cultic community; he might remain monogamous or if single abstain from sexual encounters he might earlier have had. For women, it was often more difficult, given their frequent subordination in male-dominated monetary and sexual economies (see for example Schoepf 1992; also Obbo 1993 and Susser and Stein 2004). The cultural and personal resources for changes that did emerge from these networks of suffering and witness were gradually shared with others in a growing and heterogeneous complex of discourse.

TACT, SUSPICIONS, AND ACCUSATIONS

The same "absences of AIDS" and uncertainties of diagnosis I encountered in Brazzaville were also evident to me during fieldwork in Congo's northern Sangha Province, a thousand kilometers by river from the capital. People in the north often stated to me that there was no AIDS there, despite studies that showed adult HIV seroprevalences of 4 percent and higher in the main towns (Congo 1994). Hospital patients had no way to be tested for HIV even if they were suffering from apparent symptoms of AIDS, as, with the state's deepening fiscal crises, the few test kits that had once been available had not been resupplied.

Further, in northern Congo as in Brazzaville, I found the same profound caution around elaboration of the epidemic in public discourse. I learned to introduce myself carefully and speak with circumspection, to avoid premature or sudden references to the topic, and to be especially careful in reference to any individual. My own affiliation with the national AIDS control program and the time I spent in hospitals and clinics were not necessarily reassuring to everyone. Individuals who were visibly ill might risk being identified and stigmatized as *sidéens* (persons with AIDS) as a result of their association with me. Further, as Philip Setel noted in northern Tanzania, the appearance of foreign experts and equipment that signify AIDS can seem "virtually the same thing as importing the syndrome itself" (1999: 244).

Alongside such suspicions of European and Euro-American outsiders like myself went interpretations of some modern social institutions—including biomedical clinics—as Western-controlled, exploitative, and potentially lethal. Such interpretations have a long history in central African societies, as elsewhere, arising in part from centuries of trauma and exploitation. They may be expressed within rumors of expropriation of body substances (White 2000), as when in north Congo I was told that colonial authorities had been believed to make aspirin from the crushed bones of seized Africans. Or they may be cast in idioms of occult forced labor, as among BaKongo in the 1960s, for whom hospitals were perceived as staging grounds for Africans taken through death to work under the ocean in slave factories producing Western goods (MacGaffey 1972: 58).[4]

Contemporary mistrust of biomedical authority in some regions of central Africa has been heightened by media campaigns that described contaminated needles as means of HIV transmission, as Susan Whyte (1997: 221) recounts from her research in rural Bunyole in eastern Uganda. Those suspected of transmitting the virus thus included health workers as well as traders and prostitutes. To these suspect social categories might be added "foreigner" and, in particular, "American."

Indeed, many in Congo and beyond believed or suspected that AIDS had originated in the United States and was being brought to Africa by Americans,[5] and at least some people wondered if I might be spreading the disease through my fieldwork. In north Congo, local residents asked me directly if I was giving injections of any kind during my stay. I found the topic more confrontationally handled in southern Cameroon during this time. Their vigorous denials of the existence of AIDS alternated with accusations of Western conspiracy and genocide. A Peace Corps volunteer told me that men would shout angrily at her "AIDS! You brought us AIDS!" on the streets of Douala.

Critiques of international medicine's role in the AIDS epidemic took similar shape in Congo during this time. In Brazzaville, a major weekly journal reviewed approvingly a book that claimed AIDS had been launched in trials of hepatitis-B vaccines in 1978 by a Columbia University professor with connections to the Soviet Union. The anonymous author of this review seemed to concur with the book's claim that the pandemic was biological warfare against "undesirable populations"—first homosexuals and then nonwhite and poorer peoples of the world.[6]

The arguments made in the review and in the book were homologous to those of sorcery accusations, attributing conscious malevolent intention to conspirators harnessing forces that bring illness to others. Whatever the correctness of these attributions, the claims made do accurately index several problematic issues in international biomedical practice and opinion in relation to HIV and AIDS. In particular, they condemn some medical experts for wanting to understand AIDS as a disease originating in stigmatized and exotic practices in rural Africa and accelerated by supposed African "promiscuity."[7] They also assert that AIDS may have been introduced into Africa by contaminated immunizations organized by the World Health Organization (WHO)—a possibility explored recently by a number of Western researchers as well.[8] The author of the review commented that such contaminated vaccines should be no surprise, saying that although the WHO presents itself as a humanitarian organization, it "often tests new medicines on poorer populations."

HIV TESTING AND ITS (NON)DISCLOSURE

The suspicions and accusations I have described are not only reactions to the violence and exploitation experienced by many Congolese populations over the past few centuries, brutal though these have been. Attempts to identify the social origin of affliction, and more specifically to discern evil intention and capacity, represent fundamental processes in contemporary central African systems of therapy.[9]

These practices and perceptions have created specific problems for programs of HIV antibody testing and disclosure in Congo, as in some other African contexts. They have played crucial roles in personal as well as collective diagnoses and in individual as well as international contexts. In what follows I examine how the HIV antibody test procedure has been conjoined with these regional logics of divination and diagnosis to create unique dilemmas and problems for those involved. I begin with problems encountered in implementing testing and counseling in clinics in Brazzaville and in other central and east African medical centers.

In Congo in the early 1990s, as HIV testing became more widely understood among some of the populations at risk, an increasing number of professionals began to inform their patients of test diagnoses. A few individuals came forward publicly with seropositive identities on television and radio and at public functions in Brazzaville to mobilize organizations and services for persons with HIV and AIDS.

But where testing was offered, it created a set of ethical dilemmas. To begin with, many people said they would not want to be tested or to learn their test results.[10] They questioned the wisdom and usefulness of knowing one's condition, citing the lack of a cure and equating seropositivity with illness and imminent death.[11] They also feared that knowledge of their condition would not be properly contained and could lead to stigmatization and abandonment, as test results were seldom available anonymously and clinic records were often openly discussed among staff.

Clinicians themselves were divided as to whether patients should be informed of a seropositive test. "Much better to let them be, to let them rest tranquilly," I was told by more than one physician. "It will only upset them, make them sick or sicker—or perhaps even provoke their suicide if their family and friends do not support them."

It has long been clear that HIV test disclosure can prove constructive in settings in which relatively high standards of medical care, counseling, and confidentiality were provided together with testing, as research in other cities of central and east Africa had already shown. In Kigali, the capital of Rwanda, more than 95 percent of approximately fifteen hundred women in a prospective cohort study chose to be tested for HIV and to receive medical care and counseling for them and their families (Allen et al. 1991).[12] Other clinically based studies in Zaire, Uganda, and Kenya by the early 1990s reported willingness to participate and a reduction in risk behavior (Kamenga et al. 1991; Moses et al. 1991; Muller et al. 1992; Green 2003: 197).

Only a few venues in Congo offered these high standards of confidentiality and private counseling. Notable among them was Brazzaville's national Outpatient Care Center for HIV infection in Brazzaville, established at the Central University Hospital there in 1994. When I visited the center the following year, its relative privacy, new equipment, and spotless facilities seemed to me in striking contrast with the heavily used main wards of the hospital and with the dilapidation of other state-sponsored health facilities I had visited. However, even a year after its opening, only handfuls of self-selected individuals were choosing to be tested and counseled there, and these tended to be individuals at relatively lower risk.[13]

In other settings in Congo where HIV antibody testing was conducted, profound reservations about its value and impact were common. As Marc-Eric Gruénais has documented in an important series of studies, the test was available only in a few other arenas: for blood screening, for anonymous serosurveillance in selected regional sites, for confirmatory diagnosis of severe illness in larger hospitals, and—especially in Brazzaville—by prescription request of a physician to one of four laboratories (see Gruénais 1993: 212 ff.; also Gruénais 1994). Although Brazzaville had been the first African city to systematically test all blood donations for HIV antibodies, beginning in 1986, a decline in donors followed over the next half decade, as very few people wanted to be tested. In the early 1990s, few donors returned to get their HIV test results; for example, at the National Blood Bank only 4 people in one year—of more than 350 seropositive individuals—chose to be informed and counseled. Many regular donors who were seropositive were not informed (Gruénais 1993).

More generally, there were very few independently initiated patient requests for testing in Brazzaville at this time, and these were usually to obtain credit or a visa. Gruénais estimated that only two or three out of every hundred nonanonymous tests were asked for voluntarily (1993: 210). Instead, most tests were given to sick people on entry to the hospital, usually without notification, and 30 to 70 percent tested seropositive. Often a partner was brought in also for a test without being told its nature either. Perhaps half of the tests were followed by services that informed patients of their results (Fassin 1993).

Didier Fassin (1994) saw these practices of nondisclosure as reflecting in part the challenge posed by AIDS to the legitimacy of the state (see also Dozon and Fassin 1989; Ashforth 2002). As I will explore in what follows, however, these silences also reflect tactics of speech and secrecy in daily life, regionally specific modes of inquiry into misfortune, and the effects of economic and family contexts of modern clinical practice.

SHARING DIAGNOSES: DILEMMAS
AND CONSEQUENCES

The delicacy of conversation involving possible AIDS diagnoses have been described by Susan Whyte in her accounts of her fieldwork in rural eastern Uganda. She writes that talk about serious illness that might be AIDS is "careful and subtle" among those closest to the person affected, noting that "a family with AIDS speaks carefully and acts hopefully, while more distant acquaintances of the sick person may engage in straight talk" (1997: 217).

In clinics in Brazzaville, as noted above, physicians and others feared that HIV test results would disrupt a couple or family, or would "enfeeble" the ill person psychologically and hasten their death. Many Congolese physicians felt the disclosure of such a serious diagnosis should only be made within a developed relationship, sometimes established over the course of hospitalization. Discussing the diagnosis with relatives could help temper accusations of sorcery within the family, but did not necessarily prevent such accusations. Gruénais (1993: 218) notes that this was particularly true with AIDS, where remissions could give the impression of efficacious care by various healers and procedures.

Informing the family about diagnoses is an especially serious dilemma in these contexts because of the frequent scarcity of resources available for therapy. A diagnosis of AIDS can lead to the withdrawal of resources from the sufferer if death from the syndrome is seen as inevitable. Thus, although Congolese clinicians often had confidence in the solidarity of the family in emotional support for the ill person, they also feared that some families would not spend scarce money for care for a person with a diagnosis of AIDS (Gruénais 1993: 217–18). But in their work in northern Tanzania, Julian Harris and colleagues (2003) also noted that any grain of hope for the ill person could ruin a poor family through the expenditures they would undertake, leading in some cases to the loss of schooling of other family members and the malnutrition or even death of children.

In the teaching hospital studied by Harris and colleagues (2003), Tanzanian physicians at a major teaching hospital often withheld diagnostic information from patients, while in many cases discussing the illness carefully and indirectly with family members. In explaining their practice, physicians at this hospital cited not only patients' cultural beliefs about illness, but also the difficult choices faced by many in regard to allocation of scarce economic resources to care. Many foreign physicians initially opposed to this withholding of information came to change their minds as they saw the often deleterious impact of direct disclosure on patients' families. When family members were made aware of diagnoses of serious illness, they were often encouraged to make the final decision about disclosure to the patient.

When disclosure was made to the patient, many physicians preferred a roundabout approach over several encounters, allowing the physician to assess comprehension and response as the patient gradually digested diagnostic and prognostic information. This mzunguko counseling method (from kuzunguka, "to circle around," in Kiswahili) embedded these clinical encounters within dominant local forms of social intercourse that prescribe extended greetings and indirect discussion before difficult topics are raised. Harris and colleagues see this method as "sensitive to the desire and readiness of patients to be informed or to remain ignorant of their diagnoses and prognoses," while respecting patients' autonomy and recognizing the often-key role of families in treatment decisions (2003: 912; see also Beyene 1992). This jibes with C. O. Davis's formulation of therapeutic knowledge "not as a closed totality, but as a living resource which adults learn from and teach each other, and with which people can try to live up to the undecidability of the vital moment" (2000: 19).

FAMILY AND THERAPY IN COMPARATIVE CONTEXT

Such observations give context and support to the argument made by David Armstrong (1987) and others that the change in mid–twentieth century practices of medical disclosure in the West was not the lifting of a century-long silencing of death, as Philippe Ariès (1974) had famously proposed. Rather it was a transformation in locally practiced biological discourse that, through medical ethics, now required the confession of the clinician and encouraged the dying person qua subject to speak.

Deborah Gordon and Eugenio Paci (1997) have described such practices as components of an emergent US-based "autonomy-control narrative" actualized by explicit disclosure, a narrative problematized by their field research in Tuscany, Italy, as well as by many other local studies in North America and elsewhere. Gordon and Paci, like Harris and colleagues and others (see Russ and Kaufman 2005), posit family relationships as a primary matrix within which these clinical politics are played out. In the Tuscan context, Gordon and Paci see the common practice of nondisclosure of cancer diagnoses as situated within a contrasting cultural narrative of "social embeddedness" that confers group protection through the cultivation of ambiguity and indirect speech about illness. They describe "a world of secrets and silences, of cultivated vagueness, manipulated hope, and institutionalized 'middle knowledge'" (see Weisman 1972).

In contrast, the extreme individualism of the autonomy-control narrative, with its informed consent and advance directives, risks undermining the social spaces and available existential options through which the individual finds his or her place within the life of an often hierarchical and unified family. Such a narrative is geared instead to ends of self-sovereignty and the elimination of uncertainty. To parse these conflicting imperatives anthropologically and ethically, Gordon and Paci call for comprehension of the particularity of local worlds from which greater individuality within family and therapeutic relationships can be sought.

John Janzen and William Arkinstall are among those who have pursued such research in KiKongo-speaking contexts similar to those of much of Brazzaville and the southern Republic of Congo today. Their joint studies in Lower Zaire found that illness-related decisions were handled collectively by a "therapy management group," distinct from the "lay referral system" proposed to function in Western societies to initiate medical consultation. This therapy management group was composed of family members and others who supported a patient in his or her quest for effective treatment. Janzen and Arkinstall described a pluralistic situation among BaKongo in which "loosely affiliated cults, services, clinics, and specialists must be mediated [by the group] within a broader structure of rights and organization of decisions shared by therapy, litigation, and ceremony" (1978: 134). Such procedures implied "the temporary surrender of the sufferer's individual decision-making rights," they wrote, as "the sufferer and his advocates select from optional and alternative remedies that, in consecutive episodes, create a total course of treatment" (137–38).

In many Western milieux the sufferer's family is often imagined primarily as a potential haven of common purpose and support. Comparative research into therapy management has shown, however, that households and families are complex composites of social groups that often conflict in their manipulation of knowledge and their setting of priorities in the care of an ill person (Nichter 2002: 82–83). Further, in Congolese circumstances, as in many other societies, the family is also widely understood as a potential source of danger to the sufferer. Members of the family may be responsible for the affliction as well as for its care; disclosure of illness in the sufferer implies that one of them may then be identified as its agentive cause. The disturbed social relations and malevolent intentions that may underlie such illness must be addressed if the sufferer is to find relief. Thus the quest for therapy among BaKongo described by Janzen and Arkinstall is integrated both with ceremonial and cultic hierarchies and with traditional courts of arbitration (1978: 134).

DANGEROUS CAPACITIES AND FULL DISCLOSURE

Simon Bockie (1993), writing of the BaManianga of the lower Congo (the BaKongo group of which he is a member), contrasts BaKongo and Western treatment of persons with AIDS. In the West, as Bockie sees it, effort is spent tracing origin, placing responsibility on segments of a population, and isolating pollution. In contrast, among BaManianga, Bockie states, a person with AIDS is not blamed and isolated, but instead is embraced by the community as a victim of misfortune. As a result, he says, clinical depression and suicide are almost unheard of.

However, as Bockie notes, suspicion may arise that "some antisocial force" is responsible for the illness, and this may lead to accusation of those who may have caused this misfortune through occult action. These are the "only true outcasts," as Bockie puts it; "those who willfully choose to go outside traditions and values determined by the ancestors" (1993: 38). The act of publicly establishing the identity of such individuals and their actions could be said to represent therapeutic "full disclosure" in BaKongo medicine. Such identification can be established through consultation through an *nganga ngombo* (a specialist in divination);[14] in the past this was sometimes done through a poison ordeal. Whatever its means, this identification is in some ways the inversion of Euro-American full disclosure in HIV testing and counseling policies. Indeed Bockie sees these latter as failing to identify the source of affliction and instead blaming, isolating, and demoralizing the victims of ill fortune.

Further, the HIV test procedure itself may be understood by some as a diagnosis of occult capacity for malevolent action. As in divination or as in postmortem autopsy for witchcraft substance found in the belly (*kundu*, in KiKongo, with parallel terms in other equatorial Bantu languages), the test may reveal internal body components and capacities that are potentially dangerous to others. Such lines of interpretation do not necessarily sustain or recognize certain Euro-American distinctions between material, spiritual, and intentional attributes of a person.

Thus a positive HIV antibody test makes an individual vulnerable to a form of accusation in which this marker of a physical state is also seen as a sign of potential malevolent intention. Katherine Fritz's research, like Whyte's also based on fieldwork in eastern Uganda, confirms this. She describes "interpretations, popular in contemporary Uganda, of asymptomatic, serostatus-aware, HIV-infected individuals as clear dangers to their communities" (Fritz 1999). These individuals were often perceived to harbor destructive intentions, and to purposefully infect others.

Whyte has commented on such stories, also in a Ugandan context: "There are all kinds of rumours and remarks about 'victims' who do not want to die alone and entice unsuspecting men and women into playing sex. . . . Such rumours of bad-heartedness were almost always anonymous; unnamed 'victims' were posited. Rarely did I hear of specific individuals who intentionally tried to kill people and were publicly confronted about it" (Whyte 1997: 220).

In my own fieldwork, I found staff at Brazzaville's Outpatient Care Center suggested to me that in most cases, as best they could judge, individuals diagnosed seropositive had acted responsibly to reduce risk to others. I was told by others not affiliated with the center, however, that the Congolese National Blood Bank discouraged and carefully restricted disclosure of serostatus (partly explaining the low rate of return by those tested to get their results), because once informed they were infected, many individuals would respond by seeking to pass the virus to others. I was assured that numerous such cases existed. A man diagnosed as seropositive, for example, might say to himself "I have my money, and I'm going to use it to have multiple partners before I become too ill." At the root of such actions, people told me, was an unwillingness to "die alone."

At the community level, as Whyte has argued in relation to eastern Uganda, programs of testing thus created not only awareness of risk—a goal of those implementing the testing—but an "increased consciousness of invisible danger [that promoted] suspicion and a special combination of rumour, gossip, insinuation, and worry" (1997: 218–19). Indeed, heightened levels of sorcery accusations and subsequent killings of elders were reported in certain northern provinces of Congo during my fieldwork, as more and more young people sickened and died of mysterious wasting diseases (see LeClerc-Madlala 1997, Ashforth 2002, and Stadler 2003 for comparable situations in South Africa).

Yet anthropological researchers have long emphasized the desperate need for more open discourse and access to accurate knowledge as crucial in response to the epidemic in African communities as elsewhere. Philip Setel has written from his work in Tanzania that "the least that any AIDS-prevention program can do is to ensure that young people have the knowledge necessary to save their lives and the material means and the social support to put the knowledge into practice" (1999: 246). Christine Obbo has described dominant male and elite voices in Uganda as silencing and overriding others in discourse and discussion on sexuality and AIDS, especially those she characterizes as "muted voices of women" and "silent voices of girls in need of awakening" (1993: 80). Like Brooke Schoepf (1995), who has advocated frank and open dialogue on sexuality, gender, and AIDS risk, Obbo has called for "new forms of discourse . . . [that use] culture as a tool to negotiate societal survival while at the same time exposing . . . class, gender and self-serving indifference" (1993). The place of diagnostic technologies in such new forms of discourse seems a particularly problematic and crucial one.

CONCLUSION: HOPE, SECRECY, AND THE AMBIVALENCE OF KNOWLEDGE ABOUT AIDS

In studies spanning more than a decade, Mary-Jo Good and colleagues have explored the constitution of hope in biomedical clinical settings, in the United States but also more recently in east African medical centers (M. D. Good et al. 1999; see also M. D. Good et al. 1990). In their research published in 1999, Good and colleagues examined ethical dilemmas faced by physicians in Tanzania and in Kenya brought by the need to provide appropriate counseling and palliative care to the large numbers of patients with AIDS. They saw physicians as challenged to develop new means of communication and therapy in the face of "unhealthy" silences in practices of disclosure and counseling. One response at the Tanzanian center was to start a program to explore the teaching of counseling in physician training. A contrasting Kenyan approach at the National Hospital in Nairobi created a multitiered system with separate private fee-for-service treatment offices that created a "political economy of hope" founded in social inequality.

The social location of hope, therefore, and its relation to speech and silence, remains problematic in these communities facing AIDS. The broader dimensions of this question, as has been shown above, go beyond the clinic across communities and regions of Africa and elsewhere. To many people in rural eastern Uganda, again according to Susan Whyte (1997), seropositivity meant not only stigma, but hopelessness. Understanding their problems as AIDS did not create possibilities for social support and plans for action that were available through other interpretations of misfortune, which instead emphasized disturbed relationships. It was only "saved" Christians, and "those urbanized and educated [into] the national 'enlightened' discourse of 'living positively,'" who were likely to embrace diagnoses of HIV seropositivity and AIDS. Divination, in contrast, never pointed to the disease and allowed people to remain instead "in the subjunctive mode of possibility and hope" (Whyte 1997: 212–16, 223; see also Whyte 2002).[15]

Thus the apparent silences around AIDS evoked at the beginning of this paper can be understood as evidence of other contexts of possibility, negotiated within complex dynamics of family and community. A related theme emerges from Maud Radstake's research in Ghana, in which she found that secrecy and denial were "strategic choices" made by individuals with AIDS to allow them to keep options open to maintain relationships and cope with their illness. Secrecy—although a crucial barrier to the provision of home care from outside the household—was a prerequisite to family care, a care based on reciprocity rather than solidarity and responsibility (Radstake 2000, reviewed by Mill in 2003).

Given these contradictory realities, what possibilities exist for forms of knowledge, speech, and diagnosis that could help more people to escape infection with HIV or to cope more fully with its effects? Obviously, well-managed testing, effective treatment options, and a decrease in stigma can play a major role in shifting attitudes over time—as happened in the United States with many cancer diagnoses. Across many societies, HIV testing has stimulated activist groups who work to transform the circumstances and conditions of research and care. The emergence of antiretroviral combination therapies in the late 1990s has transformed the stakes of testing wherever these have become available, as shown, for example, in Vinh-Kim Nguyen's research (2005) in Cúte d'Ivoire and Burkina Faso, and in South Africa's revolutionary Treatment Action Campaign and AIDS Law Project (ALP 2007).

However, as Edward Green (2003: 128–34) and Brooke Schoepf (2000), among others, have cautioned, we must also keep a clear sense of the limits of treatment in the majority of African contexts. Despite sharply increased national and international commitments to public financing of diagnosis and care, in 2006 less than a quarter of Africans in need of antiretrovirals were receiving them, with the numbers "dwindling to less than five percent" in rural areas (Farmer and Garrett 2006) and to an estimated 4 percent, for example, in the Democratic Republic of Congo (PANA 2007). In the Republic of Congo, Minister of Health and Population Alain Moka went so far as to put the number of people receiving adequate treatment nationwide in 2003 as "about 100" (IRIN 2003) of the roughly 130,000 people estimated to be seropositive (4.2 percent of the population) (Gouala 2004). In Congo, as elsewhere, these problems of HIV/AIDS care are conjoined with those of other public health burdens such as malaria, tuberculosis, typhoid, and malnutrition, reflecting in part the disruption brought by the 1997 civil war and its aftermath (IRIN 2007; M'Boussa 2002; Mikangou 2003; Reuters 2007).

Given these circumstances, many of the problems of knowledge and action discussed in this chapter seem likely to remain salient in many African milieux. Taken together, these conditions of illness and options for care give weight to Katherine Fritz's observation (1999; see also Fritz 1998), based on her work in eastern Uganda, that "the Euro-American value of full disclosure, as embodied in voluntary counseling and testing programs, faces challenges that have been only vaguely recognized by practitioners of public health.'" Indeed, the dilemmas that have attended much HIV testing and disclosure in Congo have been shaped not only by economic constraints, lack of effective treatment, and stigmatization, but also by widely shared understandings of human capacities that offer alternative explanations of illness, by tactics of speech and conversation that protect vulnerable persons, and by potential courses of therapy embedded in familial dynamics and regionally specific social institutions. For medical personnel to address the perceived causes of suffering while respecting and protecting the patient and the family, they have had to engage circumstances and conceptions of person, responsibility, and misfortune unfamiliar or obscure to clinic workers in some other societies. These continue to problematize the possibilities for AIDS awareness and treatment, and especially for HIV testing, in this region of Africa as elsewhere throughout the world.

NOTES

1. In Brazzaville, seroprevalence among pregnant women rose from 3.5 percent in 1988 to 7.3 percent in 1990 and 8.3 percent in 1991 (WHO 1992). In other Congolese towns where similar sentinel-site serosurveillance was conducted, rates in 1990 ranged from 2.4 percent to 11.2 percent. Lower rates were reported in smaller towns and villages of the region.

2. The risk involved in procreation was heightened by the common belief that semen is necessary for the proper growth of the fetus and should be acquired by the woman through repeated intercourse during pregnancy (Schoepf 1995: 41).

3. In Kigali, Rwanda, men stressed repeatedly that it had been firsthand experience with AIDS—seeing or knowing a person, often a family member or friend, who was ill or had died of AIDS—that had brought them to change their own risk

behavior (Eaton 1991: 7–8). Susser and Stein (2004: 134) make a similar observation based on studies in southern Africa.

4. See Rugalema (2004) and Heald (2002) for discussions of local interpretations of biomedical discourse on HIV and AIDS in eastern and southern Africa.

5. Douglas Feldman in 1987 reported half of his informants in Kigali, Rwanda, as saying that AIDS came from America (1987: 97). This, together with similar trends in African news coverage early in the epidemic (Lear 1990), indicates the wide currency of these perceptions.

6. *Aujourd'hui* (1993b). The author of the unsigned article reviews these claims as they are reportedly made in a "recent book by Doctors Robert Strecker and [Alan] Cantwell." I have not been able to locate the reviewed book, but other books by Cantwell (1988, 1993) apparently develop similar themes. See Farmer (1992) for a detailed discussion of the relation between local and transnational accusations that sets them in a context of economic and political exploitation.

7. One article in the *Review of Infectious Diseases*, for example, discussed "cultural practices" contributing to the transmission of HIV in the following order: female circumcision and infibulation, promiscuity, female infertility, homosexuality and anal intercourse, bloodletting and blood brotherhood, injection doctors and scarification, and contact with nonhuman primates (Hrdy 1987).

8. Hooper (1999) argues that the emergence of HIV stemmed from oral polio vaccine given to more than a million people in the then Belgian Congo in the late 1950s. See Martin (n.d.) for key documents relating to Hooper's claims and their critics.

9. The degree to which sorcery and witchcraft accusations have come to dominate in circumstances where other inquiries and remedies have been employed (involving especially charms, cults of affliction, and the propitiation of ancestral and nature spirits) is an open question in equatorial African communities. See Andersson (1968), Janzen (1982), MacGaffey (1986), Vansina (1990), Geschiere and Fisiy (1995), and Hersak (2001), among others, on these issues. Hersak cautions against the "pervasive tendency . . . to amalgamate sources from various sectors into a single Kongo universe, devoid of seeming contradictions . . . [flattening] the rich fabric of specificity and diversity . . . into 'uniform, but fictive, custom'" (2001: 616–21).

10. Similarly, Whyte (1997) writes about the widespread reluctance of individuals to be tested in eastern Uganda and the potential socially destructive consequences of this procedure, especially away from islands of high-level clinical intervention in capital cities. Letters to Ugandan newspaper health advice columnists in the mid-1990s evidenced the letter writers' preference not to learn their HIV serostatus (Whyte 1997: 214).

11. This, of course, did not address questions of how informing oneself could better protect one's partners and family. It also did not fully consider potentially life-prolonging treatments of opportunistic infections that were available to some at that time.

12. Patients enrolled received not only counseling, but also free medical care for themselves and their immediate families for the duration of the study, jointly administered by the Rwandan Ministry of Health and the University of California, San Francisco.

13. This dearth of voluntary patients is reported at a similarly well-equipped Center for Outpatient Treatment supported by the Red Cross in the city of Pointe Noire on the coast (*Le Moustique* 2004).

14. See Janzen (1982: 14–15) for a typology of divination in this region of Africa.

15. Byron Good has raised similar issues in his examination of the subjunctivizing elements of illness stories, in which narrators are "deeply committed to portraying a [world] in which healing was an open possibility" (1994: 153).

REFERENCES

AIDS Law Project and the Treatment Action Campaign (ALP). 2007. Submission to Human Rights Commission on Healthcare Services: 17 April 2007, Annexure 3. ALP, 17 April. www.alp.org.za/modules.php?op=modload&name=News&file=article&sid=359.

Allen, S., et al. 1991. Human Immunodeficiency Virus Infection in Urban Rwanda: Demographic and Behavioral Correlates in a Representative Sample of Childbearing Women. *Journal of the American Medical Association* 266 (12): 1657–63.

Andersson, E. 1968. *Churches at the Grass-Roots: A Study in Congo-Brazzaville.* London: Lutterworth Press.

Ariès, Philippe. 1974. *Western Attitudes toward Death.* Baltimore: Johns Hopkins University Press.

Armstrong, D. 1987 Silence and Truth in Death and Dying. *Social Science and Medicine* 24 (8): 651–57.

Ashforth, A. 2002. An Epidemic of Witchcraft? The Implications of AIDS for the Post-Apartheid State. *African Studies* 61 (1): 121–43.

Aujourd'hui. 1993a. Le tuberculose tue à Mossendjo [Tuberculosis Kills in Mossendjo]. 8 November.

———. 1993b. Afrique et SIDA [Africa and Aids]. 29 November.

Beyene, Y. 1992. Cross-Cultural Medicine, a Decade Later: Medical Disclosure and Refugees—Telling Bad News to Ethiopian Patients. *Western Journal of Medicine* 157 (3): 328–32.

Bockie, S. 1993. *Death and the Invisible Powers.* Bloomington: Indiana University Press.

Cantwell, A., Jr. 1988. *AIDS and the Doctors of Death: An Inquiry into the Origin of the AIDS Epidemic.* Los Angeles: Aries Rising.

————. 1993. *Queer Blood: The Secret AIDS Genocide Plot.* Los Angeles: Aries Rising.

Congo, Republic of. 1994. *Bulletin epidemiologique semestriel* [Weekly Epidemiological Bulletin]. Brazzaville: National AIDS Control Program.

Davis, C. O. 2000. *Death in Abeyance: Illness and Therapy among the Tabwa of Central Africa.* Edinburgh: Edinburgh University Press.

Dozon, J.-P., and D. Fassin. 1989. Raisons epidemiologique et raisons d'état: Les enjeux socio-politiques du SIDA en Afrique [Epidemiological Reasons and Reasons of the State: The Sociopolitical Stakes of AIDS in Africa]. *Sciences Sociales et Santé* 7 (1): 21–36.

Eaton, D. 1991. Perceptions of HIV and AIDS among Men of Kigali, Rwanda. Working paper, Center for AIDS Prevention Studies, Project San Francisco/Rwandan Ministry of Health.

————. 2001. Men's Lives and the Politics of AIDS in the Republic of Congo. PhD diss., University of California, Berkeley.

————. 2004. Understanding AIDS in Public Lives. In *HIV/AIDS in Africa: Beyond Epidemiology,* ed. Ezekiel Kalipeni, Susan Craddock, Joseph Oppong, and Jayati Ghosh. Malden, MA: Blackwell.

————. 2006. Diagnosing the Crisis in the Republic of Congo. *Africa* 76 (1): 44–69.

Farmer, P. 1992. *AIDS and Accusation: Haiti and the Geography of Blame.* Berkeley: University of California Press.

Farmer, P., and L. Garrett. 2007. From "Marvelous Momentum" to Health Care for All: Success Is Possible with the Right Programs. *Foreign Affairs* 86 (2).

Fassin, D. 1993. HIV Testing and Disclosure in Brazzaville, Congo. Workshop on the social sciences and AIDS in Africa, Abidjan, Cúte d'Ivoire.

————. 1994. Le domaine privé de la santé publique: Pouvoir, politique et SIDA au Congo [The Private Sphere of Public Health: Power, Politics and AIDS in Congo]. *Annales Histoire et Sciences Sociales,* no. 4: 745–75.

Feldman, D. 1987. Public Awareness of AIDS in Rwanda. *Social Science and Medicine* 24 (2): 97–100.

Fritz, K. E. 1998. Women, Power and HIV Risk in Rural Mbale District, Uganda. PhD. diss., Yale University.

————. 1999. Dangerous Times: Local Interpretations of Asymptomatic HIV Infection in Contemporary Uganda. Paper presented at the American Anthropological Association annual meeting, Chicago.

Geschiere, P., and C. Fisiy. 1995. *Sorcellerie et politique en Afrique: La viande des autres.* Paris: Karthala. Trans. J. Roitman and P. Geschiere as *The Modernity of Witchcraft: Politics and the Occult in Postcolonial Africa* (Charlottesville: University of Virginia Press, 1997).

Good, B. 1994. *Medicine, Rationality, and Experience: An Anthropological Perspective.* Cambridge: Cambridge University Press.

Good, M. D., et al. 1999. Clinical Realities and Moral Dilemmas: Contrasting Perspectives from Academic Medicine in Kenya, Tanzania, and America. *Daedalus* 128 (4): 167–96.

Good, M. D., B. Good, C. Schaffer, and S. Lind. 1990. American Oncology and the Discourse on Hope. *Culture, Medicine, and Psychiatry* 14:59–79.

Gordon, D., and E. Paci. 1997. Disclosure Practices and Cultural Narratives: Understanding Concealment and Silence around Cancer in Tuscany, Italy. *Social Science and Medicine* 44 (10): 1433–52.

Gouala, Joseph. 2004. HIV/AIDS Spreading in Congo, Particularly among Women. *Agence France-Presse*, 12 February. www.aegis.com/news/afp/2004/AF040244.html.

Green, E. 2003. *Rethinking AIDS Prevention.* Westport, CT: Praeger.

Gruénais, M.-E. 1993. To Speak or Not to Speak: Stakes of Disclosure of Seropositivity in Congo. Workshop on the social sciences and AIDS in Africa, Abidjan, Cúte d'Ivoire.

———. 1994. Qui informer ? Médecins, familles, tradipraticiens et religieux au Congo. *Psychopathologie africaine* 26 (2): 189–209.

Harris, J., et al. 2003. Disclosure of Cancer Diagnosis and Prognosis in Northern Tanzania. *Social Science and Medicine* 56 (5): 905–14.

Heald, S. 2002. It's Never as Easy as ABC: Understandings of AIDS in Botswana. *African Journal of AIDS Research* 1:1–10.

Hersak, D. 2001. There Are Many Kongo Worlds: Particularities of Magico-Religious Beliefs among the Vili and Yombe of Congo-Brazzaville. *Africa* 71 (4): 614–40.

Hooper, E. 1999. *The River: A Journey to the Source of HIV and AIDS.* Boston: Little, Brown and Company.

Hrdy, D. B. 1987. Cultural Practices Contributing to the Transmission of HIV in Africa. *Review of Infectious Diseases* 9 (6): 1109–19.

Integrated Regional Information Networks (IRIN). 2003. Congo: Media Professionals Create National HIV/AIDS Awareness Network. *IRIN PlusNews*, 29 August.

———. 2007. Congo: Boost for Anti-Malaria Campaign. 21 March. www.irinnews.org/Report.aspx?ReportId=70849.

Janzen, J. 1982. *Lemba, 1650–1930: A Drum of Affliction in Africa and the New World.* New York: Garland.

Janzen, J., and W. Arkinstall. 1978. *The Quest for Therapy: Medical Pluralism in Lower Zaire.* Berkeley: University of California Press.

Kamenga, M., et al. 1991. Evidence of Marked Sexual Behavior Change Associated with Low HIV-1 Seroconversion in 149 Married Couples with Discordant HIV-1 Serostatus: Experience at an HIV Counselling Center in Zaire. *AIDS* 5 (1): 61–67.

Lear, D. 1990. AIDS in the African Press. *International Quarterly of Community Health Education* 10 (3): 253–64.

LeClerc-Madlala, S. 1997. Infect One, Infect All: Zulu Youth Response to the AIDS Epidemic. *Medical Anthropology Quarterly* 17 (4): 363–80.

MacGaffey, W. 1972. The West in Congolese Experience. In *Africa and the West*, ed. P. Curtin. Madison: University of Wisconsin Press.

————. 1986. *Religion and Society in Central Africa: The BaKongo of Lower Zaire*. Chicago: University of Chicago Press.

Martin, B. N.d. Polio Vaccines and the Origins of AIDS: Some Key Writings. www.uow.edu.au/arts/sts/bmartin/dissent/documents/AIDS (accessed 21 September 2004).

M'Boussa, J., D. Yokolo, B. Pereira, S. Ebata-Mongo. 2002. A Flare-up of Tuberculosis Due to War in Congo Brazzaville. *The International Journal of Tuberculosis and Lung Disease* 6 (6): 475–78.

Mikangou, Lyne. 2003. Les Brazzavillois 'achètent les maladies' dans la rue [In Brazzaville They 'Buy Illnesses' in the Street]. Santé-Congo, Interpress Service News Agency, 9 January. www.ipsinternational.org/fr/ (site discontinued).

Moses, S., et al. 1991. Controlling HIV in Africa: Effectiveness and Cost of an Intervention in a High-Frequency STD Transmitter Core Group. *AIDS* 5 (4): 407–11.

Le Moustique. 2004. Les voleurs d'espoir [The Stealers of Hope]. 16 April. www.afrioo.com/lemoustique (site discontinued).

Muller, O., et al. 1992. HIV Prevalence, Attitudes and Behaviour in Clients of a Confidential HIV testing and Counseling Centre in Uganda. *AIDS* 6 (8): 869–74.

Nguyen, V.-K. 2005. Antiretroviral Globalism, Biopolitics, and Therapeutic Citizenship. In *Global Assemblages: Technology, Politics, and Ethics as the Anthropological Problems*, ed. A. Ong and S. Collier, 124–44. Malden, MA: Blackwell.

Nichter, M. 2002. The Social Relations of Therapy Management. In *New Horizons in Medical Anthropology: Essays in Honour of Charles Leslie*, ed. M. Nichter and M. Lock, 81–111. London: Routledge.

Obbo, C. 1993. HIV: Men Are the Solution. *Population and Environment* 14 (3): 211–43.

Panapress (PANA). 2007. Four Percent of AIDS Infected Persons in DR Congo Receive ARVs. 4 April. www.panapress.com/dossindexlat.asp?code=eng001.

Radstake, M. 2000. *Secrecy and Ambiguity: Home Care for People Living with HIV/AIDS in Ghana.* Leiden: African Studies Center. Reviewed by J. Mill in *Social Science and Medicine* 57 (2003): 765.

Reuters. 2007. Congo (Brazzaville) Troubles. AlertNet, 26 March. www.alertnet .org/db/crisisprofiles/CG_TEN.htm?v = in_detail.

Rugalema, G. 2004. Understanding the African HIV Pandemic: An Appraisal of the Contexts and Lay Explanation of the HIV/AIDS Epidemic with Examples from Tanzania and Kenya. In *HIV and AIDS in Africa: Beyond Epidemiology,* ed. E. Kalipeni et al., 191–203. Malden, MA: Blackwell.

Russ, A. J., and S. Kaufman. 2005. Family Perceptions of Prognosis, Silence, and the "Suddenness" of Death. *Culture, Medicine, and Psychiatry* 29 (1): 103–23.

Schoepf, B. 1992. Women at Risk: Case Studies from Zaire. *The Time of AIDS,* ed. G. Herdt and S. Lindenbaum. Newbury Park, CA: Sage.

———. 1995. Culture, Sex Research and AIDS Prevention in Africa. *Culture and Sexual Risk: Anthropological Perspectives on AIDS.* ed. H. T. Brummelhuis and G. Herdt, 29–52. Amsterdam: Overseas Publishers Association/Gordon and Breach.

———. 2000. Theoretical Therapies, Remote Remedies. In *Dying for Growth: Global Inequality and the Health of the Poor,* ed. Jim Yong Kim et al. Monroe, ME: Common Courage Press.

Setel, P. W. 1999. *A Plague of Paradoxes: AIDS, Culture, and Demography in Northern Tanzania.* Chicago: University of Chicago Press.

Stadler, J. 2003. Rumor, Gossip and Blame: Implications for HIV/AIDS Prevention in the South African Lowveld. *AIDS Education and Prevention* 15 (4): 357–68.

Susser, I., and Z. Stein. 2004. Culture, Sexuality, and Women's Agency in the Prevention of HIV/AIDS in Southern Africa. In *HIV and AIDS in Africa: Beyond Epidemiology,* ed. E. Kalipeni et al., 133–44. Malden, MA: Blackwell.

Vansina, J. 1990. *Paths in the Rainforest: Toward a History of Political Tradition in Equatorial Africa.* Madison: University of Wisconsin Press.

Weisman, A. 1972. *On Dying and Denying: A Psychiatric Study of Terminality.* New York: Behavioral Publications.

White, L. 2000. *Speaking with Vampires: Rumor and History in Colonial Africa.* Berkeley: University of California Press.

Whyte, S. 1997. *Questioning Misfortune: The Pragmatics of Uncertainty in Eastern Uganda.* Cambridge: Cambridge University Press.

———. 2002. Subjunctivity and Subjectivity: Hoping for Health in Eastern Uganda. In *Postcolonial Subjectivities in Africa,* ed. R. Werbner, 171–90. London: Zed.

World Health Organization (WHO). 1992. Statistics from Serosurveillance of Pregnant Women in Africa. *AIDS and Society* 3 (2).

TO LIVE WITH WHAT WOULD
OTHERWISE BE UNENDURABLE, II

Caught in the Borderlands of Palestine/Israel

Michael M. J. Fischer

I

From the Balkan frontline trenches in Bosnian writer-director Danis Tanović's 2001 film *Ničija Zemlja* (*No Man's Land*, in which three incapacitated Serbian and Bosnian soldier-enemies are trapped together in a no-man's-land in a situation that the United Nations is incapable of mediating)[1] to the International Red Cross helicopter drops of prostheses to Afghans crippled by land mines, running on crutches to catch the humanitarian aid in Iranian writer-director Mohsen Makhmalbaf's 2001 film *Safar-e Qandahar* (*Journey to Qandahar*)—somewhere in the space between these Western and Eastern poles of the Middle Eastern theater sits the *Maus* cartoonist Art Spiegelman slumped over his drawing table, threatened on one side by a man with drawn curved sabre and on the other by a man with drawn gun, equally terrorized by al-Qaeda and by his own government (Spiegelman 2004). Such is the space in which we now (again) must find a way to live. Gilles Deleuze provides a nicely enigmatic harmonic for this modality of existence and a temporary fold from which the anthropologist might speak: "We have to manage to fold the line and establish an endurable zone in which to install ourselves, confront things, take hold, breathe—in short, think . . . to live with what would otherwise be unendurable" (Deleuze 1995: 111, 113).

. . .

Borderlands are folded over and crossed again, and recrossed. Membranes of the border are of varying porosities, closures and openings, subversions and states of exception, checkpoints and circumventions, surveillances and (in)securities, orders and disorders, fears and displacements, with the Real gazing back from holes in the defenses. Communicative and linguistic in- and recursions come through Arabic and Hebrew—distinctively differing Palestinian dialects and sociolects of Ramallah and Hebron, the Arabics of Algerian-returned PLO Kastel forces and Israeli Druze commanders, the Hebrew idioms of Mizrahi Israelis, and the Hebrew of "Insider Palestinians" who have learned their Hebrew in Israeli prisons and schools—but also occasionally through Cuban Spanish, GDR German, and the Russian of Palestinians trained in the former Soviet bloc, the Russian and Amharic of recent immigrants to Israel, Ladino, Judeo-Arabic, Yiddish, Polish, German, English, and American of other waves of immigrants to Israel, as well as the Arabic of Israeli Muslims, Christians, and Circassians, the literary Hebrew of Anton Shammas, and the literary Arabic of Sami Michael and Samir Naqqash. Where in these borderlands are the tent posts, the orientations, for humanitarian and human rights interventions?

II

We live (again) in an age in which the very institutions of humanitarian intervention are suspected of complicity, when the humanitarian industry all too often follows military intervention, like brigades of prostitutes and merchants in the wake of the armies of History, providing jobs and succor, but destroying local initiative, creating new vortices of power and intrigue, before moving on to the next urgent call, the next crisis, the next firestorm of emotion and outrage fanned by a restless telemedia machine that turns its theater lights and thundering and weeping program music from the elections in Poland to Tiananmen Square in Beijing, from Bosnia to Gaza, Rwanda to Chechnya, Colombia to Kashmir.

I want to turn the mirror back upon three of these theater lights: the sovereign subject (or political order, transnational infrastructures, stuttering religious revivalisms, and global civil societies or moral orders); the returns to subjectivities (the emotional and personal order of selves and ethical actions); and the constraints on a politics of democratic pluralism in a world of telemedia frenzy phantasmagoria, traumatic memory, psychological displacements, and repetitions of ideological scripts. For purposes of this volume, I will focus attention primarily on the second of these: the returns to subjectivity, returns in both senses of returns, to the unstable grounds of certitude or witnessing, and returns as in payoffs, or second-order rhetorics, the performativities of rhetorics of subjectivities. I want to ask what the method of ethnography of social contexts can do, using a series of sites as crucibles. But at least a word first on the two other theater lights, in the context of the 1990s and early twenty-first century, is in order, given that the Palestinian-Israeli borderland is also part of shifts in a larger world reordering.

Palestine joins Kosovo, Albania, Afghanistan, Sudan, and now Iraq in becoming an exemplar of the late-1990s shift from pre-1970s paradigms of state-led modernization (Western, socialist, and third-world varieties; and their dependency theory critiques) to emergence of global regimes of governance of North-South relations through networks of NGOs, donor governments, military establishments, and private companies. In various accounts of these shifts a contrast is drawn between increasing density of economic, technological, political, and military interactions between North-North networks (North America, Europe, and East Asia) and international humanitarian aid and riot control in North-South networks (Castells 1996, 1998; Duffield 2001; Fassin 2002; Malkki 1995; Mbembe 2001; Pandolfi 2002). Among the key features of these shifts are: (1) a logic of consolidation and exclusion (rather than expansion and inclusion); (2) "black holes" of the excluded generating innovative and networked global criminal economies; (3) increased competition for resources, including control of the state, utilizing older ethnic and tribal cleavages, banditry, and genocide; (4) transformation of the nation-state from buffer between domestic and external economies to agency for adapting domestic economies for the global economy; and (5) selective incorporation of the South by populations needing to show themselves fit for consideration (Duffield 2001). There is a dovetailing between first-world governments' insistence upon security as now more endangered by underdevelopment than by interstate conflict; and humanitarian aid organizations' shift to conflict resolution, social reconstruction, and transformation of societies into not just liberal economic market relations but also democratic, pluralistic, political institutions.

"In studying the new wars," says Mark Duffield (2001: 6) at the outset of his survey of the merging of development and security, based in part on his long experience with the Sudan, "one is largely reliant on the contribution of political economy and anthropology." Anthropology, here, I take it, is the ethnography of social contexts, to crucibles of which in the Palestine-Israeli borderlands, I turn.

III

I want to begin with the returns to subjectivity: the payoffs and feedbacks among the registers of the political, psychological, linguistic, and bodily selves that we often turn to as witnesses in situations of trauma, as agents in judgments of ethical action, and as partners in creating those elementary forms of social life that we apperceive in friendship, hospitality, parenting, conversation, and gaming. I want to invoke two ethnographic situations from one of the most traumatic of on-going world conflicts: the first from a psychiatrist in Gaza, the second from an ethnographer of joint Palestinian-Israeli patrols in the years from May 1994 (Oslo I) to September 28 and 29, 2000.

First, Gaza psychiatrist Dr. Eyad el-Sarraj speaking at Tel Aviv University on June 18, 2003:

Both sides are so exhausted and frightened that it seems maybe the talks this time will hold. [The *hudna* or cease-fire collapsed a few weeks later.] We don't trust [Israeli prime minister Ariel] Sharon or Hamas. We in Gaza are in prison. The last two and a half years, each side has seen the ugliest side of the other. Neither side recognizes that the other can live with them peacefully. Israelis just want the Palestinian problem to go away. The occupation has lasted thirty-seven years, but has never been so ugly as the past two and a half years. Twenty-four percent of children under twelve dream of becoming martyrs. Stone-throwing kids of the first Intifada have become the suicide bombers of the second Intifada. There is radicalization of women, more so than of men, and women are the carriers and motivators of the culture of a society. In the first Intifada, Israelis practiced systematic humiliation of fathers: 55 percent of children witnessed beating of their father. The identification of a boy is with the power of the father. If the power of the father is not what he can identify with, he will switch to another source of power. In games we see boys identifying with and playing the roles of Jewish soldiers. There is also increasingly violent behavior towards other children. As they grow up Hamas takes the role of the father. I believe in every case of a suicide bomber there is a traumatic experience that has transformed them.

In the first Intifada, the *individual* was traumatized: stones thrown were responded to with rubber bullets and breaking of bones. In the second Intifada the *community* was traumatized: the noise of fighter planes, helicopters, drones, loudspeakers, breaking of the sound barrier puts the population into a state of chronic panic. Any sound is first thought to be maybe an F-16 even if it turns out to be only a washing machine. I myself have to shut off my refrigerator at night in order to get some sleep. After the attempt to assassinate [Hamas leader, Dr. Abdel Aziz] Rantisi, we saw some fifteen F-16s high in the sky—but it turned out to be only a cloud moving, and then we saw stars behind. Many children do not want to go to school for fear that when they return, there will be no home or parents, especially in Rafah where there have been many house demolitions. It is the psychopathology of Israelis to be so short-sighted, a form of paranoia, and a tribal psychology of revenge, especially among women. The level of aggression and violence among Palestinians increases: many are accused of being spies for Israel, which means also that their daughters cannot marry.

The celebration of martyrs is a form of denial: we have not had any opportunity to grieve for those who died, or for loss of land. Israelis need to go through such a grieving process too. The only way to build a peace movement is to have such self-insight. Why do families beat children? It is a habit, a routine, but it creates a culture of fear. The first Intifada was also a situation of children rebelling against their fathers and against all authority.

People are ready to die for country, and keep their homes clean, but the streets are dirty: the streets don't belong to them, they belong to the outside, to the Israelis, before them to Jordanians, to the Greeks, the Romans. The feeling is that public institutions do not belong to us, so it is OK to steal from the government. We are tribal: the state is always foreign and alien (including Arafat); the new jeeps and Mercedes cars of the elite are exactly like those of the Israelis. I myself was arrested three times by Arafat. The question of revenge is decided by the community: an honorable family will pursue revenge unless there is public apology and public taking of responsibility. The only honorable response then is to say yes. Public apology and public taking of responsibility would be good for Israelis because they too would become whole and reconciled with themselves. During the first Intifada a mayor in the north of Israel said we don't want Palestinians here, and if they are to be here they should be tattooed on the shoulder—the reaction reminds of the Nazis. When I was in Palestinian prison, I overheard a prison interrogation, the Palestinian interrogator started screaming, and then he started screaming in Hebrew, identifying with the aggression of the oppressor. I believe in one state, all equal before the law; I believe in the right of return of Jews who have biblical roots to the land, but I too have a right of return.

Salim Tamari, professor at Bir Zeit University and New York University, used his prerogative as chair of the session to respond, clarify, and focus some of the rough edges: "Sarraj is a mesmerizing speaker, but he essentializes as if Palestinians were all one community. Regarding public space: where civil society is strong, and where there is a tax base, the streets have become cleaner. In times of disorder, people turn inwards and protect themselves and their family. We need to rethink the concept of the state as based on territory and sovereignty. I don't think a one-state solution is the answer because it would extend the Israeli state, and mean giving up independence for Palestinians. I think we need to find a hybrid constitutional arrangement: if we guarantee mobility for Palestinians, and restitution or compensation, [the call for a Palestinian right of] return will be filtered." Tamari speculated about expanding the territorial pie so that Palestinians and Israelis would not be locked into a zero-sum game. For instance if the European Union could be expanded to include Palestine and Israel, there might be more psychological and political space for maneuver. (In 1994 in Barcelona there were discussions about Israeli accession to the EU, and the Europeans proposed that the way to this would be by including both Palestine and Israel. Once Turkey is brought into the EU, this may again become a viable possibility. In the meantime, Tamari may have been gesturing toward renewed talk of not a one- or a two-state solution, but a three-state solution among Jordan, Palestine, and Israel.)[2]

What I wish to draw attention to here is not the political debates on the Palestinian-Israeli struggles, but the mobilization of psychoanalytic and psychotherapeutic discourses. El-Sarraj understands his task at the Gaza Community Mental Health Program, established in 1990 to treat traumatized children, battered women, and adult (male) torture victims, as treating mental illness—not individual illnesses (as with a chemical imbalance), but illnesses that have family dynamics and also political dynamics. He wants at the same time to make the therapeutic setting a pedagogical site for democracy. Therapeutic sessions are, he points out, sometimes the first time that fathers are made to, and learn to, listen to their children. People have to be taught democracy in a context where there has been none. "Our mental health problems are the result of the political and economic situation. Our society has been dominated by extremism . . . violence has become endemic in our culture, anything else is seen as surrender. I oppose this both as an activist and a psychiatrist. [Moving away from violence] is very hard to implement because it threatens the establishment on both sides. There are many examples around the world where nonviolence has been successful, like India and South Africa. We have a just cause, and I believe we can win our struggle through taking the moral high ground" (el-Sarraj 2003).

Many of the same nightmares (of schools being bombed or of having parents killed while one is away at school)—with refusals to go to school, psychosomatic fevers and distress—happen also to Israeli children, something el-Sarraj and his international colleagues are aware of. Indeed el-Sarraj is involved in an unusual project to train psychotherapists with members of the Psychology Department of Tel Aviv University as well as seven other universities around the world (Tunisia, Australia, United States, and United Kingdom), as well as in a research collaboration on children and violence with the Department of Social Medicine at Harvard. Joint projects between Palestinians and Israelis at the moment are always fraught, sometimes amusingly, but not trivially so.[3]

The structural, psychotherapeutic, affect-attentive approach of these psychiatrists seems more promising than short, direct first-person testimonials, the technique relied upon by so many journalists, ideologues, and propagandists on all sides. Subjectivity, perhaps, one might say, is not usefully located merely in the enunciative function, particularly where traumatized subjects can mainly articulate laments. A minor test case is to read two accounts of the April 2002 invasion of Jenin, one a collection of bewildered accounts of helpless people with no effective agency edited by Ramzy Baroud (2003), the other an account based on interviews with mainly reservists who were called up from their lives, wives, and small children to perform the operation with as little loss of life to themselves and to civilians as possible (Goldberg 2003). The two accounts are hard to reconcile, except that in Baroud's list of the fifty-seven dead Palestinians half are identified as fighters of either Hamas, Islamic Jihad (including its local twenty-four-year-old leader, Mahmud Tawalbe), the al-Aqsa Brigade, or the Palestinian Security Forces, who refused to leave the Jenin camp with the majority of residents and chose to fight.[4] Readers will believe one, not the other account; neither will persuade or elicit much more than exasperation from the other side. Documentary film has similar problems: editing procedures are so well recognized that few who are not predisposed to the message of the filmmakers take these works at face value.

In highly charged arenas, the feedback among the four registers of subjectivity (each with their split or doubled natures)[5]—citizen subjecthood or political agency; self- or personhood and subjectivity; discursive/enunciative position; and somaticized responses—is required in the struggle "to authorize the real." Testimony, first-person witnessing, subjective-emotional certitude alone do not do the job for either mental health or social governance.[6] Indeed many of the most politically conscious in South Africa refused to participate in the Truth and Reconciliation Commission hearings on the grounds that they refused to be considered victims. They thereby remind us that more forms of agency exist than witnessing and testifying, and that witnessing and testifying are themselves genre forms within hierarchies of power and adjudication.

IV

Much more could be said about the psychiatric discourse that el-Sarraj begins to place before us, but I want to turn first to another venue, crucible, and microcosm of "living with what would otherwise be unendurable": the joint Palestinian-Israeli patrols of the post–Oslo I period, and particularly of the period after the 1996 Tunnel Incident that reset the game.

I draw here on a remarkable ethnographic dissertation by Deborah Heifetz-Yahav (2002), who managed to gain permission both from the IDF (Israel Defense Forces) and the Palestinian Authority to hang out with these joint patrols from 1997 until they came to an abrupt end. The joint patrols were set up by the Oslo Agreements as a confidence-building device to put security cooperation on public display. As such they were an effort to turn a theater of war into a theater of peace. At times, she writes, it seemed to the men involved a theater of the absurd, "an absurd show," or "a game of make-pretend friend-ships." But it was also a serious space of testing, of emotional labor, of "as if equals" roles inscribed in asymmetric relations of power, where the contradictions were the materials of mobilization, and where through emotional labor and local competences relations of power could be reversed, not only between Palestinians and Israelis, but also between Jewish Mizrahi veterans of the border patrol and Druze commanders. At issue in the daily tasks was a constant negotiation of different conceptions of masculinity, nuances of nonverbal behavior, emotion management, choreography of movement and touch, mirroring of posture and gesture, and acquiring the moves of the other's masculinity. Performing these moves built functioning work units; getting them wrong set off conflict and violence.

The exercise was in turn ritual, game, and dramaturgy. It was a *ritual process* of transformation: of physically embodying the as if equality that was to be modeled and built up over time. It was a male *game of provocations and score keeping,* attempting to shift relations of control, but always attempting to keep the loser of any particular interaction in the continuing tournament. It was a serious *game of "face."* Both personal and national honor were the stakes, with respect, reproduction of honor, and the need to avoid unanswerable humiliation of the other as the moves and countermoves. The game was one of mobilizing and leveraging the contradictory struggles of equality and inequality to realign power among not just dyads of men, but men in groups, the groups themselves set within larger structural contexts. The *theater* or *dramaturgy* used a variety of props including flags, uniforms, guns, and jeeps. The Israelis had small-fireproof and bulletproof jeeps with locked doors and wire mesh across the windshields, cramped and alienating to both those inside and out; the Palestinians had roomy, open Chevrolet jeeps flown in from U.S. Operation Restore Hope in Somalia. Among the distinctive features of these patrols was the rudeness and demeaning insistence by Palestinian Israelis that Palestinian policemen had no authority to ticket or arrest them for violations ranging from illegal parking in Ramallah to drug trafficking and smuggling, because they were Israeli citizens and by the Oslo rules not subject to Palestinian authority.

The joint patrol mechanism has a history going back to (1) the Israel-Egypt Mixed Armistice Commission after the 1948 war and (2) the 1979 joint military patrols that monitored the buffer zones during the withdrawal of Israel from the Sinai desert. Those agreements were again expanded into (3) a sixty-page manual for the Israeli-Lebanese Joint Patrols that were agreed to in 1983 as part of the Israeli withdrawal plan from Lebanon, and even included the SLA (the South Lebanon Army, which the Lebanese side at first did not want to integrate, stigmatizing them as collaborators); both Israel and Lebanon signed the treaty but Syria blocked it, according to a Palestinian negotiator, because Syria was not included in the treaty agreement. The Palestinians meanwhile had experience first with (4) PLO-Jordanian joint patrols in 1969–71, but when the PLO attempted a coup d'etat against King Hussein, Jordan responded with what became known as "Black September": thousands were killed by the Jordanian army, some two thousand guerrillas and noncombatants were evacuated to 'Ajlun and the Jordan Valley, and on April 16 the PLO was completely defeated and removed to Beirut. The PLO had further experience with (5) joint patrols with the Falangist Party in 1974. So while both Israelis and Palestinians had some experience of doing joint patrols with enemy forces, they did not have the experience yet with each other.

The 1990s Palestinian-Israeli joint patrols were remarkable, not least because they also sociologically mirrored the complexities of each side. At the extreme the same Palestinians who once had been Intifada activists throwing rocks, Molotov cocktails, and bombs were working joint patrols with the same Israelis who had chased, interrogated, and imprisoned them during the first (1987–93) Intifada. But on the Palestinian side, the commanders were all from the Kastel Force, that is "Outsiders" who had returned in 1994 from Algeria; these were well-educated, trained military men, but they had not lived in the West Bank and Gaza since 1948, or interacted with Israelis under occupation or through the labor force in Israel; they tended not to know Hebrew. Their men, by contrast, tended to be "Insiders," also often college educated, looking for work and a salary, and often knowing at least some Hebrew. The tug-of-war between Insiders and Outsiders for power and control that structures the Palestinian Authority was thereby also reproduced here. On the Israeli side, the men who served on the joint patrols were from the Border Police, that is, "fighter units" known to be the most aggressive units of the IDF, trained to do the work of breaking into houses at night to surprise and seize suspected terrorists. Over half of these (55 percent) were Jewish Israeli-born Mizrahim (of Middle Eastern origin, often from lower socioeconomic and less educated backgrounds, and mostly non–Arabic speaking despite their parents or grandparents being Arabic speakers). Not only were they caught in the contradiction between their military and now constabulary duties, but they increasingly felt devalued in the context of the joint patrols. Most of the commanders of the joint patrols on the Israeli side were Druze, valued for both their Arabic and their cultural competence in the masculinities of the Palestinians. Druze and the other Israeli minorities (Bedouin, Christians, Muslims, and Circassians) comprise 30 percent of the Border Police; immigrants from Russia and Ethiopia are 10 percent. As with the Palestinians, there was also a division between many of the commanders and the "veterans" of the first Intifada, the commanders having served in Lebanon instead of the West Bank, as had their Palestinian counterparts.

In 1996 the game of the joint patrols was reset through the Tunnel Incident. The Likud government of Benjamin Netanyahu, despite warnings that it would be explosive, decided to open the exit of the 491-meter-long Hasmonean tunnel under the Muslim Quarter in Jerusalem. Violence erupted first in Ramallah and then for three days in Gaza and the West Bank: fifty-nine Palestinians and fourteen Israelis were killed including several Israeli border police and one of its commanders. None of the Palestinian joint patrolmen were injured or killed. It was a test for the joint patrols. The Palestinians thought they performed well; the Israelis thought the Palestinians had not performed well, accusing some of them of shooting at Israelis. The patrols were temporarily stopped, but they started up again a few months later. It was after this that the Israeli joint patrolmen donned bulletproof vests and were ordered to lock their jeep doors and bar their windshields and windows. The Palestinians argued that their men had performed well: without the joint patrols the violence would have escalated even more, only a few of the patrolmen engaged in armed battle with the IDF, and most resisted the prodding and humiliation from their own people. Moreover, in Nablus, after forty-one Israeli soldiers had been trapped inside Joseph's tomb, stripped of their cell phones, Palestinian joint patrol officers had given them cell phones and traded information with them throughout the incident.

In short, the Palestinians felt empowered by their performance: they felt they had acted professionally, had demonstrated to their own people that they could fight, that they had performed in a manner very different from the collaborationist SLA, and specifically that they could act from strength facing the Israelis eye to eye, gun to gun. Many of the Israelis, by contrast, believed that the PNA (Palestinian National Authority) had sent out directives for violence against them, that they awoke one morning to find their professional partners cold if not belligerent; their fears were reinforced that they could not trust their joint patrol partners.

At issue here are not the objective facts so much as the subtle choreography of emotion, the dynamics of fear and distrust, the failures of incorporating or embodying the masculinity moves of the other. The joint patrols, writes Heifetz-Yahav (2002), were "like a throbbing crystal ball," they "signaled a pulse," and they "revealed that the Intifada was inevitable should the forces of asymmetric access to resources remain unchanged."

The end for this particular experiment came in late September 2000. On Thursday, September 28, Ariel Sharon, then a member of parliament, marched onto the Temple Mount with armed guards to assert the right of Jews to freely be on the site of the ancient temple of Judaism. At six o'clock the next morning, Friday, September 29, a Palestinian five-year veteran of the joint patrols turned on his twenty-seven-year-old Israeli colleague, shouted "Allah o Akbar," and shot him point-blank. His Palestinian colleagues attempted to stop him, but he threatened them with the gun and succeeded in escaping into Area A (Palestinian-controlled area). Within two days, the joint patrols were terminated, and the second or al-Aqsa Intifada began to escalate with its suicide bombers, reoccupations of Palestinian areas, and closures.

While one can read this end to the joint patrols as one of a small-scale experiment being overwhelmed by the structural asymmetries in which it was embedded, one can also see it as one of many such efforts to find spaces where work on interaction, conversation, engagement, familiarity, and understanding proceeds. Heifetz-Yahav (2002, 2003) judges the patrols themselves as a success in stabilizing a transitional period, in reducing levels of violence; what failed was that there was no end to the transition, that a temporary confidence-building measure could not itself create a political settlement.

I was, at the end of the summer of 2003, privileged to be part of a proposal-writing working group of Palestinian and Israeli environmental scientists where again a substantive task of importance to both sides provided a ritual, game, and dramaturgical space in which many of the same complicated dynamics between Palestinians and Israelis and among the factions on each side were exercised. Many of these participants too had known each other for years if not decades, familiar antagonists, who increasingly knew how to push the hot buttons of the "other" but also were genuinely puzzled and exasperated at some of the reactions to things said, or more often, not said but acted out.

V

The provocation that I would like to take away from these two kinds of ethnographic settings has to do with the challenges suggested by the literature on UN peacekeeping and transnational humanitarian intervention. Again, I draw from the work of Deborah Heifetz-Yahav (2002, 2003) and her mentor Eyal Ben-Ari (1989, 1998), as well as other observers such as Mark Duffield (2001), David Rieff (2002), Mary Anderson (1996), and Michael Ignatieff (2001, 2002a, 2002b). The increasing blurring between civilian and military functions—privatized military functions, militarized humanitarian functions, intersecting information technologies, requirements for flexibility, interoperability, and adaptability—produce tensions not only between the training and ethos of peacekeeping-constabulary-relief versus those of the military, but also between the need for interorganizational interoperability and the need to maintain the distinctions and restrictions of action between military and civilian organizations. The example here of negotiating the tensions and contradictions between military and constabulary functions is particularly unnerving for the IDF. These tensions undid the American military in the Somalia Operation Restore Hope. Communication technologies provide one locus where such tensions (as well as some salutary openings) are easily observed in the recent wars of the twenty-first century. The use of cell phones by Israelis and Palestinians facilitates the deployment of better informed and less conformist soldiers, and, says Heifetz-Yahav, potentially transforms the other from an object of fear/distrust into a subject who becomes familiar/predictable, as in the example of the Nablus coordination between the Palestinian joint patrol officers and the trapped Israeli soldiers inside Joseph's tomb.

Rafal Rohozinski (2003) provides a useful catalog of communications technologies in recent wars as they cut across peacekeeping, development, and military intervention.[7] As with the cell phone example, Israel/Palestine provides multiple infrastructure warfare points of entry at the "high end" development of encryption technologies but also in less sophisticated arenas. In the airwaves warfare, Hezbollah's Al Manar broadcasting (terrestrial, satellite, news wire, and streamed video) circulates guerilla-action music videos, provides an archive of downloadable video clips, and is the venue for non-Hezbollah groups claiming responsibility for suicide attacks in Israel. Rohozinski points out that its nonstop feeding of the Arab world with incendiary media is untempered by the "stability concerns" of state broadcasting networks. In fall 2000, Israeli hackers mounted "denial of service" attacks on the Hezbollah Web site. In response some twenty groups of hackers in several parts of the Arab world (e.g., Gforce Pakistan, Xegypt, UNITY) and the United Kingdom and Brazil attacked 166 Israeli Web sites, including those of the Prime Minister's Office, Foreign Ministry, Knesset, IDF, and a major commercial ISP, Netvision. They used some sixteen attack tools. They threatened future attacks against banks, the stock exchange, and e-commerce sites. Although this round of cyberwarfare was not very damaging and petered out, Rohozinski suggests that the attacks were sufficiently threatening that they might explain why in spring 2002, when Israel reoccupied the Palestinian Territories, the opportunity was taken to destroy large numbers of Palestinian hard drives, ISPs, switchboards, and television and radio stations. At issue is not just infrastructure, propaganda, and information warfare ("incitement" in primary- and secondary-school textbooks has been a longstanding concern), but also the enormous underground economy of drugs, illicit arms, human trafficking, money laundering, and smuggling that the new information technologies support.

Infrastructure, propaganda, and information, like the psychology of displacements, affect, and trauma, are themselves among the modalities of border incursions and crossing folds, which unsettle drawn lines and provide the conflicted materials for ritual processes, dramaturgies, and just gaming that is not just gaming but gaming toward justice.

Palestine/Israel is a borderland of disorders (psychic and otherwise) where there is strong resistance to third-party intervention; where there are a series of high-pressure crucibles, loci for useful ethnographies of social context, under conditions of what Walter Benjamin called a standing state of emergency; where we are forced "to live with what would otherwise be unendurable," to find folds in the borderland in which "to install ourselves, confront things, take hold, breathe—in short, think" beyond the slogans of side taking and instead interact, talk, extend hands through the pores of the membranes, and find the humanely Real gazing back from holes in the defenses.

NOTES

This chapter follows on from a paper with the same title, but different subtitle and content, developed for João Biehl, Byron Good, and Arthur Kleinman's edited volume *Subjectivity: Ethnographic Investigations*. The first of the two "crucibles" in the present chapter is repeated from there. That paper was oriented toward more general issues of subjectivity, this chapter toward conflict, intervention, and peacekeeping. A version of this chapter was originally delivered at the International Conference on Intervention, held at the University of Montreal and at McGill University in October 2003, organized by Mariella Pandolfi. I am grateful to her for her invitation and encouragement, to the conference participants, and to Mary-Jo and Byron Good, Chris Dole, Erica James, Sandra Hyde, and the members of the Friday Morning Seminar on Medical Anthropology and Cultural Psychiatry for which this version was reworked.

1. Winner of Best Screenplay (Cannes 2001), Oscar and Golden Globe (2002); a French-Belgian-Italian-Slovenian coproduction filmed in Slovenia and Italy and submitted as the Bosnian entry for the Oscar; with beloved Bosnian comic actor Branko Duric and Filip Šovagović as the two Serbs, and Rene Bitorajac as the Serbian recruit.

2. The U.S. Geological Survey has a mission to provide water resources and hydrological training to get all three (Jordan, Palestine, and Israel) to collect information in commensurable and standard terms, and to begin to build working relations among professionals in all three.

3. The psychotherapy certificate program that operated from 1993 to 1996 grew out of a symposium in Lisbon convened by the psychotherapist Maria Belo. Ten stu-

dents each were selected from the West Bank and Gaza, Palestinian Israelis, and Jewish Israelis. The Palestinians from the West Bank and Gaza complained that they were only ten, the Israelis were twenty; the Jewish Israelis complained they were only ten, the Palestinians were twenty. More trenchant was the shock of the Jewish Israelis when two ten-year-old boys ("children of the stones") who had been injured by Israeli bullets were brought in and expressed hatred and defiance. The Israeli Palestinians helped diffuse the tension. In Gaza, el-Sarraj also has other problems: the board of the Gaza clinic proved to be troublesome, being political rather than professional.

4. It is possible that with much work the accounts could be made to seem as if they were of the same event. One gets, of course, a much better understanding of the battle itself from the much better armed and prepared attackers than from the defenders. According to the Baroud accounts (2003), the defenders who died seem mainly to have died while trying to help the injured, rather than while fighting. This seems unlikely, and the accounts given to Goldberg (2003) describe a good deal of cross fire. With Goldberg's accounts in mind, many of the actions that seem unfathomable (in these accounts) to Palestinian ambulance drivers or men asked to strip to their shorts take on rationales. That many were killed and injured and, from the Palestinian side, that many remain unaccounted for, perhaps dead, perhaps in prison is no light matter. From the Israeli side, the admitted bomb-making efforts of Mahmud Tawalbe all over the West Bank are also no light matter. War and armed resistance is not civilized.

5. See the companion piece where I spell this out (Fischer 2007).

6. Insofar as one can believe the Goldberg book (2003) as an honest account of how the reservists and soldiers he interviewed think, it is an account of the still vital core of a citizen-soldier republic that constantly debates its own actions. My own interviews with two of the reservists involved in the Jenin attack fit this pattern, as does a group interview I participated in with the June 2003 Faculty for Israel-Palestine Peace delegation with five of the five hundred refusenik reservist combat officers who are willing to serve and fight except in the Occupied Territories. One does not get a similar sense from the Baroud interviews (2003) of anything about the organization of Jenin or the Jenin refugee camp, the relations to the several armed factions, to the Palestinian Authority, or to their own life trajectories. And perhaps this simply illustrates the point: it is a portrait of the registers of subjectivities at issue.

7. In Somalia in 1993, three cellular operators provided telephone and Internet coverage for 70 percent of the country, allowing Aideed and other warlords to eavesdrop on NGO and UN traffic and to track U.S. and UN military forces, depriving them of the element of surprise. Two U.S. helicopters were shot down, U.S. forces killed, and an airman dragged through the streets; and while U.S. forces finally prevailed after killing over five hundred Somalis and injuring over a thousand, the video image of the airman being dragged through the streets proved politically devastating and caused the collapse of the UN mission. Russia, similarly, suffered

an even more devastating defeat in its first invasion of Chechnya, losing four thousand dead and 250 armored vehicles in two days. The Chechen fighters used cell phones, while the Russians were using unencrypted old radios whose reception was often blocked by high buildings in Grozny. The Chechens also pursued a skillful media war aimed at the Russian public, allowing open access to Russian reporters to their side of the war, with the result being a flooding into Russian television sets of images of dead Russian soldiers and atrocities by Russian forces, helping force the 1996 withdrawal of Russian forces. Russia learned its lesson: before invading again in 1999, it cut off phone service, targeted cellular towers and other communication infrastructure, and crafted a public relations campaign for its domestic audiences built around a rhetoric of fighting a war on terrorism and blaming Chechen terrorists for apartment building bombings in Russian cities. In the Great Lakes region of Rwanda, Burundi, Tanzania, Congo, and Uganda, the UN radio network was pirated, stolen, and subverted by the Interhamwe militias to perpetrate genocide, and by the Rwandan military in its campaign against these militias, often monitoring NGO communications to track Hutu refugees. In Bosnia, cell phones and the ability to monitor NGO, UN, and stabilization forces' (SFOR) radio are credited for the inability of NATO forces to apprehend indicted war criminals.

REFERENCES

Anderson, Mary B. 1996. *Do No Harm: Supporting Local Capacities for Peace through Aid.* Cambridge, MA: Collaborative for Development Action, Inc.

Baroud, Ramzy. 2003. *Searching Jenin.* Seattle, WA: Cune Press.

Ben-Ari, Eyal. 1989. Masks and Soldiering: The Israeli Army and the Palestinian Uprising. *Cultural Anthropology* 4 (4): 372–89.

———. 1998. *Mastering Soldiers: Conflict, Emotions, and the Enemy in an Israeli Military Unit.* New York: Berghahn Books.

Castells, Manuel. 1996. *The Rise of the Network Society.* Cambridge: Blackwell.

———. 1998. *End of Millennium.* Cambridge: Blackwell.

Deleuze, Gilles. 1995 [1990]. *Negotiations.* New York: Columbia University Press.

Deleuze, Gilles, and Felix Guattari. 1987. *A Thousand Plateaus.* Minneapolis: University of Minnesota Press.

Duffield, Mark. 2001. *Global Governance and the New Wars: The Merging of Development and Security.* London and New York: Zed.

el-Sarraj, Eyad. 2003. Talk at Tel Aviv University, June 18.

Fassin, Didier. 2002. Politics of Suffering and Policies of Order: The Moral Economy of Immigration in France. Paper presented to the American Anthropological Association meetings, New Orleans, November 20–24.

———. 2003. L'espace moral de l'action humanitaire: à propos de quelques épreuves recentes. Paper presented to the International Conference on Intervention, University of Montreal, 24 October.

Fischer, Michael M. J. 2007. To Live with What Would Otherwise Be Unendurable: Return(s) to Subjectivities. In *Subjectivity: Ethnographic Investigations*, ed. João Biehl, Byron Good, and Arthur Kleinman, 423–46. Berkeley: University of California Press.

Goldberg, Brett. 2003. *A Psalm in Jenin*. Tel Aviv: Modan Publishing House.

Heifetz-Yahav, Deborah. 2002. From Fighters to Peacekeepers: Negotiating Relations in the Israeli-Palestinian Joint Patrols. PhD diss., Tel-Aviv University.

———. 2003. Non-Mediated Peacekeeping: The Case of Israeli-Palestinian Security Cooperation. Unpublished paper.

Ignatieff, Michael. 2001. *Human Rights as Politics and Idolatry*. Princeton, NJ: Princeton University Press.

———. 2002a. Mission Possible. *New York Review of Books* 49 (20)

———. 2002b. The Rights Stuff. *New York Review of Books* 49 (10).

Malkki, Liisa. 1995. *Purity and Exile: Violence, Memory and National Cosmology among the Hutu Refugees in Tanzania*. Chicago: University of Chicago Press.

Mbembe, Achille. 2001. *On the Postcolony*. Berkeley: University of California Press.

Pandolfi, Mariella. 2002. Right of Interference, Temporality of Emergency, Necessity of Action: The Triangle of Humanitarian Biopower. Paper presented at the American Anthropological Society meetings, New Orleans, November 20–24.

Rieff, David. 2002. *A Bed for the Night: Humanitarianism in Crisis*. New York: Simon and Schuster.

Rohozinski, Rafal. 2003. Bullets to Bytes: Reflections on ICTs and "Local" Conflicts. In *Bombs and Bandwidth: The Emerging Relationship Between Information Technology and Security*, ed. Robert Latham. New York: New Press.

Spiegelman, Art. 1991. *Maus*. New York: Pantheon.

———. 2004. *In the Shadow of No Towers*. New York: Pantheon.

PART III: MADNESS, ALTERITY,
              AND PSYCHIATRY

A History of Violence and Silence

João Biehl

We colonists want to let Your Majesty know how much we have suffered, not just from our neighbors who are rowdy and conniving, but also from the very authorities of this district who have been protecting the wicked. . . . And so they insult us wherever they meet us, directing obscene words to ward us off, whipping some, throwing stones at others without any reason. . . . They cut to pieces the white clothes belonging to the peasant Nicolau Barth, which were hanging in the yard. And they cut the tails and manes of five horses.

> Letter from the so-called Mucker to Brazilian emperor Dom Pedro II, December 1873

The indignation against the Mucker is so immense that the officers couldn't hinder the corpses' mutilations by colonists and soldiers. Someone cut off the head of Robinson and brought it to São Leopoldo in a bag. Another man carried the ear of a Mucker in his hands. The persecution of the Mucker continues until all have been hunted down.

> Karl von Koseritz, *Deutsche Zeitung*, July 1874

In heaven there is no more suffering, perishing and death, there our desires are dried up into an eternal reencounter.

> Tombstone, cemetery of Linha Nova, ca. 1870

CULTURAL CATACLYSM

The body of a beheaded woman was found in May 1993 in the woods near São Leopoldo, the first German colony founded in 1824 in the southern province of Rio Grande do Sul, Brazil. As if the brutal killing wasn't bizarre enough, the stories that explained her death were equally strange—they speak to a history of violence in that region.

Local newspapers reported that very little was known about the beheaded woman's identity, aside from her dark skin, her scar from a caesarean section, and her age of roughly thirty years. No fingerprint matches could be made, and her head was not found. The local police chief, in a peculiar move, ordered a dummy to be dressed in the victim's clothes "so as to rouse the memory of the people." Someone might recall having seen a woman dressed similarly, he reasoned, and "might then contact us" (*Jornal NH* 1993).[1]

This story was also mentioned in *Zero Hora*, the province's main newspaper, in a report on the increasing number of homicides in that relatively prosperous region (ZH 1993). The report stated that the violence originated in metropolitan- area slums now occupied by the legions of unemployed migrants looking for work in local shoe factories, and that middle-class citizens were now building walls around their homes and arming themselves. One reporter went so far as to associate that "migrant violence" with a phantasmatic reoccurrence. A headline read, "Violence Is Resurrected in the Land of the Mucker." For over a century, the word "Mucker" has signified sectarian fanaticism, communal breakdown, and murderous violence in the region.

Following independence from Portugal, the new imperial authorities founded the colony of São Leopoldo for two thousand German immigrants (Hunsche 1975; Delhaes-Gunther 1980; Roche 1969; Frobel 1858; Seyferth 1990).[2] Given external market demands and the urgency to feed a growing urban population, the country needed to find alternatives to slavery and to diversify its agricultural production (Petrone 1982). Then and in the following decades, thousands of German peasants, *Lumpenproletariat*, and former prisoners were recruited with promises of land, full-fledged citizenship, and religious rights, none of which would be fully granted. In this Catholic land, Protestant baptisms and marriages were not recognized and had no legal significance; the colonists also had no rights to participate in local administrations (Hillebrand 1924; Hunsche 1979). Neither free nor enslaved, the immigrants had to invent their own means of survival, and many enlisted as soldiers in wars against Argentina and Paraguay. Available statistics say that some five million immigrants entered Brazil between 1819 and 1947 (Seyferth 1990: 11).[3]

Until the 1840s, the colonists were subsistence farmers, but that would change as agricultural products began to find their way into the thriving markets of Porto Alegre as well as those of São Paulo and Rio de Janeiro (following a coffee plantation boom). By the late 1860s, the region was prospering, attracting investments from Britain (for railroad construction) and imports from Germany (a range of industrialized goods, from nails to textiles to champagne). Lutheran and Jesuit missionaries came as well.

In its coverage of the 1993 beheading story, *Zero Hora* reported that around 1872 a group of second-generation German-speaking colonists, from various social ranks, began to be singled out as "Mucker" (meaning very religious, stubborn, and hypocritical people) by their neighbors and local authorities. For several years they had been meeting peacefully around the words of Jacobina Mentz Maurer and the herbal medicine prepared by her husband, João Jorge Maurer. According to the newspaper, the Mucker were led by "a woman suffering from psychological disturbances." Local clergy prohibited people from witnessing her trances, as she was said to be interpreting the Bible in a messianic way and engaging in adultery and civil disobedience. According to the newspaper, the ostracized Mucker sought revenge by ambushing local authorities and by burning down neighboring homes and trading posts. The report noted that the army was justifiably called in to respond to the Mucker's deadly actions and to restore order.

Military records show that the Maurers' house was attacked and set on fire on July 19, 1874. Dozens of men, women and children died in the attack, as did Colonel Genuíno Sampaio, who led the provincial and imperial troops, aided by locals. Several Mucker survived and were taken to prison. Seventeen of them, including thirty-three year-old Jacobina and her newborn child, escaped and hid in the nearby woods. Two weeks later, the group was found and killed. Soldiers and colonists mutilated the dead bodies—Jacobina's mouth was slit—and placed them in a common grave in the woods. The body of João Jorge Maurer was never found. "Mucker" became a curse word and a heuristic for violence and impunity—a continuous legend of the present (Biehl 1991, 1996a).

Omitted from the *Zero Hora* report is the fact that the military action against the Mucker was sponsored by the Germanist upper class living in the capital Porto Alegre (then Brazil's fourth-largest city) and was silently supported by the religious authorities, newly arrived in the region. Karl von Koseritz, a Freemason philosopher and politician who also directed the influential newspaper *Deutsche Zeitung* (DZ), spearheaded the anti-Mucker campaign. In reference to the Mucker, Koseritz wrote, "These swindlers don't deserve citizenship. They adore as Christ a woman who with good reason should be considered a Babylonian whore. For this band there is room either in the penitentiary or in the mad house. They have spread over society like a deadly poison. If the government does not liberate society from this monster, the inhabitants of the colonies will themselves seek justice by lynching. Deaths will come" (DZ 12/10/1873).

At the peak of the armed conflict, the *Deutsche Zeitung*'s editorial read, "The Mucker have to be banished to a land where there are still cannibals. We have to treat them humanly: at deportation we should give the Mucker guns and ammunition. They would then have the opportunity to satiate their death instinct while killing cannibals, and the cannibals would have the pleasure of having Mucker for breakfast. In this way, we would help the Mucker as well as the cannibals" (DZ 7/22/1874). Meanwhile, members of the local German Society for Gymnastics and Hunting had taken over the civic guard of Porto Alegre: "We want to prove to the Brazilian government as well as to the other nations that we by no means share the sentiments of those [criminals] who call themselves our compatriots. On the contrary, we desire to contribute to their extermination."[4]

Immediately after the war, Koseritz (under the pseudonym C. M. S.) published a report in the German magazine *Die Gartenlaube* entitled, "Jacobina Maurer, the Feminine Christ, amidst the Germans in Brazil" (reprinted in Hunsche 1974: 255–62). The Mucker events should interest the *aufgeklärte Deutschen* (enlightened Germans), he wrote:

> How could a noncultured and libertine woman as Jacobina—who does not read anything which is handwritten and only reads with difficulty what is printed—have gained so much influence over a high number of honored and hard-working men? One is tempted to believe in a certain form of mental alienation, as we can find reference in the reports of the horrendous times of the trials against the witches. . . . It is unfortunate that in spite of all the progress of humanity, an individual can still fall so deeply into the superstition of backward times. We deplore the fact that what the poet Schiller wrote still survives today: "The worst of all horrors is man in his illusion."

This chapter is concerned with the savagery of these enlightened men. Based on archival research I carried out in Brazil and in Germany, I explore the following: (1) how stories about the Mucker as mad, criminal, and bestial were choreographed; (2) how Koseritz's sensationalist master narrative informed public opinion and military action; (3) how Jacobina and João Jorge's followers managed their ordinary life problems and articulated their theological ideas; and (4) how, in the end, these colonists embodied the alterity "Mucker" into which they had been classified and learned to kill too. What were the implications of this war for ethnic identity formation and local governance?

The Mucker events form the basis of my understanding of the mobility of nineteenth-century European notions of rationality and progress: how they migrated and became culturally ingrained in the peripheries, contributing to political violence and to the redefinition of common sense. The social, religious, philosophical and political conflicts of the period were dramatized around the Mucker. Koseritz and associates used science, institutionalized religion, and the media to stigmatize ordinary pious and healing practices as fanatic and sectarian. Amid cultural cataclysm, independent colonists were remade as criminal Mucker characters. Their subsequent murder as politically dangerous, I argue, was part of the dynamic installation of a local Germanist order and of the constitution of an enlightened, albeit transplanted, German Self in the South. In this context, for reason to rule, life representations had to literally become truth in the flesh of the Other. With the violent encroachment of a German identity also emerged a sense that things could have been otherwise, that a certain way of knowing oneself and the world was now a devalued currency. Interviews with local historians and with elderly people who have knowledge of the war's aftermath helped me to sketch the ways in which the massacre lives on in the contemporary political imaginary.

"A TRIBE THAT THINKS AND TRADES IN GERMAN"

By 1875, the Ministry of Agriculture and Commerce praised São Leopoldo as an exemplary settlement to be reproduced everywhere if the country were to modernize its economy and society: "There, the German race has been working for the Empire. The Brazilian organism must continue to be lightened with new European blood, intelligence, and the fever of progress. With the ending of slavery and the generation of a free labor force, *a beneficial moral revolution is taking place in the country*. In this great laboratory of the present . . . the state's strong hand must continue to be wielded" (Souza 1875: 420, my emphasis).

For Germany, which had little success in the colonial practice of territorial annexation, the nineteenth-century settlements in South America and Africa became a testing ground for a different kind of cultural and economic imperialism (Frobel 1858; Fabian 2000; Comaroff and Comaroff 1991; Steinmetz 2004). By fostering German communities in isolated enclaves that were somewhat independent of the host country, Germany was generating specific sites from which raw materials and food could be imported, and through which markets for the export of consumer goods, technologies, and other investments could be created.

An 1874 report by the German Society for Protestants in Southern Brazil made the goals of its mission clear: "It is indeed important to have a tribe overseas that thinks and trades in German, sympathizes with us in terms of business and politics, and represents our interests in all matters. This common sense shall become obvious to all enlightened men" (Auftrag 1874: 45). We live in a world of compensations, stated Koseritz, "if Germany has the power, Brazil has the natural resources" (1897: 47). By 1903, the province of Rio Grande do Sul was importing 45 percent of its goods from Germany, accounting for 19 percent of Germany's total yearly exports (Schrader 1980: 205; see also Oberacker 1985).

While a local form of *Kultur* was being painfully inscribed in the flesh of the Mucker, in Germany Friedrich Nietzsche was publishing *The Use and Abuse of History*. In 1874, Nietzsche wrote about how the embodiment of a particular German Enlightenment presupposed the forgetfulness of one's lived experience. Imposed by the "gravediggers of the present," this forgetfulness induced a generalized moral blindness: "Men are to be fashioned to the needs of the time, that they may soon take their place in the machine. . . . Some birds are blinded that they may sing better; I do not think men sing today better than their grandfathers, though I am sure they are blinded early" (1957: 7, 44).

The Mucker events were an extension of such German experiments in the south, I argue, and the war grotesquely realized some of the very aims and cultural productions of this form of Enlightenment (Biehl 1996a). In the process, a scientifically informed history became itself a phantasm, a modern substitute for reality that even today informs public perception. On August 1, 1874, the *Deutsche Zeitung*'s editorial read, "The Mucker must be hunted like dogs and killed so that no trace of them remains. The entire population holds this opinion. The head of each one of them must be cut off without exception. Even though the band can hardly read and sign their names, these fanatics want to reform today's world according to their visions." Here we are not speaking of colonial violence, but of colonist violence, which was based on rural/urban and primitive/enlightened distinctions and their enforcements.

Before following the footprints of the hunters and makers of history so to speak, I want to relate a human encounter that has profoundly framed my understanding of the Mucker matters as a historical Real that both resists symbolization and gives occasion to what anthropologist Michael Fischer (1999) calls "ethical moments." I am a descendant of German immigrants who settled in southern Brazil circa 1860. I grew up in the colony of Kaffee Schneitz (Picada Café), speaking *ecke Deutsch* (not high German, but an oral dialect "grown in the bushes") and hearing stories about the Mucker: how they came in the middle of the night to steal animals and goods and how people slept in fear next to their rifles.

Sometime in 1991, I visited Vó Minda, my maternal grandmother (born in 1910), in the nursing home where she lived out the final days of her life. I prompted her to inquire about the Mucker from her acquaintances there. In my next visit she had something to tell me:

"João, the Mucker did not cut the tails of their horses."

"What does this mean?" I asked.

Vó Minda's answer could not have been more compelling, revealing the matter-of-factness of the story of the cut tails that, for her, held a mirror to her current isolated existence: "That is something we don't do to what is *ours*."

As I heard it, in Vó Minda's speech, the word "Mucker" circulated lonesome-ness, a remembered tie, and the presence of inconceivable violence—the voice of a body that is denied a home.

And to my surprise, when I began reading the personal letters, official peti-tions and police files of the times when the word "Mucker" for the first time appeared in history, I discovered a curious detail: Jacobina and her friends had complained to no avail that the tails of their horses had been mysteriously cut. The cutting of the horses' tails signifies the beginnings of the expulsion of these men and women from everyday life. Vó Minda and others kept circulat-ing such traces as a measure of oneself in the face of dying.

KULTUR

In Germany, the revolutionary unrest of the 1840s, allied to demographic pres-sures ensuing from the end of feudalism and the country's rapid industrializa-tion, resulted in very high emigrant outflows.[5] In spite of Brazil's still-precarious colonization infrastructure and increasing sense of outrage against that "most tentative experiment" by European governments (Assu 1873: 7), a second wave of immigration brought to the São Leopoldo colony freedom fighters and intellectuals such as Karl von Koseritz, the future leader of the anti-Mucker campaign.

Karl von Koseritz was born in 1830 in Dessau, the son of a Prussian major. By the age of fifteen, he was already taking part in local revolutionary activities. In 1851, he quit the Wittenberg *Gymnasium* and traveled to northeastern Brazil— "a disenchantment," he later wrote. "I lost my fortune in the thoughtlessness of my youth and with it I lost the paternal house and my fatherland" (quoted in Oberacker 1961: 21). He returned to Brazil in 1852 as part of the German Legion (nineteen hundred soldiers and fifty-three officers) contracted to aid the Brazilian Army in the war against Argentina, which had taken over Uruguay. Like Koseritz, the majority deserted and settled down in the southern region. These men became known as Brummer and took up key positions in the colonies (Dickie 1989; Sudhaus 1962).

By 1855, Koseritz was married to Zeferina Vasconcelos, the daughter of a large landowner in the city of Pelotas. In the following years, he worked as a bookkeeper, teacher, and school director and also contributed to local newspa-pers. In 1857, he published his *Summary of the Universal History* and the female char-acter plays *Inês* and *Nini*. In Koseritz's view, "The Brummer brought with them a new and independent spirit, stimulating what existed of German identity at that time, tuning it up, so to speak, into the leaven which made local German-ism rise" (quoted in Oberacker 1961: 17). And as the Brummer spread their democratic, scientific and moral ideals, they became catalysts for an emergent Germanist bourgeoisie that understood itself as "cultured" and "politicized" in contrast to the backward colonist descendants of the first immigration wave (Oberacker 1961: 17; see also Elias 1978).

By the mid-1860s, 15 percent of Porto Alegre's twenty thousand inhabitants were Germans or German Brazilians. Approximately two-thirds of them had come directly from Germany and were economically well-off (Gans 2004: 26). As naturalist Robert Avé-Lallement wrote in 1858, "I met many Germans of honorable heart and loyal sentiments in Porto Alegre. It seems that the majority of them live well, very well. Hard-working men can make a fortune here, infinitely more than in Germany under the same circumstances. If they saw the affliction people experience in Germany they would thank God for their tranquil and half-Germanized existence in Porto Alegre" (quoted in Gans 2004: 32).

In 1867 congressman José Joaquim Rodrigues Lopes wrote his "General Considerations on the ex-Colony of São Leopoldo" (the colony had recently become a municipality and was now administered by German physician Dr. Hillebrand), in response to the emperor's concern about the possible formation of an independent Germanic state in Rio Grande do Sul: "The population of the ex-Colony is almost entirely made up of Germans and their children . . . they amount to sixteen thousand to eighteen thousand souls. They do not show any desire to be naturalized. . . . One can say that their heart and soul belong completely to the German deity. . . . Does what I saw turn me into a visionary? So, does the current state of affairs pose a great threat for the integrity of the Empire in the future?"[6]

The press played a formative role in installing the image of a cohesive Germanist society in the south. In 1862, a consortium of businessmen founded the *Deutsche Zeitung* and two years later they hired Koseritz as the director. Correspondents, generally teachers, were hired in almost every colony, and their reports were usually published next to news from Germany and from Porto Alegre. Newspapers were distributed and commented upon at the trading posts; it was common to read them after Sunday worship services. As Germanist historian Hans Gehse argues, "Objective reporting replaced primitive gossiping, and a critical perception of and stance toward political events of interest to the German immigrant emerged" (1931: 121). These men ardently denied allegations of separatism. They were thoroughly invested in the development of an ethnic collective, "a fraternal Germanism" (as Koseritz called it), independent of German institutions and fully participating in Brazil's legal and political system (Gehse 1931; Pinsdorf 1990; Porto 1934).

This is how Koseritz defined himself circa 1870: "I am a straight adherent of Materialism and Darwinism, and I have the courage to express my opinions in a land that is essentially Catholic and metaphysical. . . . In Brazil, we do not live under a German flag. We are part of Germany through language and habits. We are linked to our fatherland with all the fibers of our heart. Politically, however, we must become full Brazilian citizens" (quoted in Oberacker 1961: 26, 53). A fierce adept of Bismark's *kulturkamp* and a spokesman of a Brazilian pro-German and anti-French intellectual movement, Koseritz published several books: *Rome in the Trial of the Century* (1870); *The Church and the State* (1873); *Earth and Man in Light of Modern Science* (1878); *Images of Brazil* (1884). In the 1880s, following changes in the electoral system, Koseritz was twice elected to the province's legislature.

Beyond centralized politics, what legitimized this Germanist bourgeoisie was the expansion of its self-image. The concept of German *Kultur* was vital for the assertion of the "spiritual" segregation of German descendants from other Brazilians, and for the assertion of moral values and obligations regarding individual conduct and the organization of family lives (Elias 1978). Local historian Carlos Oberacker states, "Koseritz was able to congregate . . . political forces for the good of a collective of German culture" (1961: 18). The purely spiritual (*das rein Geistige*) aspect of *Kultur* was transmitted through the press and the Freemason educators and newly arrived German-educated clergy. This Germanist breakthrough was also dependent on the establishment of a network of productive sites (*Gemeinde*, "communities") where new individual truths and public order could be surveyed as well as, later, on the production and extermination of a "primitive" colonist's worldview.

"THERE WAS ENLIGHTENMENT FOR ALL KINDS OF ILLNESS, NO MATTER WHAT THEIR NAMES WERE"

I stumbled on a collection of the *Deutsche Zeitung* and other writings by Koseritz in the archive of the Mentz family in 1991. The Mentzes played an important and controversial role in the constitution of *Deutschtum* in the south. According to historian Carlos Hunsche, "Liborio Mentz would be the great-grandfather of Frederico Mentz, a renowned businessman in the state of Rio Grande do Sul, and on the other side, the grandfather of the infamous Jacobina Mentz Maurer, most important protagonist of the Mucker" (1975: 21). Professor René Gertz told me that UFRGS, the province's most prestigious public university, had acquired the Mentz archive. It had never been inventoried or studied before. I found the archive dumped in an unused classroom, consisting of old library cabinets packed with books, newspapers, and magazines.

According to local historians, the Mentzes participated in a dissident religious movement in the town of Tambach, and they fled to Brazil because of religious persecution.[7] The fact that the family received Lot Number 1 in the settlement of Hamburger Berg of the new colony of São Leopoldo led some historians to speculate that Libório Mentz, a farmer and carpenter, had been favored by Empress Leopoldina (the colony's namesake, originally from Austria). In H. Schüller's imaginary-sounding account (1954: 390), Libório meets the empress upon his arrival in Rio de Janeiro, the capital of newly independent Brazil. Goethe, so the story goes, advised Liborio and his two adult sons to go to Brazil. The simple man also delivered a letter from Goethe to the empress. This letter has never been found.

The oldest son was called André and he married Maria Elizabeth Müller, who immigrated in 1825. The couple lived in Hamburger Berg and they would have eight children (Jacobina, born in 1842, was the second youngest). The couple helped to build the village's Lutheran wooden chapel and held Bible group readings in their home—the children made up a choir, which sang at worship services and funerals. The Mentzes built up a considerable patrimony and, after André's death in 1853, all children inherited land.

The Mentz children were then put under the legal protection of Frederico Schreiner, a maternal uncle and father of the future chief of police, Lúcio Schreiner, who would become one of the Mucker's fiercest persecutors (Domingues 1977: 35). As Jacobina prepared for confirmation in the local Lutheran church, she learned how to read the Bible in German. Jacobina helped her mother with domestic duties until she married João Jorge Maurer in 1866, soon after he returned from the Paraguayan war. The couple lived on the land she had inherited in the settlement of Padre Eterno (Eternal Father). In 1867, besides working with carpentry and agriculture, João Jorge started to make herbal medicine (a process he learned from the itinerant healer Buchhorn).[8] Soon he became known as the *Wunderdoktor* (miraculous doctor). After her first child was born in 1867, Jacobina started to lose consciousness from time to time. Ill health was not new to her; at the age of twelve, she had been taken to Dr. Hillebrand in São Leopoldo, who recommended that she be married as soon as possible (Domingues 1977: 39). The couple had six children, and the family participated in the local Lutheran church.

In the beginning, there was no Mucker. Around 1868, neighbors started to meet at the Maurers' house. They sang, prayed, and read the Bible together. They prepared communal meals, rested, and returned to homes. Many left with medicines. Miguel Noé, a Mucker survivor, left a report highlighting the therapeutic genesis of the movement. During Jacobina's trances, "her body abandoned all senses and reasoning. In this way, everything she spoke was communicated through her spirit. . . . There was enlightenment for all kinds of illness, no matter what their names were. Herbal infusions were made, depending on the illness's location, for rubbing as well as for drinking" (Noé 1977:

383). After three years "in perfect order," as Noé put it, "these healing practices were spoken about in other regions and sick people flowed in from everywhere." In this form of enlightenment, "there was no religion, no sacredness. There were no secondary things, only a safe and calm existence aimed at the health of everyone" (384).

. . .

"There is no true religiosity in Brazil," wrote Pastor Günther Borchard upon his arrival in São Leopoldo in 1864. Borchard and his successors fiercely campaigned to eliminate the common practice of lay priesthood and to gather congregations into a synod (see Dreher 1984). According to Borchard, "Faithless books like the Gospel of Nature and vile novels and writings on Materialism have found their way here across the ocean. Romances are more widely read than the Bible; the dance halls attract more people than the churches; the rest on Sunday is not observed." Yet "that savage disbelief found in the United States doesn't reign here . . . this battlefield is very promising for the German Protestant Church; there is no better in any other Catholic land. Here it is possible to found pure German colonies."[9]

Like the Protestants, the Jesuits also interpreted the colonists' religious practices as a deviation and dysfunction to be corrected: "The long absence of a regular healer of souls produced a sort of brutishness among the Catholic population. And since they were missing a priest, they themselves organized lay worship services. This people who had more pious feelings than common sense foolishly departed from the path of order. . . . Nobody can command him to do anything. The peasant is independent. He feels equal to every other peasant. Any words used against his family or his belongings irritates him very much . . . he uses the rudest expressions" (Schupp quoted in Rabuske n.d.: 141; see also Schupp 1912).

The practices around Jacobina's unconscious words and João Jorge's medicines emerged alongside the Germanist *Kultur* efforts. Geographic and Freemason societies, rifle clubs, church councils and choirs, and urban congregational schools—they all supported the claims of legitimacy of a *hiesiges Deutschtum* (local Germanism). Transplanted moral prescriptions were presented as the living proof of a German natural history at work: the memorialization of an ethnic past, a nonlibidinal life, hard work from childhood until old age, group separation according to religious affiliation, unconditional obedience to the foreign clergy and to the economic and legal authorities of the Germanist bourgeoisie, and racial superiority. "Outlawing" and dismantling lay priesthoods, local healing practices, and Catholic-Lutheran "mixed marriages" proved to be powerful means to institutionally ground this Germanist evolution already described as "truth" in idyllic narratives left behind by illustrious travelers.[10] As Michael Mulhall, a British journalist wrote , "Imagine yourself, reader, a country nearly as large as Belgium or Holland cut out of these Brazilian forests, where the inhabitants are exclusively German, and speak no other language ... where individuals' happiness and the welfare of the commonwealth go hand-in-hand" (1873: 105).

While increasingly involved in the region's commerce, the Germanist elite learned that upward social mobility and political power depended upon high status within the larger society, not within the ethnic and "backward" subgroups (Luebcke 1987: 29; Porto 1934). As I have been arguing, the elite's social and political evolution was also contingent on the fabrication and, later, elimination of a group of "primitive" and "mad" colonists. In the end, the "demonic" Mucker worked as an instrument for the purification of the German Spirit that was to inform the work ethic of these colonists, and as a venue for the German bourgeoisie to further integrate itself into the region's social and political status quo.[11]

In the beginning of the nineteenth century, Johann Fichte had actually envisioned such strategies of self-formation linked to Germany's nation building: "The dawn of the new world is already past its breaking. . . . I wish ... to catch the rays of this dawn and weave them into a mirror, in which our grief-stricken age must see itself; so that it may believe in its own existence, may perceive its real self, and, as in prophetic vision, may see its own development, its coming forms pass by. In the contemplation of this, the picture of its former life will doubtless sink and vanish; and the dead body may be born to its resting place without undue lamenting" (1923: 15).

"LEAVE THE TUMULT OF THE WORLD AND COME BACK"

Large segments of the colonists did not readily accept the new forms of control embedded in the teachings and administrative practices of the Germanist elite and missionaries. For many, Germanism was neither a myth of origin nor an inexorable destiny. They claimed existence on their own terms. These colonists, far from apolitical, openly expressed their concerns about corruption among public officers and about the unjust distribution of wealth, an effect of the region's modernization. The colonists who visited Jacobina and João Jorge's home held this belief particularly strongly.

Consider João Jorge Klein, Jacobina's brother-in-law, a former lay pastor and self-taught intellectual to whom Jacobina dictated several letters. In a public statement written in early 1873, Klein cited instances of public corruption: communal bridges left unfinished, public moneys misused and privately diverted—"There is need of many reforms" (Klein 1957). Later in 1873, the *Deutsche Zeitung* refused to print texts sent by Klein in which he criticized the taxation system and the cumbersome bureaucracy, which hampered wealth transfers among the colonists: "so the poor end up paying the taxes for the rich" (quoted in Sperb 1987: 243–45).

As of 1872, some of the friends of Jacobina and João Jorge started to abandon their congregational memberships, stopped selling and consuming goods at neighborhood trading posts, began to bury their dead on their own land, and assumed responsibility for educating their children. The Lutheran clergy began to berate Jacobina, João Jorge and their friends as fanatic Mucker (Domingues 1977: 78–81), and they became subject to bizarre incidents—the tails of their horses were cut. Wherever they rode, these colonists were now identified as Mucker through their mutilated animals. This literally marked the beginning of their animalization, so to speak.

I did not find the letters or personal diaries I was hoping to find at the Mentz archive. Yet the Germanist materials I encountered have dramatically changed the way I saw the civil war the Mucker had reportedly occasioned. I studied all issues of Koseritz's *Deutsche Zeitung* from 1868 to 1875 and of his *Deutsche Volkskalender für die Provinz Rio Grande do Sul* (the first yearly almanac carried the essay, "The Mucker Swindle in the German Colonies: A Contribution to the Cultural History of Local Germanism"). The Germanist elite and media had been altogether omitted from the Mucker war's history books. Yet, in reading these reports, I could not avoid the conclusion that Koseritz and associates had actively shaped the conflict through fantastic accounts, support for police raids, anti-Mucker petitions, and so forth.[12]

The *Deutsche Zeitung* also reprinted incendiary reports against the Mucker published by Jesuit and Lutheran authorities in their own newspapers (*Volksblatt* and *Der Bote*—the issues of that time are nowhere to be found). On May 17, 1873, Koseritz published news from *Der Bote* saying that several Lutheran families were leaving their congregations to found a new religion around the "prophet of the Ferrabraz"—"the Bible, newspapers and books of any sort are prohibited to them." These ex-members were comparing German pastors to the Pharisees: "They say that they don't want anything to do with Pharisees and wolves in sheep's clothing." As reported by Koseritz, the Jesuit's *Volksblatt* mentioned that Maurer was "a false Christ" and that undue lay interpretation of the Bible was a cause of that "religious madness." An anti-Mucker ecumenism had been launched. As Koseritz put it, "We are also of the opinion that the Bible can be put to dangerous use. The misreading of the Bible causes more misfortune than wars and pestilence. Instead of the Bible, people should be given natural history books."

Mucker survivor Miguel Noé described those days: "In their sermons, the clergy tried to inculcate a strong aversion towards Jacobina, saying, 'She is a witch, a sorcerer! She is a prostitute, a seducer of men, an unruly woman, a liar'" (1977: 384). In her first known letter, February 1873, Jacobina wrote to her oldest brother who was associating with people who slandered her, particularly Lúcio Schreiner, a cousin and São Leopoldo's new police chief (Schreiner's father had been the fraudulent executor of the Mentzes state): "Your charity has vanished. Where is your faith? What are your deeds? . . . The hands of men have grown tired and their hearts coward. . . . But in the name of the heavenly father I ask you: leave the tumult of the world and come back, for you wounded me in the heart which bleeds drop by drop. And what will our good mother say when she will know about it? She will then say: my heart hurts so much." In the letter, Jacobina denounced "the scribes who make unjust laws and utter iniquitous sentences, so as to twist the cause of the poor and to oppress the rights of the unhappy, judging that the widows ought to be their prey and the orphans their victims. . . . But I endure" (quoted in Domingues 1977: 86).

In a suggestive statement, Noé implies that the Mucker were aware of the powerful "shadows" that determined those events, but were unable to fight them: "At that time the government of Brazil and of the province was in a difficult situation because of the infiltration of dim shadows which wanted to interfere in governmental measures or were setting up a parallel government . . . to then seize power" (1977: 391).

Absence of documentation makes it very difficult to know the exact number of people who routinely assembled at Jacobina and João Jorge's house. Historian Janaína Amado scrutinized police reports and identified by name at least "249 rebels" (1978: 127–36). She suggested that at the peak of the conflict there were about 1,000 people directly or indirectly participating in the meetings (which at that time represented approximately 10 percent of the population of the São Leopoldo colony). Taking these 249 rebels as a matrix, Amado produced a statistical portrait of a possible Mucker constituency. Children up to thirteen years of age represented 30 percent of the total number of participants. Seventy percent of the adult Mucker were married. Nine percent of the Mucker were elderly (over fifty-nine years old). Sixty-four percent of the known Mucker were born in Brazil. The majority of the Mucker spoke only German: 57 percent were illiterate; 23 percent were semiliterate in German. Most of the Mucker were not property owners; 39.2 percent worked on lands owned by relatives. Sixty-nine percent of the adult men were peasants, 13 percent were artisans and peasants, 11.5 percent worked only as artisans or small businessmen. Regarding religious affiliation: 85 percent were Lutheran and 15 percent were Catholic.

THE ELITE'S IMAGINARY WORLD
AND FREE-SPIRITED PEOPLE

Reading Koseritz's reports led me to reconsider the ways the Mucker entered social science: as a millennial movement, nostalgically responding to the disintegration of kinship-based communities (Queiróz 1976) and acting as counter-capitalist crusaders (Amado 1978). Yet, as I saw in letters and testimonies the so-called Mucker gave to the police, they always referred to themselves by their names, denied that Jacobina was Christ and that she had named apostles, and spoke of the ordinariness of their lives and the concreteness of the circumstances and frames they were caught in. Yet their claims to truth and dignity were met by silence from authorities at all levels. While Lutheran and Jesuit missionaries portrayed the Mucker as nonreligious and amoral, as being averse to religious authority and to family values, Koseritz and associates framed the colonists as messianic and inspired by ideas of communism.

The Germanist elite was indeed concerned in constructing an imaginary world. Their denunciations of the Mucker as delirious and fraudulent were coupled with references to the life in the colonies as an Arcadian paradise, where hard work and the maintenance of the German cultural values ensured general economic well-being and public order. The Mucker became the past, so to speak, of a morbid Germanist project of social evolution and political and economic integration.

> If the peasants had learned something of the Natural Sciences and had been brought up according to some of the principles of *Aufklärung* they would certainly laugh at the Mucker's prophecies. (DZ 5/17/1873)

> One cannot be precise about the objectives of this society; but the gossip is that the whole band has bad intentions. They want to be the sole dwellers of this place. One also hears that much lead, gunpowder and brimstone is being bought. . . . The prophetic couple is very silly, but there are even more stupid people who let themselves be manipulated by them. What is worst, they destroy families . . . encouraging divorce. For this destruction they find replacement in the Mucker association, because for them everything is communism. What a beautiful moral. (DZ 6/28/1873)

> It is essential to neutralize the influence of this bunch of fanatics over thousands of families, to bring back the lost peace. . . . All this cannot and ought

not be tolerated by the state if it does not want to destroy its very existence. (DZ 5/9/1874)

The *Deutsche Zeitung* unleashed its anti-Mucker campaign in March 1873, associating this pious group first with unreason and prophecy (due to Jesuit influence) and then later with Indian black magic and African witchcraft—friends of the Maurers were "white niggers" (DZ 5/17/1873). By mentioning the figure of the Indian, Koseritz was evoking that primal immigrant fear of having family killed and property overtaken by natives living in the woods. By equating the Mucker with slaves, Koseritz (who owned slaves, like several of his fellow Germanists) was also beginning to frame them as divested of any legal rights. In the following months, Koseritz and his correspondents consistently disseminated sensationalistic news about the practices at the Maurers, creating an all too strategic epistemic murk (see Taussig 1986).

Consider this report from May 10, 1873, published by Koseritz under the pseudonym Y. Z.:

Last Sunday, a large meeting took place around the "miraculous doctor."
Some say that two hundred people of all creeds assembled there, others say
five hundred. If the police does not take adequate measures, terrible things
might happen in the future. Some say that Maurer was crowned Savior and
that he chose twelve apostles among his followers. Others say that his wife
considers herself the Savior; she mentions this while asleep, and then she
prophesies the end of the world and all kinds of possible and impossible
absurdities that only God knows. Last Friday, the end of the world was supposed to have taken place, but since this has not happened she rescheduled it
for Pentecost's day. The Maurers' followers have been making an ark like
Noah's; they butcher cattle and pigs and salt them so that they might be
fried when history reestablishes itself. From time to time, the miraculous
doctor climbs the Ferrabraz mountain (probably because the Sinai is too far
away), where—like a second Moses—he talks to God in person. Maurer
asked his followers not to go to any church, Protestant or Catholic; not to
dance on Sunday and not to play cards.

Mucker Noé characterized the participation in the meetings at the Ferrabraz as an option of free-spirited people: "Why did the withdrawal from the church take place? In order for us to reach clarity and not go on wandering in darkness. Spiritually, people were kept at a lower level, subject to the constant negative judgment of the Church and having to work for the despotic clergy. If *freedom of thought* had been allowed in the churches then each person could have said freely *whether Jacobina's enlightenments were for or against them*, and whether her healing practices were moved by great financial ambition, which was not the case" (1977: 384, my emphasis).

On May 22, 1873, Jacobina was arrested and taken to São Leopoldo in order to testify before the province's police chief. The *Deutsche Zeitung* reported what the police produced as evidence: "Their fortress is built of mysterious illusions. The rooms are contiguous; it is not necessary to get out of one in order to get into another. We inspected the dark room where Miss Christ makes her experiments . . . we found pistols, knives and the images of Christ, Pastor Borchard and Jesuit Ignatius Loyola" (DZ 6/28/1873). Later, in a plea to Emperor Dom Pedro II, the Mucker mentioned that "even though Jacobina was in an unconscious state, eight soldiers put her on an oxcart and escorted her to the city. The trip took nine hours and along the road she was constantly insulted. She was still ill when they placed her in the City Hall and exhibited her to the public."[13]

Jacobina was then submitted to a medical examination coordinated by the same doctor who had seen her as a teenager (Dr. Hillebrand was now the general administrator of São Leopoldo and surrounding colonies). In order to confirm suspicions that she was dissimulating, they "pinched her skin, pierced her body with needles and knives, and tried many other medical applications to wake her up" (DZ 6/28/1873). Police reports say that around 7:00 P.M., her head perspired and she began to murmur with her eyes still closed. Only after some of her friends chanted and kissed her she opened her eyes and asked for some water. "I have never before in my whole life heard such a cat howling," ridiculed Koseritz, who was there (quoted in Domingues 1977: 41).

Jacobina testified that meetings were held in her house during which she explained the Bible "according to inspiration from above" (DZ 6/14/1873). She kept her narrative within her conception of the legal limits of official inquiry, stressing her right as a Protestant to lay priesthood as well as the group's legal right to assembly. Her testimony was matched with that of her husband, who had been previously interrogated by the police: "Maurer said that reunions take place in his house, but with the only purpose of explaining the true meaning of the Scriptures; and that he has even invited clergy of several beliefs to attend them" (DZ 6/11/1873).

Since those religious meetings couldn't be legally prohibited, Germanist administrators and the police created, in the name of order and safety, exceptional practices. "Mr. and Mrs. Christ signed a 'vow of good behavior' and were placed under police custody" (DZ 7/5/1873). In spite of not being charged with any crime or diagnosed with any illness, the authorities kept the healer imprisoned at the headquarters of the Imperial Army and the dreamer confined to a psychiatric ward in Porto Alegre. The authorities alleged that they had done so in order to protect "the treacherous couple" from the wrath of neighboring peasants (DZ 6/18/1873).

This confinement had the effect of publicizing the Mucker as mad and delinquent. These interventions also unleashed a mechanism of self-reporting within a new matrix of what good behavior meant, legitimizing the interventions of public officers and the police when fellow colonists reported breaks in the vows. Through these laws of exception, the colonists' domestic spaces and private lives became open to frequent inspection. This framing of reality became a technology, one used frequently and effectively to gather support against the Mucker from local authorities as well as from large segments of the colonist population.

In a letter dated December 27, 1873, Carolina Mentz, Jacobina's youngest sister, used the events involving domestic animals to challenge the ways her cousin Lúcio Schreiner, chief of police, used his public office: "Don't be bothered by the familial bond which ties you to us; don't give yourself reasons to blame your modest and nowadays, often insulted relatives for your failure to obtain a higher office. We were to expect that people who live in the civilized world and consider themselves as belonging to the enlightened classes . . . would have behaved as educated men and not as savages when going into homes and meeting human beings. I requested information about Maurer's horse, injured by the men of your guard, and you replied that Maurer had loaned the horse to one of those men. Now everybody knows that you have lied" (quoted in Petry 1957: 155).[14]

In a letter to another cousin, Jacobina referred to Schreiner as in fact the "anti-Christ," as a colonist who had already lost his mind: "Lúcio, the anti-Christ, also tried to falsely influence your mind by saying that I had dishonored all the relatives and had slandered the name of your dead father. . . . Why does he so arbitrarily search for *our head?* I suppose that he does so because he himself doesn't have one any longer, he has already given proof of this" (my emphasis).[15]

As polemics grew and violence against the Mucker escalated, Freemasons, Jesuits, and Protestants engaged in a fierce debate: each party blamed the other as the Ur-cause of *Muckerei*. The truth about incidents involving the so-called Mucker and the legality of the maneuvers that led to the war were not addressed. The enemy Mucker united these parties. Through the Mucker, each party claimed institutionality and authority, thus crystallizing their ideas of religion, *Kultur*, and public order. Here, one could argue, the privileged Germanist class and priesthood did not merely recognize "the usefulness of popular belief systems in controlling people," as Max Weber would have framed such matters (1963: 89). Rather, they were profoundly dependent on the development of an "irrational religion" as a means of guaranteeing their social and psychological legitimacy.[16]

THE UNCANNY MUCKER

Sigmund Freud's essay *Das Unheimlich*, "The Uncanny" (1955), is helpful in thinking about the manufacture of the Mucker as a bestial double of the Germanist ideal ego (Biehl 1999). The uncanny, writes Freud, is a particular feeling related to something so dreadful, a shadow, trace, or a nuance, that it calls forth repulsion and distress. The etiology of the word *Unheimlich* shows that the meaning of *heimlich* (familiar) developed ambivalently, passing through the negation *Un*, until it finally coincided with its opposite: "the factor of repression enables us . . . to understand Schelling's definition of the uncanny as something which ought to have remained hidden but has come to light" (Freud 1955: 241).

Of particular interest here is Freud's emphasis on the experience of the uncanny as not being derived from revelations or apparitions, but coming about through literary artifices that produce a "double." For example, a living person to whom one ascribes evil intentions can be taken as uncanny. In this case, the harmful intentions must be perceived and carried out with the constructed help of special powers. Freud explores how fantastic narratives leave readers uncertain as to whether the characters are human beings or automatons, and as to whether one is witnessing deliriums or a succession of events that could be regarded as real. "The quality of uncanniness can only come from the fact of the 'double' being a creation dating back to a very early mental stage, long since surmounted—a stage, incidentally, at which it wore a more friendly aspect. The 'double' has become a thing of terror, just as, after the collapse of their religion, the gods turned into demons" (Freud 1955: 236; see also Freud 1961).

The reconstruction of the Mucker events challenges Freud's view that "fiction presents more opportunities for creating uncanny feelings than are possible in real life" (Freud 1955: 251; see Hacking 1999 and Greenblatt 2000). In fact, Koseritz and his associates were capable of socially manufacturing Mucker doubles. Through fantastic discursive practices, backed by the authority of natural history, media and pastoral power, and disciplinary strategies, the Mucker were carved out of simple and pious colonists who had handled matters of illness and dying on their own terms. Koseritz and fellow Germanists used a fantastic rationalism to deconstruct that culture, turning it into the negative form of a Germanist interiority understood as second nature. The "deadly magical powers" of Jacobina, a "necromancer," were to be surpassed by the media-based and paralegal powers of enlightened leaders, physicians, and professional clergy.

The Mucker worked as social technology, that is, they became the catalysts of the way free individuals were to "truly" understand themselves and relate to each other. Through the Mucker events we see the unmaking of time-honored value systems and the emergence of new forms of control and subjectivity. Here the conflicts between Self and Other were not exclusively transposed to an imaginary plane (Lacan 1991: 282). The adversaries went beyond exhibiting and bearing each other's image; they did not avoid a real struggle. In fact, they acted out a war to end each other or each other's representatives or absent enemies. This is the crucial dimension of the Mucker events: the construction and the embodiment of the Mucker is not just literary but *literal*. In order for there to be the possibility of Germanist subjects rediscovering the power of the truth in themselves, that truth must not have been first discovered or veiled, but made, inscribed, and transferred as a violent dependency.

While studying Koseritz's anti-Mucker reports, I also realized that the war's main reference books (which had informed the *Zero Hora* report on the beheaded woman) had all been, directly or indirectly, informed by this Germanist master narrative. A comparative analysis revealed that authors had either taken reports from *Deutsche Zeitung* at face value or had plagiarized Koseritz's interpretations of the events, without reference to him.

Let me give a few examples. Jesuit Ambrosio Schupp wrote *Die Mucker* (The Mucker) in 1878 (it was first published in Brazil in 1901). It remains the core bibliographic reference of the Mucker war. After a close rereading of *Die Mucker*, I found that Schupp basically emulated Koseritz's core arguments, fleshing them out with reports from local adversaries of the Mucker as well as from legal procedures that anteceded and preceded the war. For the Mucker, reasoned Schupp, "there were no sacred ties . . . relations were marked by passion" (1901: 209). Jacobina had untied "men's passions" and given crimes "the stamp of religion and piety." Further, "In the hands of a woman [the Bible] became a weapon with two edges, which would bring first the ruin of those who had been obsessed by her and, second, her own ruin" (339).

Leopoldo Petry, a historian born in the colonies, wrote the apologetic *O Episódio do Ferrabraz* (The Episode at the Ferrabraz) in 1957 "so that the name of respectful families will no longer continue to suffer the dishonor of being associated with criminals" (1957: 31). He drew from policy documents, testimonies of Mucker descendents, and a report by João Jorge Klein (according to many, including Koseritz, the "mastermind" manipulating Jacobina and the "simpleminded" colonists). According to Petry, local authorities should be blamed for unleashing the armed conflict, while colonists had been the naive prey of Jacobina's intrigues. There is no mention of Koseritz and his associates. Yet, in the end Petry concedes that he has not found a satisfactory explanation for "the mysterious force that, acting backstage, infused such a tenacious hatred against the Mucker among laborious, peaceful and orderly colonists . . . they could not rest until they exterminated the poor victims of Jacobina Maurer" (115).

Moacyr Domingues published *A Nova Face dos Muckers* (The New Face of the Mucker) in 1977. The retired colonel aimed to remove from the Mucker events "the thick veil that until today surrounds its causes and objectives" (9). In various public archives, he discovered previously unpublished governmental documents as well as letters the Mucker exchanged among themselves and with local authorities. Domingues's detailed chronology of the Mucker events are a corrective to Schupp's and Petry's "either incomplete or merely probable accounts" (9)—yet his account too remains obsessed with Jacobina's psychology: "Jacobina was victim of an inexorable process of psychological deterioration; it began in her early childhood due to a congeries of factors unleashed by an extremely rigorous education. Out of necessity she learned—without having consciousness of this—to hypnotize herself or to influence herself by suggestion: it was the crowning of a constant exercise of self-control, which has powerfully contributed to strengthen her stoicism and will" (44).

CIVIL WAR

In May 1874, amid accusations that the Mucker had ambushed a local inspector and killed an orphan in the center of São Leopoldo (crimes for which nobody was ever convicted), the *Deutsche Zeitung* increased its campaign for a military intervention against them: "Never before has the social order been so profoundly ripped apart. It is urgent to neutralize the influence of this bunch of fanatics over thousands of families. All this cannot and ought not be tolerated by the state if it does not want to destroy its very existence. A despotic state would certainly have the means to end this disorder" (DZ 5/9/1874).

There was no way out of that new reality. According to survivor Noé, throughout the colonies, even children were brandishing their knives, ready to slaughter the animal: "They heard everything from their parents. When they were holding a knife they proudly said: 'with this knife we will make sausage out of Jacobina'" (1977: 391). After the imprisonment of some of their leaders, the Mucker knew that they were facing their death and decided to take an active part in the form it took. "For now a heated struggle of life and death would take place and all were supposed to show up at the Maurers on June 24. The Mucker would not let this inhuman fraud be blamed on them. They would have been cowards if they had not defended the honor of their names" (392).

While fighting for their honor, these colonists ended up embodying the alterity they had been made into and murdered those living nearby who had conspired against them: "That night, on all paths, they went to the barbarian instruments of darkness, to the ones who had hurt them the most and ... made a bloody ending" (392). The Mucker set fire to several neighboring households and trading posts. Fourteen persons died. "The Mucker responded to the challenge put to them and made their response real," wrote Noé. "They returned to Maurer's house and waited for the last battle to take place" (392). The official celebrations of the fiftieth anniversary of the German Immigration, scheduled for the next day, were canceled.

In fact, Jacobina had announced a "final judgment" in a letter sent a few weeks before to Schreiner, her cousin and São Leopoldo's chief of police: "Soon the situation of each of us is going to be defined. Keep on feeding your instincts in your own flesh and in your blood, i.e., in your relatives. However, beware, for the Judgment Day will not tarry. And does Your Excellency not know that each day that passes can in fact be the last day of life?" (quoted in Domingues 1977: 242). Thus, before their vanquishment, the Mucker "transcended wild animals in madness and ferocity and turned that place into an image of terror," wrote Koseritz (DZ 6/27/1874). "They should be devoured by dogs, so that the honored man would not have to foul his hands" (DZ 7/15/1874).

Killing was woven into the political fabric. The railroad was now carrying the police forces and the Imperial Army to the colonies. Throughout the colonies, people who had in one way or the other associated with the Mucker had their properties invaded and destroyed, domestic animals were butchered, bodies were left unburied along the roads. "More than one thousand people gathered at São Leopoldo's train station to see the [Mucker] prisoners. . . . A mass of people rolled through the streets with shouts of joy and threats of lynching" (DZ 7/1/1874).

On July 19, 1874, after several weeks of battles and severe casualties on both sides, the president of the province wrote a telegram to the minister of justice announcing the attack on Maurer's house: "The Mucker offered tenacious resistance. Sixty to eighty of them were killed. Thirty of our soldiers were killed. Only two officers were wounded. The city of São Leopoldo is celebrating."[17] Soon, however, it would be known that Jacobina and her closest friends had escaped into the woods. Other news from the war zone mentioned that Mucker corpses were being mutilated. "The persecution of the Mucker continues until all have been hunted down" (DZ 7/22/1874).

A few weeks later, the end of the war was announced. As Koseritz wrote, the Mucker had embraced a primitive, immoral, and criminal vision of life that had to be done away with so that historical men could act. The forces of reason and law woke the Mucker up from the world of dreams and from the forms the dreamers see: "The remaining Mucker were sleeping in the arms of Morpheus inside a hut made of skinned animals and of tree bark. . . . Their slaughter was quick, even though they still offered one last and desperate resistance. Jacobina died in the arms of Rodolfo Sehn, who covered her with his body, both were penetrated by bayonets. . . . The curtain went down, the bloody drama ended. Damaged justice is restored and the citizen can calmly go back to his peaceful daily work" (DZ 8/4/1874). And in his 1875 essay on the Mucker swindle Koseritz rewrote this last scene, adding that, while dying, Jacobina "exhaled her dark soul."

The recollection of the Mucker Noé affirms autonomy till the end: "As in the last battle almost everything was over, Jacobina said that the survivors should try to take good care of themselves, that her things would have an ending, but that she would not allow them to take her life. She herself would make the ending. These were the last words she delivered" (1977: 396).

While trying to affirm their own ways of thinking and exchanging, the Mucker became a cursed object, were killed as bestial Other; their memory became the primitive nature to be forgotten and part of an evolving local German Spirit and modern political economy. The Germanist elite then created Relief Committees to reconstruct the colonies. Life had to be remade through the building of schools and cultural societies, where the natural sciences would be taught. In the words of Koseritz, "We have to introduce the children at a young age to the perennial and eternally active laws of nature . . . so that the memory of a mad and hysterical woman like Jacobina will be simply left behind" (1875: 126).

In 1878, Koseritz wrote a travel book aiming to recruit hard-working, frugal, and orderly colonists, and to attract new foreign investments for the region. The book was published by the Geographical Society Fostering German Interests Overseas.[18] He now depicted the colonies as a sanitized and nonhybridized extension of German *Kultur*. In the colonies, the true German Self could be sensed: "Language, morals and religious manners of the old fatherland were so truly preserved in the South, that upon arrival the new immigrant breathes an almost pure German air" (Koseritz 1897: 38).

DISAPPEARANCE

By inquiring into how Jacobina's spirituality and those colonists' struggles for survival entered history as the past of a morbid Germanist project of social evolution and economic integration, one tastes the truth drop by drop, like a bitter powerful medicine, as Friedrich Nietzsche envisioned it: "I mean the power of specifically growing out of one's self, of making the past and the strange one body with the near and the present" (1957: 68, 7). As I learned growing up in southern Brazil and later through this memory-building work, anyone related to the Mucker or to the thoughts, rituals, and values they were associated with—which actually meant rebellion against the monopolizers of God, science, and capital and the affirmation of an autonomous symbolic order—became socially known as *nichts*, a nothing worthy of disappearance, then and in the century that followed the war.

As reflected in today's media, the Mucker are a continuous legend of the present. Other wars for survival and for social exclusion/inclusion, and the need to explain and contain the surplus of daily violence in that society as well as the dying out of familial ties, keep giving occasion to the Mucker's phantasmatic-like return. And interestingly, while the media evoke the Mucker as the interpretive reservoir of today's events, fundamental questions such as racism and moral blindness, as well as enduring patterns of economic exploitation and the patriarchal physical capture of the other's body, remain publicly unaddressed.

The woman in the beginning of this chapter, without a head, without an identity, without anyone claiming her body, was finally buried as a nameless indigent in the local public cemetery—the aura with which the media left her was that of a licentious woman on the run, a victim but also the potential inducer of a crime of passion. To kill the Other with impunity is in the structure of this modern Brazilian scene.

NOTES

1. Serrano (1999) discusses this report.
2. In 1808, the ruling house of Portugal escaped the Napoleonic wars and moved to Brazil. After centuries of plundering, the colony was to quickly experience a modernizing makeover—particularly Rio de Janeiro, the new capital. Upon arrival in Brazil, King Dom João VI immediately signed a decree opening the ports to free economic exchange with England (Portugal's new economic and political mentor) and a law that allowed foreigners to own land in Brazil (Luebcke 1987).
3. Meanwhile, the imperial administration continued to be trapped between Britain's pressures to develop a free labor force and create a consumer demand on the one hand, and the demands of the powerful territorial aristocracies to maintain slavery on the other (Brazil was the last country in the Western Hemisphere to abolish slavery in 1888). Overall, the history of the São Leopoldo colony epitomizes the makeshift and contingent ways in which the plans for Brazil's modernization and future have again and again been structured. They are attempts to follow external models—Brazil as a "failed" American model of emigrant settlement and integration—and coexist with oligarchic modes of control and patterns of illegality. These experiments are only partially carried out, and Brazilians have to invent structures parallel to the state in order to guarantee their survival.

4. Letter from the Sociedade de Ginásticos e Atiradores Alemães to the president of the province of Rio Grande do Sul, July 2, 1874, Arquivo Nacional, Rio de Janeiro.

5. In order to compete for those immigrants with other host countries, such as the United States, Canada, Australia, and New Zealand, Brazil decided to make colonization a responsibility of local provincial governments and private companies. The province of Rio Grande do Sul, for example, adopted plans that British colonizer Edward Gibbon Wakefield had designed for Australia and New Zealand. Wakefield advocated making small properties available to immigrants at very low prices and the creation of common funds for agricultural development—in southern Brazil the plan faced fierce opposition by the large landowners (Nogueira and Hutter 1975: 31).

6. "Considerações Gerais sobre a ex-Colúnia de São Leopoldo em 1867—Exposição do Comissário do Governo em São Leopoldo, José Joaquim Rodrigues Lopes," Código 807, Vol. 16, Imigração: Coleção Memórias, Arquivo Nacional, Rio de Janeiro.

7. According to Moacyr Domingues, "There were two alleged causes for the dissidence: the fact that the official Lutherdom negated the divinity of Christ and that the doctrine's books were against the freedom of teaching" (1977: 32). Leopoldo Petry writes that "they practiced their religious acts in their homes" (1957: 44; see also Amado 1978: 116–20).

8. Domingues (1977: 69–71) suggests that Maurer and Buchhorn met in an attempt to address Jacobina's deep sleep.

9. *Die Mission unter den Evangelischen Deutschen in Südbrasilien,* January 1, 1865, Evangelisches Zentralarchiv, Berlin, 01/01/1865.

10. See Avé-Lallemant (1980) and Tschudi (1868).

11. Deviltries are at once "social symptoms and transitional solutions," argues Michel de Certeau in *The Possession at Loudon* (2000: 2; see also Freud 1961). In seventeenth-century France, deviltries signaled the end of a religious modus operandi that couldn't be spoken yet and the emergence of a new scientific discursivity, a rationalizing of state power, and a novel way of medically knowing the body.

12. In *The Cunning of Recognition,* Elizabeth Povinelli examines the role of the colonial archive in the crystallization of the liberal subject and the Australian nation-state. She writes: "Only by experiencing the horror of moral alterity could the science of man sketch a sociology of morality itself, the real of human(e) society. . . . It was in this hypermorally animated scene that reason was forced to—and writers promised reason could—discover a 'convergence,' a 'horizon' . . . a synthetic a priori where a universal idea resided connecting these human orders into human being[s]" (2002: 85).

13. Código 605, Questão Maurer, Arquivo Nacional, Rio de Janeiro.

14. Schreiner resented the colonists for not having endorsed him in a recent vote for the administrative council (the 1867 law that gave immigrants this specific right was the first step toward universal voting rights granted in the 1880s).

15. Letter from Jacobina Maurer to Mathias SchrÖder, May 29, 1874, Arquivo Nacional, Rio de Janeiro. This letter is mentioned by Petry (1957: 152). See also Domingues (1977: 244).

16. Nineteenth-century imperialism has largely rested on the authority of science. Historian Gyan Prakash (1999: 6, 14) shows that a Western-educated elite played a key role in the translation of science into governance in the British-Indian context and that the identification of irrational religious and social practices was central to the project of reordering history and values according to a modern Indian self-conception.

17. Telegram from the president of the province to the minister of justice, July 20, 1874, Arquivo Nacional, Rio de Janeiro.

18. The third edition of the book was dedicated to the memory of Koseritz, "The Pioneer of the Workings of German Culture in the South and the Loyal Son of His New Fatherland."

REFERENCES

Aguiar, Antonio Augusto da Costa. 1862. *O Brazil e os Brazileiros*. Santos: Typographia Commercial.

Amado, Janaína. 1978. *Conflito Social no Brasil*. São Paulo: Símbolo.

Assu, Jacare. 1873. *Brazilian Colonization, from an European Point of View*. London: E. Stanford.

Auftrag für die Protestantischen Deutschen in Südbrasilien. 1865. *Die Mission unter den Evangelischen Deutschen in Südbrasilien*. Barmen.

———. 1874. *Die Mission unter den Evangelischen Deutschen in Südbrasilien, Fünfter Bericht*. Barmen.

Avé-Lallement, Robert. 1980. *Viagem pela Província do Rio Grande do Sul 1858*. São Paulo: Editora da Universidade de São Paulo.

Barman, Roderick. 1988. *Brazil: The Forging of a Nation, 1798–1852*. Stanford, CA: Stanford University Press.

Biehl, João. 1991. Jammerthal, o Vale da Lamentação: Crítica à Construção do Messianismo Mucker. Master's thesis, Universidade Federal de Santa Maria.

———. 1996a. Jammerthal, the Valley of Lamentation—The Mucker War: A Contribution to the History of Local Germanism in Nineteenth-Century Southern Brazil. PhD diss., University of California, Berkeley.

———. 1996b. Uma Tribo Que Pensa e Negocia em Alemão. In *Nós, os Teuto-Gaúchos*, ed. Rene Gertz and Luis A. Fischer. Porto Alegre: Editora da UFRGS.

———. 1999. Jammerthal, the Valley of Lamentation: Kultur, War Trauma, and Subjectivity in Nineteenth-Century Brazil. *Journal of Latin American Cultural Studies* 8 (2): 171–98.

Certeau, Michel de. 2000. *The Possession at Loudon*. Chicago: University of Chicago Press.

Comaroff, Jean, and John L. Comaroff. 1991. *Of Revelation and Revolution: Christianity, Colonialism, and Consciousness in South Africa*. Vol. 1. Chicago: University of Chicago Press.

Cunha, Euclides da. 1976. *Um Paraíso Perdido: Reunião dos Ensaios Amazúnicos*. Petrópolis: Vozes.

Delhaes-Günther, Dietrich. 1980. Colonização Européia no Rio Grande do Sul durante o Século XIX (Causas do êxito e Limitações). In *III Colóquio de Estudos Teuto-Brasileiros*. Porto Alegre: Editora da UFRGS.

Dickie, Maria Amelia Schmidt. 1989. Dos "Senhores do Sul" aos Brummer: A Trajetória da Construção Social do Trabalho (RS, 1824–1880). Unpublished ms.

Domingues, Moacyr. 1977. *A Nova Face dos Muckers*. São Leopoldo: Rottermund.

Dreher, Martin. 1984. *Igreja e Germanidade*. São Leopoldo: Editora Sinodal.

Elias, Norbert. 1978. *The History of Manners*. New York: Pantheon Books.

Fabian, Johannes. 2000. *Out of Our Minds: Reason and Madness in the Exploration of Central Africa*. Berkeley: University of California Press.

Fichte, Johann Gottlieb. 1923. *Addresses to the German Nation*. Chicago: Open Court Publishing Company.

Fischer, Michael. 1999. Emergent Forms of Life: Anthropologies of Late or Postmodernities. *Annual Review of Anthropology* 28:455–78.

Foucault, Michel. 1991. Governmentality. In *The Foucault Effect: Studies in Governmentality*, ed. Graham Burchell, Colin Gordon, and Peter Miller, 87–104. Chicago: University of Chicago Press.

Freud, Sigmund. 1955. The Uncanny (1919). In *The Standard Edition of the Complete Psychological Works of Sigmund Freud*, vol. 17, 217–52. London: Hogarth Press and the Institute of Psycho-Analysis.

———. 1961. A Seventeenth-Century Demonological Neurosis (1923). *The Standard Edition of the Complete Psychological Works of Sigmund Freud*, vol. 19, 609–708. London: Hogarth Press and the Institute of Psycho-Analysis.

Frobel, Julius. 1858. *Die Deutsche Auswanderung un ihre Culturhistorische Bedeutung*. Leipzig: Franz Wagner.

Gans, Magda Roswita. 2004. *Presença Teuta em Porto Alegre no Século XIX (1850–1889)*. Porto Alegre: UFRGS Editora.

Gehse, Hans. 1931. *Die Deutsche Presse in Brasilien vom 1852 bis zur Gegenwart*. Münster: Aschendorffsche Verlagsbuchhandlung.

Giddens, Anthony. 1990. *The Consequences of Modernity*. Stanford, CA: Stanford University Press.

Greenblatt, Stephen. 2000. *Hamlet in Purgatory*. Princeton, NJ: Princeton University Press.

Hacking, Ian. 1999. Making Up People. In *The Sciences Studies Reader*, ed. Mario Biagioli, 161–71. New York: Routledge.

Harrison, Austin. 1904. *The Pan-Germanic Doctrine: Being a Study of German Political Aims and Aspirations*. London: Harper.

Hillebrand, João Daniel. 1924. Relatório Apresentado ao Governo da Província em 1854. *Revista do Arquivo Público do Rio Grande do Sul* (Porto Alegre).

Hunsche, Carlos Henrique. 1974. Dez Novas Fontes, Desconhecidas e Inéditas, sobre o Episódio e o Epílogo dos Mucker no Rio Grande do Sul. In *Anais do I Simpósio de História da Imigração e Colonização Alemã no Rio Grande do Sul*, 247–62. São Leopoldo: Rottermund.

———. 1975. *O Biênio 1824/25 da Imigração e Colonização Alemã no Rio Grande do Sul (Província de São Pedro)*. Porto Alegre: A Nação/Instituto Estadual do Livro.

———. 1979. *Primórdios da Vida Judicial de São Leopoldo*. Porto Alegre: Escola Superior de Teologia São Lourenço de Brindes.

Jornal NH. 1993. Delegado Tenta de Tudo para Identificar Mulher Decapitada. May 27, p. 37.

Klein, João Jorge. 1957. Sobre a História dos "Mucker" nos Anos de 1872 a 1874. In *O Episódio do Ferrabraz*, by Leopoldo Petry. São Leopoldo: Rottermund.

Koseritz, Karl von. 1875. Der Mucker Schwindel aus der Deutschen Colonie (ein Beitrag zur Culturgeschichte des Hiesigen Deutschtums). In *Koseritz Deutsche Volkskalender fur die Provinz Rio Grande do Sul—1875*. Porto Alegre: Walther Rühn.

———. 1897 [1878]. *Rathschläge fur Auswanderer nach Südbrasilien*. Berlin: Allgemeine Verlags-Agentur.

Lacan, Jacques. 1991. *The Seminar of Jacques Lacan. Book 1: Freud's Papers on Technique, 1953–1954*. Ed. Jacques-Alain Miller. Trans. John Forrester. New York: W. W. Norton & Co.

Lando, Aldair M., and Eliane C. Barros. 1976. *A Colonização Alemã no Rio Grande do Sul: Uma Interpretação Sociológica*. Porto Alegre: Editora Movimento.

Luebcke, Frederick C. 1987. *Germans in Brazil: A Comparative Study of Cultural Conflict during World War I*. Baton Rouge: Louisiana State University Press.

Mulhall, Michael G. 1873. *Rio Grande do Sul and its German Colonies*. London: Longmans and Green.

Nietzsche, Friedrich. 1957. *The Use and Abuse of History*. New York: Macmillan Publishing Company.

Noé, Miguel. 1977. História do Ano de 1874. In *A Nova Face dos Muckers*, by Moacyr Domingues, 383–98. São Leopoldo: Rottermund.

Nogueira, Arlinda Rocha, and Lucy Maffei Hutter. 1975. *A Colonização em São Pedro do Rio Grande do Sul durante o Imperio (1824–1889)*. Porto Alegre: Editora Garatuja and Instituto Estadual do Livro.

Oberacker, Carlos H. 1961. *Carlos von Koseritz*. Porto Alegre: Anhambi.

————. 1985. *A Contribuição Teuta à Formação da Nação Brasileira*. Rio de Janeiro: Presença.

Petrone, Maria Thereza Schorer. 1982. *O Imigrante e a Pequena Propriedade*. São Paulo: Brasiliense.

Petry, Leopoldo. 1957. *O Episódio do Ferrabraz*. São Leopoldo: Rottermund.

Pinsdorf, Marion K. 1990. *German-Speaking Entrepeneurs: Builders of Business in Brazil*. New York: Peter Lang.

Porto, Aurélio. 1934. *O Trabalho Alemão no Rio Grande do Sul*. Porto Alegre: Estabelecimento Gráfico Santa Terezinha.

Povinelli, Elizabeth. 2002. *The Cunning of Recognition: Indigenous Alterity and the Making of Australian Multiculturalism*. Durham, NC: Duke University Press.

Prakash, Gyan. 1999. *Another Reason: Science and the Imagination of Modern India*. Princeton, NJ: Princeton University Press.

Queiróz, Maria Isaura Pereira de. 1976. *O Messianismo no Brasil no Mundo*. São Paulo: Alfa-úmega.

Rabuske, Arthur. n.d. A Contribuição Teuta à Igreja Católica no Rio Grande do Sul. *Estudos Leopoldenses* 28: 131–50.

Roche, Jean. 1969. *A Colonização Alemã e o Rio Grande do Sul*. Porto Alegre: Globo.

Schrader, Achim. 1980. Da Imigração de Pessoas à Transferência de Tecnologia: Mudanças nas Relações entre a Alemanha e o Brasil. In *III Colóquio de Estudos Teuto-Brasileiros*. Porto Alegre: Editora da UFRGS.

Schüller, H. 1954. *Die Erste Kaiserin von Brasilien*. São Leopoldo: Rottermund.

Schupp, Ambrosio. 1901. *Os Muckers*. 2nd ed. Porto Alegre: Selbach-Mayer.

————. 1912. Die Deutsche Jesuiten-Mission in Rio Grande do Sul (Brasilien). São Leopoldo: Instituto Anchietano de Pesquisas. Unpublished ms.

Serrano Pereira, Lucia. 1993. A Violência Ressurge na Terra dos Mucker. *Revista da Associação Psicanalítica de Porto Alegre* 4 (9): 89–93.

————. 1999. O Imigrante e o Laço Social. In *Psicanálise e Colonização*, ed. Edson Luiz André de Souza, 169–79. Porto Alegre: Artes e ofícios.

Seyferth, Giralda. 1990. *Imigração e Cultura no Brasil*. Brasilia: Editora UnB.

Souza, João Cardoso de Menezes. 1875. *Theses sobre Colonização do Brazil—Projecto de Solução às Questões Sociaes, Que Se Prendem a este Difficil Problema—Relatório Apresentado ao Ministério da Agricultura, Commércio e Obras Públicas*. Rio de Janeiro: Typographia Nacional.

Spalding, Walter. 1965. Naturalizações: 1833 à 1864 em Porto Alegre. *Revista do Instituto Histórico e Geográfico Brasileiro*, no. 169.

Sperb, Angela T. 1987. Autos do Processo dos Mucker. In *ais do IV Simpósio de História da Imigração e Colonização Alemã no Rio Grande do Sul*, ed. Telmo L. Muller, 239–48. São Leopoldo: Museu Histórico Visconde de São Leopoldo/Instituto Histórico de São Leopoldo.

Steinmetz, George. 2004. The Uncontrollable Afterlives of Ethnography: Lessons from "Salvage Colonialism" in the German Overseas Empire. *Ethnography* 5 (3): 251–88

Südhaus, Fritz. 1962. *Deutschland und die Auswanderung nach Brasilien im 19. Jahrhundert*. Hamburg: Hans Christian Druckerei und Verlag.

Taussig, Michael. 1986. *Shamanism, Colonialism, and the Wild Man: A Study in Terror and Healing*. Chicago: University of Chicago Press.

Tschudi, Johann Jakob von. 1868. *Reisen durch Südamerika*. Leipzig: F. A. Brockhaus.

Weber, Max. 1963. *The Sociology of Religion*. Boston: Beacon Press.

Zero Hora (ZH). 1993. Violência Ressurge na Terra dos Muckers. July 12, p. 44.

The *Asylum* and Marginality in Rural Ireland

A. Jamie Saris

So deep was she in this thought that she did not notice the
entrance of old Marse Prendergast, who lived in a cabin just
across the road. Marse was a superannuated shuiler[1] and
a terror in the valley. The tears had been summoned to her
eyes by the still unchanging quality of Ned's tone. They
were at once detected by the old woman.
  "Still crying, are ye, Nan Byrne, for Henry Shannon that's
dead and gone?"
  This was a sore cut, but it was because of its severity that it
had been given. Marse Prendergast's method was to attack the
person from whom she desired an alms instead of making an
approach in fear and trembling.

Brinsley MacNamara, Valley of the Squinting Windows

This piece is a sustained reflection on three types of marginality found in
Kilronan, a market town and its environs containing about sixteen hundred
people found in the Sligo-Leitrim area of Ireland. The three terms I am investigating—"character," "unrespectable," and "mental patient"—all overlap in the
life of one of my consultants who has been connected to the mental hospital in
Sligo town, about eighteen miles away, for much of his adult life. My main purpose in this piece is to try to think clearly about the implications of the simultaneous presence of these seemingly different forms of subjectivity, all of
which show a different aspect of the local presence of the mental hospital, different legacies of a "colonial" history, and what this state of affairs might say to
ideas derived from postcolonial contributions to anthropology and related disciplines, such as "subaltern history." Not so well hidden beside the trail of this
excursion is a longstanding argument of mine that the really interesting aspect
of the power exercised by states (colonial or postcolonial) is not to be found in
their existence as imagined entities, nor in their production as the effects of

individual actors, but in their reality as concrete institutions possessed of particular technologies and histories in a specific time and place (Saris 1996, 1997, 1999, 2000).

PURPOSE

Tomás O'Connor gives the sense of understanding his mission in life. He possesses that distinctive gait generally associated only with purposeful individuals. Forward-leaning, energetic, yet dignified, his pace is smooth and nothing short of ground-devouring as he walks upward of eighteen miles a day around Kilronan and the surrounding countryside.

My first impression of Tomás, when I made his acquaintance in 1990, was of a sturdy, medium-sized man whose shock of white hair made him look older than his (then) fifty-four years. He and one of his sisters, Bridie, occupied a farm of about twelve acres roughly six miles east of Kilronan. Little cultivation was happening there when I arrived on a grey January day. The two larger fields were let to a neighbor for grazing, and the two outbuildings hard by the farmhouse showed the effects of decades of indifferent maintenance. At one time, however, the farm generated enough resources (if just enough) to support nine people. Into the late-1990s, Tomás was still tending a small kitchen garden of spuds and cabbage of about a third of an acre, more out of a conviction that it was right to grow one's own food than for any real need to subsist.

By the time I had met Tomás, he had spent roughly half his adult life in the asylum in Sligo town, wherein he had been hospitalized several times over the course of twenty-five years under diagnoses as diverse as "agitated depression," "personality disorder/borderline schizophrenia," and "bipolar disorder." For the last ten years, he has been visited regularly by the new regime of community psychiatry to which Ireland, along with nearly every other nation on the globe has subscribed. According to his own terse reports when questioned directly (by me or the professionals with whom he interacted) about his current state of health and happiness, he has adapted well to the community, enjoying the interaction with the townspeople and the space that the outside provides for his avocation for wandering. On the other side, both the brother and sister are looked upon with some pity by many in the area and were pointed to as an example of severe rural poverty by most of the state professionals with whom they were in contact. Tomás, due to his long association with the asylum, received the Disabled Person's Maintenance Allowance (DPMA), a weekly welfare payment made to those with disabilities, slightly larger than the dole paid to the unemployed. At times, moreover, this household was also the recipient of aid from the Society of St. Vincent De Paul, a

Catholic charitable organization run and largely controlled by the solidly middle class in the town.

WANDERING

For the ten years or so of this research, on most days, wet or fine, Tommie was awake not long after sunrise, rarely needing the prodding of his sister to get out and about. He was almost always out of the house by eight in the morning. Generally, he would set his face toward Ballycullen, a small village near Kilronan. He knew that there are a couple of places there where he could get morning tea, and the more circuitous route guaranteed that he would not arrive early at the Kilronan Day Hospital where he would have to interact alone with the staff (the other clients usually arrived a little after ten).

If tea was to be had in Ballycullen from one of the merchants or a friendly house, he would stay a moment or two chatting (in his own truncated fashion), while drinking a brew that was more sugar and milk than anything else. If the weather boded ill, he would head straight from there to the day hospital, risking some long moments with the staff to get out of the wet and to see what the crack (from Ir. *craic*—fun, conviviality) promised to be like in the town that day. If the weather looked fine, he would make no effort to arrive at any particular time in the town. Some days, he would make a long loop on a little-used road that passes behind Dromduff, a height commanding this area. If he was late enough in the morning, on the way he would see the dark sockets of the caves that sit high up the sheer side of the mountain, the erstwhile home of rebels and bandits at various times in this area's colorful history. Sometimes, however, he would go in the other direction, toward the old parish center of Castlecormack, now little more than an out of the way village, but home to the ruin of one of the oldest abbeys in the area.

If the day stayed fine, Tommie had an uncanny ability to gauge the distance and velocity of his morning perambulations to arrive just before dinner in the day hospital. On the way, he would wave at the odd passing vehicle or accost fellow travelers as they became more frequent on the road into town. During his dinner, he said little, occasionally acknowledging greetings, but concentrating on satisfying his hunger with the same efficiency as his pace had devoured the landscape that morning. After dinner, he would generally walk some more, perhaps on the opposite side of the town from where he lives, toward Kilcastle, an old gentry mansion or "Big House," which has been in the same family for more than four hundred years. For many years previous to my residence in Kilronan, it was the decaying home of "Old Man Hamilton," a difficult older gentleman retired from more than thirty years in colonial service in Africa. At the time of my work and beyond, his son and daughter-in-law were trying to revive the decaying mansion's fortune by marketing it as an upscale bed and breakfast serving organic produce grown on the still extensive demesne. Occasionally, Tommie would stay in Kilronan or try to be back early enough to enjoy a couple of pints with some of the lads, particularly on mart day when there are many farmers in the town, some of whom would be willing to stand him a round. Usually, though, he would be home by half-past six, as his sister generally had little patience for his being late for tea.

PRODUCTIONS OF PERSONHOOD

Above all else, in and around Kilronan, Tomás O'Connor is known for his "speeches," monologic or, more rarely, dialogic attempts to offer his opinion on the town, the people, and the activities in which they engage. Most of the time, he willingly interrupted his rambles to accost both strangers and friends, anyone really whom he considered a likely audience. As a newcomer to the town, I was initially cautioned "to pay him no heed," for fear that I might accidentally take offense at something he said. In truth, Tomás is not incapable of giving offense, but he rarely does so directly, and, as my experience with him grew, it seemed to me that he rarely does so "accidentally," at least in the strict sense of that term.

One of my first experiences of one of "Queer Tommie's speeches" was one he delivered to one of Kilronan's solicitors, whose father and father's father had been providing legal advice to the citizens of the town since the early part of the twentieth century. As the solicitor left his office, within earshot of many farmers who were streaming into the pub next door with the closing of the cattle mart for the day, Tommie offered the younger man a bit of advice.

"That's the point, sir," simultaneously accosting and blocking the path of the surprised professional, who seemed to be in a hurry to be somewhere else. "To earn your keep by the sweat of your brow. That's what we all should be doin'. I wouldn't be a stockbroker, no sir. They're with lots of money, but are they any happier, do ye think. You think about that, now."

The solicitor left hurriedly, before Tomás could develop his line of argument further. He was confused, I think (and relieved, I later reasoned), because Tomás' speeches can be much longer affairs. Most of the farmers, on the other hand, out of sorts as they were, for cattle prices had been frankly bad for the past several months (and had been no better that afternoon), chuckled as they passed the pair. They had clearly enjoyed the spectacle of poor Queer Tommie doling out advice to the solicitor, who is (by his own lights at least) one of the most "respectable" members of the town. I, too, had chuckled at the scene, not quite understanding all the implications of Tomás's argument, but still quietly enjoying the discomfiture of the well-dressed professional and the amusement of the cloth-capped farmers.

As my experience with these farmers grew, however, I realized there was an edge to this laughter that I was not able to appreciate at the time. In general, the small farmers whom I came to know in the coming months and years have little liking for professionals who do not obviously earn a living with their hands (the best gloss that I can put on Tomás's notion of "stockbroker").[2] And, although they admire their status and their power, they have less liking still for solicitors, whom they consider to partake of the essence of firearms—useful when a dispute arises but dangerous in themselves. In any event, the consensus in the pub on that fair spring evening was that Queer Tommie had made a point about the nature of work, and much of the subsequent discussion, centered as it was on the dark days that had descended upon the price of cattle, was punctuated and relieved by examining and reexamining the nature of the solicitor's trade. This discussion led to further talk of how the country was out of the hands of the farmers now and in the grasp of "the money boys" from Dublin. In this fashion, a seemingly unmotivated outburst by a deinstitutionalized, seemingly delusional "client" (who, in the event, was absent during most of the evening as he had to leave the pub early because of a dire warning from his sister to be home in time for tea) in many respects set the agenda for the next two hours of conversation.

NARRATING PERSONS

How do we understand someone like Tomás O'Connor? He wanders through the detritus of several colonial and postcolonial regimes—physical things, like castles, clinics, and churches. Indeed, the very landscape that he walks on every morning bears the ruts of various conquests and the resistances these aggressions provoked. More importantly for my argument here, his social life is also defined, at least in part, by venerable and robust bureaucratic structures, like state psychiatric services and public welfare support networks that have roots in both a colonial past and recent postcolonial history. Indeed, these structures, both physical and conceptual, are part of the "stuff" of colonial and postcolonial history for this locality, helping to locate Tomás, his area, even Ireland itself within a set of familiar, even hoary, oppositions: traditional vs. modern, irrational vs. rational, personal vs. political, or, indeed, serving as the subject of history vs. being its active agent (Saris 1996, 1999, 2000, and 2005). Examining Tomás's relationship to various marginal subject positions does more than merely erode such static binarisms, however. It also allows us to glimpse ethnographically how various cultural orderings of history, in Sahlins's apt phrasing

(2004), structure the experience and the interpretation of both consciousness and practice. In this way, understanding individual subjectivity and intersubjective relationships around ideas of marginality forces us to understand an enormous amount of "history," which, at the same moment, delineates important aspects of "culture."

Perhaps, it is best then to read our original question at first prosaically, that is, how do we interpret Tomás's curious utterances and avocation for wandering? I will try to answer this question from a variety of perspectives, but I want to make it clear from the beginning that Tommie's life can be refracted through several conceptual prisms.

There are, for example, a wide variety of Irish literary clues available to help us make some sense of Tomás. In *Valley of the Squinting Windows*, by Brinsley MacNamara, Marse Prendergast (introduced in my epigraph) is, like poor Queer Tommie, a sort of local institution. She is one of the harsh arbitrators of the unhappy moral universe of Garradrimna, a literary setting based on a largish village/smallish town in Westmeath. Marse terrorizes the respectable sorts in the valley, because she is in no way respectable, and she wields a weapon of gossip that all are hungry to hear, yet of which all fervently pray not to be the subject. The participants in this system, MacNamara shows, despise and fear one another. Nonetheless, they continue to reproduce a social existence with which no one is terribly happy, but in which Ms. Prendergast has an important role and voice. Finally, of course, the novel ends in tragedy. Leaving aside the fundamental pessimism that MacNamara hangs miasmically over his little valley, the point I want to emphasize is Marse's interesting ability to be at once marginal and necessary to her social environment.

Marse is endured, even occasionally supported, by Nan Byrne and the other unfortunate inhabitants of the valley precisely because of her ability to scandalize them. *Is beo fear tar éis a bhuailte, ach ní beo tar éis a cháinte*, the Irish proverb goes. "A man is alive after being beaten, but he is not alive after being satirized" (Ir. *cáinim*—I satirize, I criticize, I censure) (also see Partridge 1978: 22). In Gaelic Ireland poets had two functions: to praise and to censure (Coleman 1991; also O'Brien 1981 and O'Madagáin 1985), a verbal connection that can still be commonly found in the language. Indeed, one can still hear such pairings (in English) around Kilronan (and many other parts of Ireland) as, "If you want blame, marry; if you want praise, die."

The censuring/satirizing function of poets was particularly feared because the verses created would be remembered in local speech and repeated long after the poet had left the scene.[3] Like remembered gossip, such talk would "do the rounds," potentially becoming sedimented in local historical consciousness. It is usually possible to get up after a beating, for example, but, through the magic power of words, the successful savaging of the social person in local talk, that is the verbal attack on a reputation, potentially infinitely reproducible, was not so easily shrugged off.

While obviously not a poet, Marse's utterances are nonetheless accorded some respect because of her penchant for wandering, her ability to pick up on local gossip, and her willingness, indeed eagerness, to share what she knows. The fact that she does not have a reputation to protect in the usual sense and is therefore "outside" of respectable society makes her even more dangerous as a conduit of reported speech—having no local reputation to worry about, she is out of range of retributive gossip. Furthermore, far from diminishing the effect of her speech, Marse's remove from regular society seems to add a certain weight to her words. It seems to me that this seemingly conflicted ability of Ms. Prendergast in an admittedly created, fictional setting is more than a literary device.[4] I find MacNamara's portrayal in this work of Prendergast's importance as both a teller of stories and the subject of other stories to ring very true to my own experience of the lives of certain marginal individuals in Kilronan. In short, his novelization of how a semi-itinerant old lady, who spends much of the day talking to herself, interacts with her social milieu in a literary setting shares some significant similarities with the way in which many of my "character" consultants exist today in Kilronan.

At the same time, the question that began this section, "How do we understand someone like Tómas O'Connor?" is more complicated than it might otherwise appear because even its posing forefronts certain interpretative frames and deemphasizes others. For example, the current state of play of cosmopolitan psychiatric knowledge formally assimilates the more bizarre aspects of Tómas's behavior to the gruntings of an epileptic during a seizure, that is, as the meaningless by-products of a lesioned or badly wired brain. On the other hand, anthropologists have long understood such eccentrics as both bearers and broadcasters of some of the symbolic tensions in their environment (e.g., Comaroff and Comaroff 1992: 155–80), a sort of magnifying glass on meaningful local dynamics and contradictions. My sense of Irish tourism, moreover, is that (at least American) visitors to a small market town would find the friendly cloth-capped eccentric a welcome part of their "Irish experience." My point is that there is no Archimedean point from which to explain the idiosyncrasies of Tómas's social existence or the nature of his agency. As bystander, clinician, or ethnographer, we are implicated in developing a story that presupposes a relevant past and points to a probable future, as part and parcel of a present frame of reference.

Thus, we might have meant by our initial question something like, how do we understand the local frames of reference through which Tomás is understood? (Hanks 1990: chaps. 1–2; Goffman 1981). This version of the question leads in some interesting directions. Sociologically, for example, individuals like Tomás O'Connor are at the confluence of distinct but overlapping traditions of deviance, all of which have existed in Ireland for some time. First, and most obviously, Tommie is a deinstitutionalized psychiatric patient, intimately familiar with the asylum and the panoply of associated "helping mechanisms" that can be found in similar form in many places in the world. At the same time, he has various marginal local existences. He and his family are "unrespectable," an object of pity for many in the town, even as he is a target of scorn for others. He is also a town "character," a locally tolerated (even occasionally celebrated) eccentric who fits comfortably in a pattern of banter that surrounds those who give "color" to Kilronan. These subjectivities can only be indifferently arranged along a linear narrative, conforming to a model of modern versions slowly supplanting older survivals. Indeed, their current mutual constitution confounds any watershed sensibility in considering colonial and postcolonial history.

To begin, then, both "unrespectable" and "character" are important signposts in Kilronan's moral world that are difficult to render across divides of dialect. In the town, for example, there are some full-time characters who never come to the attention of asylum professionals, but many of my "deinstitutionalized" friends were able to fulfill this role. Ultimately, what makes a character is a certain provocative air to the unusualness of a person—a sometime subtle, sometimes gross transgressing of tacit boundaries in ways that (importantly) encourage local speculation and narration. On longer acquaintance, this unusualness starts to look like locally valued attributes cartoonishly enhanced—conviviality merges into a willingness to accost, "liking a few pints" overlaps with being "overfond of drink," "being up for a bit of crack" is near neighbors with sometimes frightening Dionysian excess. As importantly, these differences are taken up in narrative by the character himself and/or the life of the character is such that narrative deliberation about him or her leads to the consideration of much broader questions.

Clearly, "character" is a complex term. It can be (and often is) used pejoratively. Indeed, it can be used to tag an entire area as different in an undesirable way. As a respectable banking friend of mine in Sligo town observed to me about Kilronan as I was getting ready to move to my new home in 1989, "I was based in Ballytubber [a slightly more prosperous town about ten miles away from Kilronan], and I guess I took to thinking like them [about the Kilronan area].

There's something strange there; there are a lot of characters about. Maybe it was because we were only open on mart day and saw a lot of them that had just come down the mountain to sell their cattle. Whatever it was, I didn't like it."

At the same time, the term is also never far from positive valuation. Appropriately contextualized, the observation that "Ah, your man there's a character" suggests that the individual in question is something of a libertine, in the older less sexual sense of this term, *i.e.*, not one to let social conventions get in the way of a little crack. The personalities of such individuals are very often the necessary kindling to light up a memorable "big night."

Similarly, "respectability" and "unrespectability" are difficult concepts to move across dialects, but this is also one of the local divides that Tomás most evidently crosses when accosting the town solicitor and lecturing him about the nature and value of various forms of work. This separation between the respectable and the unrespectable has only occasionally been touched upon in Irish ethnography (see Silverman 1987 and Peace 2001), despite the ubiquity of this phrase in Hiberno-English. Nonetheless, I believe that this division is crucial to understanding the question of why certain townlands and families use and are the recipient of the services of formal bureaucratic structures, like the asylum, in relatively large numbers.

On the one hand, "respectability" correlates with class status broadly defined, that is to say, the "higher up" a person or family considers themselves the likelier they are to be conscious of the process of being respectable and to take steps to see that their respectability is not infringed by either their own doing (e.g., making sure to properly maintain their farm, car, house, and/or dress) or by the doings of others (e.g., vigorously defending one's reputation from verbal assaults). But respectability is by no means the exclusive property of the better-off in Kilronan. There are many people from humble backgrounds in the town and from tiny farms out in the country who treat their family's respectability as a prized possession, jealously guarding it from real and perceived threats. Even in cases where little tangible property is owned and no job is available, respectability can still be claimed and evidenced in such diverse ways as careful attention to dress or a widely accepted reputation of being willing to work if such an opportunity becomes available (see also Silverman 1987: 14).

In practice, then, the idea of "being respectable" has something of the psychological reality of a sense of "social shame," and those in and around Kilronan who clearly lack both a reputation for being respectable and a desire to reclaim such social territory enjoy the freedoms and burdens of the outcast (Scott 1985). It is, moreover, a tacit local truism for the respectable that respectability obeys relatively strict genetic laws. While the respectable can be brought low by previously hidden faults in breeding, the truly unrespectable can rarely expect to move in the opposite direction. Like Calvin's status of "elect," then, respectability is a station that can be lost, but rarely aspired to. The more centered one is in respectable areas in and around Kilronan, moreover, the more geographically mappable becomes the notion of respectability, such that particular townlands and areas are self-evidently unrespectable by virtue of such traits as density of genealogical concentrations that render charges of "inbreeding" ever more locally persuasive in historical memory, poverty of means, and regular contact with such formal bureaucratic mechanisms as the asylum and the police.

Tomás O'Connor, then, lives at the intersection between these differing, often competing, models of inclusion and exclusion. Such models presuppose certain relationships between the *intention* of his speeches and acts and their *intension*, that is, the set of postulates that gives them their meaning. These relationships, in turn, revolve around the implicit and explicit presence of the mental hospital in Sligo town in Tommie's life. Tómas is at once a deinstitutionalized long-term psychiatric patient, a subject of incomprehension and some pity, as well as a local character, someone possessing a certain license in his speech and behavior because of his sometimes provocative insights into the workings of this social setting. The presence of the mental hospital in Tommie's life, his relative poverty, and some of his speeches also tend to mark him as unrespectable.

Meanwhile, other persons with longstanding reputations for eccentricities have moved in the opposite direction, coming into contact with the asylum as its technologies have been dispersed into the countryside that the institution has traditionally served. All these individuals are marginal sorts who are often talked about. At the same time, some of these persons stake a claim to (or are conceded) the role of commentator on many processes in the town, either feeling free to offer their observations on aspects of everyday life or living an existence that itself attracts commentary and speculation. And, while none of these persons with whom I am acquainted commands the sort of outright fear with which MacNamara surrounds Marse in her literary habitat of Garradrimna, characters like Tommie can, at times, enjoy a curious authority.

Characters and stories about characters, then, mutually imply one another. Characters provide much of the grist that is ground into stories told by some who are themselves characters. The appearance in specific functions in stories is, in turn, one of the earmarks of characterhood. Characterhood, moreover, exists both largely outside of, and absolutely dependent on, respectability. In my experience at least, characters come from the ends of the social spectrum, rather than the middle. Most are from the lower end of the nonrespectable, many with obvious eccentricities. Some come from old gentry families, like

Old Man Hamilton (now, alas, deceased), existing in narrative memory in much the same sort of way as do my less respectable character informants. In this sense, stories about characters help to reproduce, from one perspective, what Turner calls "communitas." Implicit in all the stories I would hear about what "poor Queer Tommie" did today, was a "we" and an "our." Like Simmel's stranger, then, the character, from one point of view, at the shifting limits of a collectivity, is used to mark the collectivity's center.

NARRATING TOMÁS

Tomás O'Connor's social existence, then, can only be understood through the intersection of the different marginalities of mental patient, character, and the unrespectable. This branch of the O'Connor family, for example, exists in narrative memory around Kilronan as having been "non-" or "unrespectable" for at least the last three generations. They have relied on various government schemes to get by; they are prone to trouble with the law (rumoredly with violent Republican sympathies); and, crucially, they inhabit a social genealogy known to include uncles and cousins who died in both the asylum and the "Community Home" (the postindependence, pre-1970s instantiation of the old Union Workhouse). Tomás and his family, then, have never really existed in the functionalist stasis of the type portrayed by Arensberg (1937) and Arensberg and Kimball (1940), insulated from regional, national, and transnational influences, "a livelihood little connected to the outside world" (Arensberg 1937: 42). Tomás's father, for example, Séan O'Connor, was a marginal farmer of marginal land, more an occasional rural wage earner with a farm than a Jeffersonian yeoman. Through political patronage (jobbing), he gained a string of Council jobs to supplement the income on a farm that was almost always in financial difficulties. He also worked seasonally on the construction sites in England, where two of his sons still live (and another met his death under suspicious circumstances, the exact nature of which was never revealed to me).

Around Kilronan today, Séan's son serves as an often elusive target, at which any number of names and narrative nets can be cast. All these stories elucidate the interdigitated issues of his characterhood, his unrespectability, his poverty, and his mental illness. Most of the hospital nurses whom I came to know in Sligo town, for example, pointing to his agitated wanderings and his "incomprehensible speeches," saw in him an example of "deinstitutionalization" run amok, a rural Irish instance of the urban American phenomenon of "sidewalk psychosis." They muttered darkly among themselves that despite being unready to fend for himself he was turned out of the hospital by a society less interested in "caring" than in cutting back and/or redirecting Health Board expenditures.

Furthermore, they are contemptuous of how many psychiatrists who have known Tommie for many years are, in the current political climate of Irish psychiatry, now inclined to gloss over or ignore certain symptoms, such as his constant wandering and incomprehensible speeches that, little more than ten years ago, were the very stuff of his illness in the hospital.

Nurses in the "community," on the other hand, while seeing in his constant wanderings and occasional ejaculations a continuation of his behavior in the asylum, are nonetheless convinced that he can be "managed on the outside" and refer to him as a moderate success story, insofar as he has been able to be "maintained in the community." They can now point to more than a decade of success, interrupted by three short in-patient periods, in this regard. If kept on his primary medication (lithium), they feel his behavior will remain within the realm of the acceptable and that rehospitalization can be avoided. Most of their contact with him is to check his blood levels for evidence of the drug and admonish him with warnings of the dire dangers of forgetting to take it.

Many inhabitants of his old and new home of Kilronan also mention Tommie in passing, or more rarely at length, relating a recent exploit, such as the distance away from town that they might have encountered him or his latest foray in accosting someone. Generally, everyone acknowledges his unusualness, but they rarely attribute it to anything more severe than a "fondness for drink." Others point to the extreme poverty of another sister of his, "Attracta," also acquainted with the asylum and its associated social services, and mutter darkly of a "weakness in the blood" in that line of the O'Connors. The seeming poverty of the family's circumstances merges with the ubiquitous genetic idiom discussed above, and rumors of dark deeds done by another family member across the water in England substantiate this family's unrespectability. During much of my time in Kilronan, Tomás seemed to relish especially the reputed Republican sympathies of his family. In the early 1990s, after reports of Provo actions in the north, for example, he had a habit of finding those in the town who seemed to have disapproved of him the most, and with a broad smile he would give them a thumbs-up sign and a cheerful, "We're winning!"[5] Such displays tended to disconcert his interlocutor.

Generally, however, those in the town employ relatively mild terms, such as "touched," "queer," "odd," and, more rarely, the clearly pejorative "not the full shilling" when describing Tomás (see Saris 1999, 2005). Most townspeople, moreover, at least tolerate his eccentricities. During his daily perambulations, for example, he was often the recipient of informal charity—free sweets from the news shop or a complimentary jar from one of the pubs. For me, the true nature of such indulgences proved elusive. In the end, they cost little, and most people dealt with Queer Tommie in a special way, granting dispensations for activities that would be considered almost outrageous if they came from another source. Furthermore, such gifts, at least insofar as the complimentary pints were concerned, seemed to have had something in the nature of an investment in them. Many of Tomás's speeches—everything from public exhortations to make Kilronan "a grand town once again" to his surprisingly sophisticated analyses of social change in the town—provided the grist for many of the local gossip mills. As often as not, they resulted in an extra round being called to ponder some of the ideas contained in his latest outburst.

To add to this sea of names and narratives in which Tomás effortlessly swims, the mythopoetically inclined researcher can also develop some perfectly viable constructions of Tomás's life based on some very old themes in Irish history and culture. Tomás's reputed fondness for drink and the occasional authorization he enjoys with respect to commenting on aspects of life in Kilronan, for example, are quite consonant with cultural models of the creation of powerful poetic utterances in Irish sources. Indeed, the idea that some sort of altered state of mind is necessary for the production of poetry (in the sense of both Jakobson 1963: chap. 7 and Friedrich 1986: 35–46) is deeply embedded in Irish culture. Such utterances are seen to be somehow outside the ken of normal human life, requiring an ecstatic state to be successfully accomplished.

Irish folk tradition is also quite strong as regards abnormal mental states of poets while composing. Drunkenness is often presented as the standard mood of creativity, and this may in part account for the reputations of many poets in folk tradition as inveterate topers. . . . Direct evidence of intoxication through drinking is difficult to find in archaic Irish sources, but the Irish word for "drunkenness" ("meisce") signified both "intoxification" and "inspirational ecstasy" in Old Irish [Old Ir. *mescae*]. (Ó'hÓgáin 1979: 57–58)

This connection in Irish culture between ecstasis and the production of powerful speech (in the sense of blessings and curses) has also been investigated by Taylor (1990, 1995). Among other things, this connection should caution us against the too-easy reading of the seeming separation of *meisce merachta* and *meisce lenna* (the intoxification of madness and the intoxification of ale) in the Brehon Laws as evidence for the proposition that the ancient Gaels recognized insanity as a self-evident species (Kirkpatrick 1934: 6; Scheper-Hughes 1982: 83). More importantly, however, the variety of narratives that surround Tomás should encourage us to understand how and why such characters can freely interact with their social environments.

Finally, Tomás is also a moving target. A site of excess, he is partially covered by all the narrative nets cast at him, while, at the same time, he retains a social agency that has the potential to subvert any and all of these frames. This is the case because Tomás, of course, ultimately narrates himself. He literally walks and talks his social environment into being and, through these activities, both stakes a claim to his "characterhood" while constructing a cultural space in which he can interact as a social person. Tomás's personhood, then, exists in a cycle of movement, meeting, and story. Movement provides Tommie with the raw material of narrative as well as the possibility of an encounter. An encounter provides the possibility of an audience for one of his speeches, which, in turn, can become the raw material for another narrative at a later date. In this way, Tommie is far removed from the invisibility that is the sine qua non of the very marginal in many other places, such as the United States. Even the caution given to the newcomer, "Pay him no heed," acknowledges Tommie's presence in the very act of trying to contain it.

POSTCOLONIAL PSYCHIATRY?

Clearly, the presence of the asylum looms over Tomás's life, but in unexpected ways. The historical memory of the O'Connors' unrespectablity, for example, is in part strung on the local knowledge of the asylum in this genealogy. Even more interesting, Tomás's current existence as a character-narrator and a narrative character is bound up with a profound institutional transformation, that is, a now almost two-decade-long dispersal of the asylum's technologies away from a nineteenth-century building and toward "the community." This transformation is itself a complex interplay between the local historical arbitration of power, national and international concerns, and what we might call the micropolitics of institutional dispersion. This "stuff" of colonial and postcolonial history forms the backdrop to, while providing the raw material for, Tomás's current social existence.

When the Irish mental hospital service deinstitutionalized according to an imported French model of "sectors" (The Psychiatric Services 1984), it cast about for obvious "centers" wherein to coordinate these area activities and, as often as not, settled on older command-control points from a colonial past. Kilronan was established as a strong point by Anglo-Normans worried about the hostile countryside that was the north of Connacht in the early fourteenth century. In the middle of the confiscated lands of one of the more important clans in this region at that time, an earl built a castle, not far from an abbey patronized by the old owners of the district. Tomás passes both of these romantic ruins in his daily perambulations. This castle was, in its time, a magnificent fortification that served its string of owners well in the intermittent struggles that characterized Ireland for the next three hundred years.

The offer of at least some protection attracted permanent settlement near the shelter of the castle walls. It also attracted the attention of the forces of the English reconquest of Ireland, a Cromwellian adventurer eventually destroying the fortification in the late 1600s. Because of all this "history," however, the developing village that survived the castle's demise, in the middle of the eighteenth century, presented itself as a logical place for an "improving" landlord to situate one of the most modern flax mills in the British Isles. About eighty years later, even after the disappearance of the flax trade, when the train line was laid, Kilronan again presented itself as a logical site for a railway station because, by that time, it was an economic center in its own right in an otherwise impoverished countryside. Ironically, the town's former glory eventually contributed to its developing a reputation as a "mental illness blackspot" in the twentieth century, after record keeping had became more routinized and new etiological theories diffused into the area through the professional class that ran the institution. Patients, and then clients, from well outside the town, continued to list Kilronan as their address, an administrative epitaph to faded economic centrality, but now a signpost in another discourse that pointed to a very serious problem.

The site for the production of all this knowledge, that is, a "colonial" mental hospital, was eventually declared obsolete (The Psychiatric Services 1984), culminating in the increasing dispersal of its staff and services from the early 1980s. Yet, thanks to the endurance of the ruts of power, even in the late twentieth century, well after almost all of Kilronan's pretensions to being a center of any sort had largely vanished, it was chosen as a "logical" place to house a day hospital and three group hostels as part of this process of deinstitutionalization.

This decision had important local effects, besides redeploying potential characters in the environment. There is a connection, for example, between the town's recent "revival" and the situating of these "community" institutions in and near it. To be sure, the economic situation in the Republic of Ireland has been much improved in recent years as the recession of the 1980s waned and, from about 1993 onward, the so-called Celtic Tiger has roared from strength to strength. Nonetheless, the infusion of cash and custom that the day hospital and hostels represent at the very least cannot have harmed this local recovery. On average, Tomás, along with thirty-odd other people per day, use this service. According to my calculations in the late 1990s, based on tallying individual expenditures for items like sweets and alcohol and Health Board expenditures for providing dinner for the clients, this population is directly responsible for upward of £1200 (about ˇ1,500) per week in direct trade in the town. This figure *does not* include the considerable custom that local builders and subcontractors earned in getting the physical structures of the new psychiatric regime up to modern building and fire codes. In the first half of the 1990s, for example, more than £500,000 (about ˇ650,000) was spent in and around the town in fixed capital costs. These figures also do not take into account the occasional sizeable purchase that one of the "deinstitutionalized" clients makes after careful husbanding of his or her Disabled Person's Maintenance Allowance (DPMA). Thus, far from ending it, the closing of a physical structure has propelled the relationship between the asylum and the community into a newer, perhaps even more intimate phase.

CONCLUSION

We are thus confronted with several (theoretically productive) ironies in the social life of Tomás O'Connor in Kilronan. The asylum, from one point of view a historically transformative institution, firmly rooted in a colonial "civilizing" mandate, has, in its internationally influenced decline, played a small part in stabilizing a "traditional" form of locally recognized, even occasionally celebrated, marginal subjectivity—the town character, a category, whose roots in a narrative, mythopoetic logic, at clear odds with the rationality of the mental hospital, are easy to trace. Similarly, the presence of the mental hospital in the O'Connors' remembered genealogy is one of the elements that indexes the "traditional" division between the respectable and the unrespectable in Tomás's life. Finally, a poststructural change par excellence, the decline of a total (and totalizing) institution, helps to revive a "traditional" structure, that is, a community, whose existence the asylum has, in various ways, engaged all along.

What is postcolonial about all this? It would be tempting, for example, to let a term derived from another great underanalyzed British colonial apparatus, "subaltern," assimilate Tommie's existence. In Guha's (1983) virtual equation of "subaltern" with a special sort of stubborn popular resistance to the colonial project (which has endured in much postcolonial theorizing (e.g., among many others, Chatterjee 1993; Gibbons 1996; Lloyd 1993, 1999; Guha and Spivak 1988), Tomás could be seen as an embodiment of this popular struggle. His comments, his mimicries, and his silences could then be unpacked under the big conceptual tent of "resistance." Indeed, I could easily find, in nineteenth-century records of the mental hospital, vignettes of folks that would resonate with my description of Tomás's life, from his penchant to wander to his eagerness to accost.

It seems to me that such an interpretation constrains unduly the interaction between the roles of the character, the mental patient, and the unrespectable. More importantly, it obscures what theoretical and ethnographic insights we can draw from the broader question of what marginality means in present-day rural Ireland. Both Tomas's subjectivity and intersubjective environment exist, like Freud's description of Rome, at several sedimented/superimposed levels (see Das 2001 for a similar argument with regard to notions of trauma). The unrespectable character (connected in some fashion to the mental hospital) condenses several strands of history, in the broadest sense, all at once. To be sure, it is in part a postcolonial precipitate, a sort of return of the repressed of a grim post-Famine property-holding rural society. Indeed, we could understand Tomás as the last trickle of a stream of what Jones and Malcolm (1999) call "inconvenient persons" who ended up dramatically swelling the Irish District Lunatic Asylum System in the nineteenth and early twentieth centuries (see also Saris 1997). But characters are also clearly connected to older models of powerful poetic utterance that construct a profound relationship between the roles of interloper and interlocutor. Finally, many characters in modern-day Kilronan exist simultaneously as a late-modern product of radical institutional transformation, that is, as deinstitutionalized "clients" of a decentralized state mental health service.

Thus, Tomás's social existence reminds us that colonial encounters and the resistances they provoke, postcolonial contradictions and the unsatisfactory results that they often inspire, need to be analyzed beyond moments of violence and in high literature. It is through the presence of specific colonial apparatuses in everyday life, the various changes that they effect, and the various changes in turn wrought upon them that both colonial and postcolonial histories need to be examined (see also Chatterjee 1993). Understanding this quality of the quotidian is less an issue of getting to the myth "behind" history than looking at the historical structures (both physical and conceptual) that a variety of myths (both local and cosmopolitan) have created and that exist as social facts in the lives of the people in whom we are interested. Certain institutions, insofar as they exist as relatively enduring parts of a social-cultural field, are one of the bridges between the personal and political, accommodation and resistance, and the cultural organization of history and the historical production of culture, among other ostensibly opposed perspectives on ethnographic data. An institution, such as a mental hospital, geared toward a certain understanding of marginality and surviving, even thriving, under several different historical regimes serves this purpose especially well. Tomás, then, at once character, unrespectable, and mental patient, evidences the continuing influence of a modern bureaucratic structure at this locality, as well as the latest moment in an ongoing process of the indigenization of both the means and ends of this institution.

NOTES

1. Probably from the Irish *siúlóir*, meaning "walker" or "itinerant wanderer."

2. Of course, the first sense in which Tómas uses the term "stockbroker" is its literal farm meaning—a dealer or wholesaler of animals. He is also intrigued by its more urban meaning derived from the financial markets, absorbed over the years through a ubiquitous American and British television presence. Thus, he speaks easily of "yuppie stockbrokers" in Dublin, meaning that class of well-off professionals who seem to earn a very good living without the use of their hands.

3. This theme of the strange, irreverent power of popular poetic utterance is brilliantly explored by Yeats in the short story, "The Crucifixion of the Outcast" (1959: 147–58).

4. I use the term "fictional" advisedly here because the Westmeath community in which McNamara lived, Delvin, was so incensed by what they took to be an attempt to render faithfully their social existence that copies of *The Valley* were burned and the author's father, a National School teacher, was the object of a successful boycott (see O'Farrell 1990).

5. It is difficult to convey to an international audience how inappropriate such a comment was, especially when I recorded it in the early 1990s. At one level, Tómas indexes a conflicted local history with this comment, that of now-fading memories of the postindependence civil war in Ireland between the Treaty and Anti-Treaty factions, which was acute in and around Kilronan. Families, such as his own, whose Anti-Treaty sympathies from this period are "remembered," often possess a historical consciousness of being of greater interest to the Gards (the police) than their fellows. Indeed, in their unguarded and angry moments, some small-farmer acquaintances of mine from Tómas's area will use the phrase "Free State bastard" as a term of abuse for the Gards, an expression of distaste for the guardians of a political unit that had been dead for more than half a century on my arrival to Kilronan. More broadly in Ireland, for most of the latter half of the Troubles in the north of Ireland (assuming that the Good Friday Agreement indeed marks their resolution or serious abatement), most people in the republic simply tended to avoid the subject. Incidences where civilians died tended to provoke public displays of disgust (if connected to the IRA) or of concern that the political situation needed to be resolved (if the killing was effected by the British state or Loyalist paramilitaries).

REFERENCES

Arensberg, Conrad. 1937. *The Irish Countryman.* Cambridge, MA: Macmillan.

Arensberg, Conrad, and Solon Kimball. 1940. *Family and Community in Ireland.* Cambridge, MA: Harvard University Press.

Chatterjee, Partha. 1993. *The Nation and Its Fragments: Colonial and Postcolonial Histories.* Princeton, NJ: Princeton University Press.

Coleman, Steve. 1991. Fonn, Féile agus Filíocht: Poetry in an Irish Speaking District. Proposal for dissertation research, University of Chicago.

Comaroff, John, and Jean Comaroff. 1992. The Madman and the Migrant. In *Of Revelation and Revolution*, 155–80. Chicago: University of Chicago Press.

Das, Veena. 2001. *Remaking a World. Violence, Social Suffering, and Recovery*. Berkeley: University of California Press.

Friedrich, Paul. 1986. *The Language Parallax*. Chicago: University of Chicago Press.

Gibbons, Luke. 1996. *Transformations in Irish Culture*. Cork, IRL: Cork University Press in association with Field Day.

Goffman, Erving. 1981. *Forms of Talk*. Oxford: Blackwell.

Guha, Ranajit. 1983. *Elementary Aspects of Peasant Insurgency in Colonial India*. Delhi: Oxford University Press.

Guha, Ranajit, and Gayatri C. Spivak, eds. 1988. *Selected Subaltern Studies*. New York: Oxford University Press.

Hanks, William F. 1990. *Referential Practice: Language and Lived Space among the Maya*. Chicago: University of Chicago Press.

Jakobson, Roman. 1963. *Essais de Linguistique Générale*. Paris: Les éditions de Minuit.

Jones, Greta, and Elizabeth Malcolm. 1999. *Medicine, Disease, and the State in Ireland, 1650–1940*. Cork, IRL: Cork University Press.

Kirkpatrick, T. 1934. *A Note on the Care of the Insane in Ireland*. Dublin: University Press.

Lloyd, David. 1993. *Anomalous States*. Berkeley: University of California Press.

———. 1999. *Ireland after History*. Cork, IRL: Cork University Press.

MacNamara, Brinsley. 1918. *Valley of the Squinting Windows*. Dublin and London: Maunsel & Co., Ltd.

O'Brien, M. C. 1981. The Role of the Poet in Gaelic Society. In *The Celtic Consciousness*, ed. R. O'Driscoll. New York: George Braziller.

O'Farrell, Padraic. 1990. *The Burning of Brinsley MacNamara*. Dublin: Lilliput Press.

Ó'hógáin, D. 1979. The Visionary Voice: A Survey of Popular Attitudes to Poetry in Irish Tradition. *Irish University Review* 9 (1): , 44–61

O'Madagáin, Brendan. 1985. Functions of Irish Songs in the Nineteenth Century. *Béaloideas* 53: 130–216.

Partridge, Angela. 1978. *A Hundred Irish Proverbs and Sayings*. Dublin: Folens.

Peace, Adrian. 2001. *A World of Fine Difference: The Social Architecture of a Modern Irish Village*. Dublin: University College Dublin Press.

The Psychiatric Services. 1984. *Planning for the Future*. Dublin: The Stationery Office.

Sahlins, Marshall. 2004. *Apologies to Thucydidies: Understanding History as Culture and Vice Versa*. Chicago: University of Chicago Press

Saris, A. Jamie. 1996. Mad Kings, Proper Houses, and an Asylum in Rural Ireland. *American Anthropologist* 98 (3): 539–54.

———. 1997. The Asylum in Ireland: A Brief Institutional History and Some Local Effects. In *The Sociology of Health and Illness in Ireland*, ed. Anne Cleary and Margaret P. Tracy, 208–23. Dublin: University College Dublin Press.

———. 1999. Producing Persons and Developing Institutions in Rural Ireland. *American Ethnologist* 26 (3): 690–710.

———. 2000. Culture and History in the Half-Way House: Ethnography, Tradition, and the Rural Middle Class in the West of Ireland. *Journal of Historical Sociology* 13 (1): 10–36.

———. 2005. Reconsiderando los Estereotipos: Imágenes de Irracionalidad en la Obra del Columnista del Irish Times, John Waters [Rethinking Stereotypes: Images of Irrationality in the Work of the Irish Times Columnist, John Waters]. *Revista de Antropología Social* 14:281–309.

Scheper-Hughes, Nancy. 1982. *Saints, Scholars, and Schizophrenics*. Berkeley: University of California Press.

Scott, James. 1985. *Weapons of the Weak: Everyday Forms of Peasant Resistance*. New Haven, CT: Yale University Press.

Silverman, Marilyn. 1987. "A Labouring Man's Daughter": Constructing "Respectability" in South Kilkenny. In *Ireland from Below: Social Change and Local Communities*, ed. C. Curtin and Wilson T. Curtin. Galway, IRL: Galway University Press.

Taylor, Lawrence. 1990. Stories of Power, Powerful Stories: The Drunken Priest in Donegal. In *Religious Orthodoxy and Popular Faith in European Society*, ed. Ellen Badone, 163–84. Princeton, NJ: Princeton University Press.

———. 1995. *Occasions of Faith: an Anthropology of Irish Catholics*. Dublin: Lilliput Press.

Yeats, William B. 1959 [1897]. *Mythologies*. New York: Macmillan.

Postcolonial Conundrums, Madness, and the Imagination

Stefania Pandolfo

A young man and a woman sitting on a bench in the waiting area of the psychiatric emergency room, a crowded hallway in the old modular compound at the edge of the hospital grounds. The man is wearing jeans, has slightly long hair and the look of a university student. He is pale and tense, moves restlessly, and gazes through the room with a sense of imprisoned rage. The woman is older, wears a jilaba and a headscarf. The man was brought that morning by an ambulance of the Protection Civile, on a police order, RP, "requisition de police."

The head nurse keeps an eye on the patient, for until the psychiatrist on call decides on his hospitalization or his release, the patient is held by the police on garde à vue. *They came from Tiflet, the head nurse tells me, a town that was once just a weekly market where tribal populations met, which became an army station during the colonial period and is today a growing urban sprawl in the rural hinterland of Rabat. The woman is the patient's mother—it is she who filed the police complaint. I try to imagine what exasperation, what lack of issue, led the mother to that resolution. I am waiting for Dr. R., a young woman psychiatrist, with whom I have agreed to share the day on call.*

Some years later, this text is written in the margin of the encounter that took place that day, in light of encounters that followed with other patients and in different circumstances, but in the wording and concrete features of a particular life, as that life presented itself to me that morning in the emergency room. My reflections, in the form of a circumstantial commentary, address questions raised by the young man himself in his speech and related to his perception and imagination of "modern times" in its confrontation with a "cultural home" he experiences as unlivable. It is a confrontation that takes place on the battlefield of his own body and life, but that by its nature concerns a whole society—as in a way a society, and the possibility of a common life, are called in by his speech. Spoken from the midst of his uncanny experience (which is partly inaccessible to his interlocutors), his questions point to the tear of a failing transmission—the inability to inhabit a tradition. They voice the violence of cultural identity in the postcolonial nation and an essential homelessness, which is that of his madness but is also, in a different sense, the experience of his generation. Yet, at the same time, his questions bear witness to a struggle for existence and creative elaboration, for a possibility of resymbolization, fought on the very ground of the ER interview. Punctuated by a reiterated request for a lawyer, "a lawyer who may speak in my behalf and defend my right," his discourse is a paradoxical appeal to the law, the law of the state and the institution of psychiatry, in a plea to be recognized as a subject.

July 1999—it was my second summer of fieldwork at the Hospital Arrazi in Salé, Morocco, still somewhat the beginning. Since then I have been working with psychiatrists and patients, in the services, through the daily staff meetings and in the ER, in the attempt to grasp the experience of illness between different and sometimes incommensurable and antagonistic vocabularies of the self and to seize the specificity of utterance in that unstable intermediate space where speech is at once silenced and produced.[1] On one side is the psychiatric institution, with its diagnostic and therapeutic apparatuses, its styles of reasoning, its codes and its debates, the socialization of the residents into a mode of being, an academic hierarchy, and of the patients into their psychiatric illness. On the other side are the etiologies and therapeutic techniques associated with trance and the jinns in the practice of Qur'anic healers and in the experience of patients, often the same patients, outside the hospital. The question of culture was felt at the hospital as a central and a troubling one, pointing to a malaise difficult to locate, spoken in terms of the "cultural factor" in psychopathology, in the expression of symptoms and the themes of delusion, in the beliefs of patients, as a problematic attachment to a lingering and ineffective cultural tradition. It was the reason why I had been welcomed, an anthropologist, as an observer and an interlocutor. Yet despite this critical concern, approaches inspired by ethnopsychiatry or transcultural psychiatry were looked upon with diffidence, due to a feared folklorization of culture and to the colonial history that had constituted Moroccans into "cultural subjects," as against the universal subject of the Métropole. But difference, the *différance* of oneself, resurfaced with uncanny reminders: as the enigma of a word, for instance, jotted down in French by the resident on call in the admission report as an approximate translation of something the patient said in Arabic or Berber to describe an affect or a vision (French is the language of hospital files and all reports, as well as of the staff meetings and all medical school instruction); a word that returned as a puzzle during the staff discussion of the patient's case, materializing the chasm of institutional translation. What did the patient actually say in Arabic? What was the spiritual entity evoked? How do you express suicidal feelings, or speak of pleasure, in Arabic? A chasm of cultural-linguistic translation doubled the chasm of experience, bringing it as if to visibility—the experience of madness, and the inadequacy of all translation, within and beyond the perception of psychiatry.

From one fragment of life, or encounter, to another, during my time at the hospital I attempted to apprehend a scene marked by an urgent request (by the patients for listening, for recognition, for care) and, at the same time, by the impossibility of fully inhabiting the psychiatric institutional references as well as the cultural reference itself—the collectively sanctioned sites and vocabularies of healing. This is a central theme in the narratives of the women and men I met in the hospital and is a crucial site of reflection in my work. It exposes the conundrum of an attachment impossible to dissolve and of an ambivalence impossible to reduce to an unproblematic belonging; a conundrum that dispossesses the subject of the capacity to invoke the authority of the reference from which it draws its identity, all the while being seized in its matrix and its passion.

I understand this double impossibility as a complex effect of the repression of indigenous medical practices and of the understanding of illness and the body steeped in the unconscious archives of the subject under colonial and postcolonial rule. (I take "repression"—with Freud—in a literal/symbolic sense: violent political censorship, involuntary forgetting, psychic obliteration). The government of health played a crucial role in the establishment of the Moroccan colonial state; territory and subjects were conjured through sanitation, by way of vaccination campaigns and the work of mobile medical military units, while the exercise of "indigenous healing" was made punishable by law. At independence the postcolonial state inherited the colonial medical infrastructure and the legacy of the modernizing project, but failed to develop an effective social medicine. Despite the vision of late colonial and early postcolonial medical reformers, several among them psychiatrists, little efforts were made by the postcolonial state to provide health care for the growing number of impoverished and displaced populations. The result is today the de facto exclusion of large sectors of the Moroccan population from concrete access to health care— a realization that makes any claim to health rights essentially empty.

On this complex and ambiguous scene there is on the one hand the predicament of Moroccan psychiatry, with its colonial legacies as well as a history of early postcolonial experiments in deinstitutionalization and alternative care. It is a history that accounts for certain indeterminacy in diagnostic criteria, allowing for flexibility and some inventiveness in the margins of institutional practice; a history that is specifically modernist, in that it registers the experience of a rift, a desire for an elsewhere—in the form of a hospital "bed." On the other hand there is the continuing presence of other therapies and understandings of illness within a vernacular and a now increasingly revivalist theological framework, other practices, largely unrecognized and rendered incommensurable on the grounds of the hospital and in the larger discourse of national public health but that today foretell the possibility of different futures. The growth of Islamic healing in particular, in its multiple approaches and dimensions (spanning from the treatment of jinn possession in the path of God's law [ᶜilâj al-sharaᶜi] to Islamic psychology [ᶜilm al-nafs al-islami] and its debates with the natural sciences) registers a crucial shift in the existing coordinates, calling for a relegitimation of the grounds of belonging in terms of a renewed actuality of concepts, interpretations, and therapeutic interventions drawn from the ethical and theological traditions of Islam. So much is expressed in the hiatuses, the silences, of encounters in the psychiatric ER.

Before turning to the ER interview, some context is helpful to situate the institutional history, elucidate the terms of the questions, the actors at play, and the stakes.

Hospitalization by RP is not uncommon at this hospital, one of two main psychiatric hospitals and schools of psychiatry in Morocco, where what psychiatrists call les pathologies lourdes, "serious psychiatric disorders," are routinely addressed. This is consistent with the 1959 royal decree regulating psychiatric treatment in Morocco, the law still in use today. Issued three years after the independence of Morocco, the decree (dahir) of Psychiatry is a modernist law of humanitarian inspiration, conceived with the explicit intent of protecting the rights of patients against the possibility of familial and political abuses. By this law all decisions concerning issues of mental health and the hospitalization of patients are put under the responsibility of psychiatrists. The law mandates the establishment of mental health centers in all provinces, limits hospitalization to three weeks, renewable up to a maximum of six months, enforces and regulates detailed clinical records in the hospital files, and states that hospitalization takes place "at the request of the patient, or of a public or private person acting in the patient's interest, or in the interest of Public Order." A family member or a public official may request hospitalization by filing a police complaint: but the final decision rests with the psychiatrist.[2]

In the wording of the law, specialized medical knowledge—the ability to discern "anomalies of behavior" and attribute a meaning to them—is at once a judicial tool and a guarantor of the patient's freedom. Its modernist mission is attached to the responsibility of each individual physician, called to the ambivalent task of incarnating the law. As Gyan Prakash (1999) has suggested for the case of science in colonial India, psychiatry is constituted by this law under the ambivalent sign of surveillance and freedom.

Protecting the rights of patients in 1950s Morocco implied that patients be conceived in their individuality as subjects of care solely qualified by their (psychiatric) illness, understood as exclusively their own—not as the expiation of a past or collective history, not as the expression of an interpersonal or societal malaise, not as the effect of an external agency: a premise health practitioners themselves understood to be a fiction—and the site of a struggle. The 1959 Dahir of Psychiatry is a biopolitical document. Patients, les malades of this law, are subjects of human rights in as much as they can be represented as stripped of all attachments and relations, culture and belief, reduced to the "bare life" of their illness—outside of any prior inscription of living in a form of possible collective life, a symbolic order, with its intergeneration exchanges and its transference of memory and oblivion, which alone can provide a sense of ground and the possibility of choice, and creative improvisation (Arendt 1971; Agamben 1998).[3]

Yet in a context in which psychiatric care touches a small fragment of the population, and this not just because of a much debated cultural reluctance, but also due to the scarcity of institutional means (a total of some three thousand beds in specialized psychiatric hospitals located in the major cities, for a population of thirty-one million, and a dissemination of Centres de Santés in rural areas, understaffed and underequipped and operating in conditions of chronic emergency),[4] the biopolitical project of the dahir takes on a specifically local dimension, one that is both utopian and exemplary. It institutes the site of an elsewhere by ambiguous contours, in rupture with the cultural institutions, where a recourse is possible in moments of despair; but also a force, which can seize one by the legitimate and arbitrary violence of the state, as in the case of the youths from poor urban neighborhoods brought to the ER by the police at night.

A patient's file at a morning staff meeting. Overnight admission, a young man brought to the emergency room at 4:00 A.M. by the police. Had checked himself in at the police station of Taqaddoum at 3:00 A.M. Taqaddoum means "progress." It is an underprivileged neighborhood at the outskirts of the old colonial center of Rabat. The youth declared to the police that he intended to commit suicide. He was drunk.Was put under arrest, handcuffed, and taken to the psychiatric ER.To the psychiatrist on call he told a confused story that hinted at his rage and guilt toward his family, his father, of whom he refused to speak, his mother, remarried, and who in her helplessness to help her son paid for the wine with which he got drunk, and a girlfriend, the only person who understood him, but who had left to join her family who had migrated to Italy. He had studied until the fourth year in high school, then had dropped out, in a moment of rage for which he blamed his family. He spoke of the growing sense of failure over the previous months, his inability to find a job, his reality of chomeur.[5] Buried in his room, "I have become a woman, they provide for my food."The resident who admitted him stressed his sense of impotence, emasculation, his ideas of destruction and ruin. Long discussion about the case, used by the senior psychiatrist of psychodynamic orientation to lecture the residents about the importance of listening for existential sense in the trajectory of a person's life.The steps taken by the patient were unusual, a powerful request for help, a request for authority, for the law.What was the sense of that recourse to the police? he asked.The police as a symbol of power, of violence, castration. The patient made a recourse to the law as the site of symbolic mediation: but the law handcuffed him literally, and he felt let down, was furious.The patient's spectacular search for help suggested that the problematic of the subject was not psychotic, the psychiatrist said (that is, there was an attempt to express something symbolically through an act or a symptom, here perhaps to send a message to his family), inciting the resident who took the case to actively listen for sense.The next day the young man was discharged.The resident who had taken the case (reluctantly, because such patients are difficult, they need time, affect us, and there is no time) said that upon awakening the patient was sober and denied the truth of anything he had said the night before, attributing it all to the effect of alcohol. I met the young man with the psychiatrist, his words were impenetrable; I felt like asking more, but didn't. He was coherent and reasonable, and the young psychiatrist signed his discharge, said that there was no reason to hold him at the hospital, it would be an abuse.There was a thick pile of patients' files on the table, we were in a small lounge inside the men's locked ward, patients waiting outside the door, walking in the door, asking for attention, much more visibly ill than that young man.

Reflecting on questions of public health in the *banlieues* of French cities and in the context of irregular migration, Didier Fassin (2001, 1999, 2000) argues that the biopolitical reduction of being to "bare life," to the silence of a suffering body, grants to the excluded an ultimate and paradoxical recourse to the law. He names this agency "biolegitimization," a right issued from the loss of all rights and communal affiliations, and shows how the biopolitical operation is literally incarnated by migrant subjects of irregular status, for whom illness becomes the only possible ground of appeal in their request for inclusion. In Fassin's view biolegitimization is not a tactic of resistance, but a strategy of power on the shifting terrain of European late capitalist and postnational societies. Its rules are dictated by the ideological and juridical reconfiguration of the republican state, which reproduces inequality and racial exclusion as it promotes the values of *égalité* and which has come to confer an absolute moral primacy to the nonproductive life of the suffering foreign body. In a context in which eligibility to basic rights is argued and granted on the basis of an incurable illnesses (such as AIDS or lead poisoning), one must question the ideological-legal structure of a democratic state to which migrants gauge their bodies in a mortal exchange. But furthermore and unlike the case of Europe, in the situation I attempt to apprehend, becoming a biopolitical suffering body does not grant a paradoxical juridical inclusion. The appeal to the institution of care must be understood differently, in a space of impossibility that is also the ground for the imagination of life. This chapter traces a comparably paradoxical gesture of appeal, an appeal to the law of the state, the "constitution of the king," but an appeal that does not provide an access to citizenship because it rejects existing ties and affiliations and is instead spoken in an ambiguous utopian zone, where creation and loss are intertwined in the singularity of a marginal life.[6]

Overshadowing the phrasing of the 1959 *dahir* is a century-long colonial narrative characterizing the indigenous culture and family structures as obstacles to the development of individual responsibility and European-style citizenship. Leaving little room for uncertainty, discontinuities, experiential discrepancies, and for the recognition of historically different ways of being a subject, this narrative stresses the fundamental role of the patriarchal family in Islam, the overarching weight of the group, the force of a collective imaginary that makes it impossible for the individual to exist qua individual, and the weight of a religious law where the sacred is the voice of the group (see, for instance, Berthelier 1994; Igert 1955; and Pandolfo 2000). Superimposed on that narrative, however, and orienting the spirit of the 1959 law in an opposite direction, is an institutional reflection on the question of anomie in the context of colonization and modernization: a preoccupation with the crisis of traditional structures, and the unavailability of alternatives, in terms of which the new sciences of psychiatry and social psychology were situating themselves in Morocco in the 1940s and '50s.

In the writings of J. L. Roland (1957) a French psychoanalyst who became the first director of the Service Central de Psychiatrie et d'Hygiène Mentale at the Moroccan Ministry of Health at independence, as well as the first director of the newly created Hospital Arrazi in Salé, the focus is on processes of anomie in colonial modernity. The causes of mental illness are sought in the destructuring effects on the Ego of traumatic socioeconomic transformations: the rural exodus, rapid urbanization and overpopulation; the compression and promiscuity of living space in poor urban neighborhoods, where intimacy is systematically violated, producing in subjects a sentiment of intrusion bordering on psychosis; the crisis of paternal authority; the "dissociation of the family"; the growth of aggression and self-destructive behavior caused by the unconscious guilt of having violated ancestral rules; the stress of bilingualism with the colonial language; the formation of an urban lumpen proletariat; the spread of alcohol and crime. The biopolitical production of "patients" is presented in this reading as the result of a historical process of uprooting, the effect of catastrophic social change, comparable to the production of refugees in a war. The task of psychiatry becomes that of understanding and healing these ruptures, without looking back to the past, in the imagination of a new society.

In the spirit of its modernist inception, the hospital has grown as a site of treatment, education, and research, taking an active role in the public debate on pressing social issues; but it is also as a space where the postcolonial *parti pris* of a technoscientific modernity precludes the recognition of vocabularies of illness other than those of psychiatry, and to a certain extent psychoanalysis. This is a political choice consistent with the modernizing strategies of Maghribi postcolonial states, which are today full of consequences and not free of disquiet.

In *La psychanalyse à l'épreuve de l'Islam* (2002), psychoanalyst Fethi Benslama interrogates the psychic consequences, for Maghribi and Middle Eastern subjects, of the destruction of traditional forms of belonging in the successive violence of colonization, modernization, and nationalism, with particular reference to the contemporary reinvestment of Islamic religious identities. He diagnoses a process of subjective revocation (*révocation subjective*), a collective regression to archaic forms of psychic life, which he relates to the gravity of the present social crisis and to what, in his view, is its most prominent psychopathological symptom: the quest for narcissistic reparation under the sign of what he calls a "return to the Origin." In Benslama's reading, which extends a Lacanian understanding of psychosis to collective phenomena, this process results in the disclosure of a chasm, a terrifying void, which is "filled," he argues, with the psychotic fantasy of a return to an original identity—a return in which the subject dissolves. Contemporary religious movements, and the Islamic revival in particular, would be an instantiation of that kind of delusion. This chapter engages critically, if indirectly, with the questions raised in Benslama's text and attempts to displace them, at once ethnographically and theoretically.

How to think the aftermath of the subject of psychoanalysis without necessarily resorting to the categories of psychopathology? How to address the present sociocultural, political, and spiritual sea change without surrendering to comforting psychosocial diagnoses? How to cultivate the disposition of a subject open to the risk and enigma of alterity, or in T. Asad's words, "of subjects who can open their minds to something that is strange, or uncomfortable, or distasteful" (Asad 2002)? Some directions are found in the Freudian approach itself. Identification, underpinning the processes of modern mass society as well as the formation of the Ego, is "more ancient" than the covenant in speech; it is a "passage through the Other" in which the "I" is both founded and revoked. In the instability of that "passage" is located at once the risk of radical loss and the ethical possibility of coexistence (see Lacoue-Labarthe and Nancy 1997; Borch-Jacobsen 1993) Developing this line of thought would lead, among other things, to questioning the irreducibility of the boundary between subjectivity and psychosis, exploring the troubling and unstable interfaces of subjectivity and depersonalization, as was pursued in European phenomenological psycho-analysis and is recently attempted, on the basis of different premises, in American cultural psychiatry.[7]

In relation to these questions, the story of Reda,[8] the young man I was to meet in the emergency room, provides a number of unexpected answers. As with many youths at the onset of psychosis, or simply someone whose "skin" is less impermeable, Reda takes it upon himself to articulate a malaise larger than his own, that of a collectivity of which he becomes an echo. From the rage of the torture he feels, inflicted on him by a cultural home he experiences as unlivable, Reda moves to a creative interpretation of his madness, opposing to that intrusion, to that shrinkage of vital space, something other than a search for identity: a "creation" that transforms alienation from within the space of madness itself. His answer displaces the terms of the question and suggests that if we pay attention to the concrete specificity of particular lives, and the philo-sophical possibility of other forms of life, we may glimpse the inception of a renewed *kulturarbeit*, a novel articulation of unspeakable cultural truths—here, in the margins of a psychiatric encounter.

SHADOW THEATER OF MODERNITY

As is often the case in the emergency room, there is tension in the room. Dr. R. is opening the official seals, reading the letter from the police. Then she looks at the man and asks his name. The mother replies that his name is Reda and that he's thirty. But Reda is not listening. He complains loudly about her, his mother, speaks French and addresses Dr. R. directly. Says that his mother doesn't under-stand him, couldn't possibly understand him, she is illiterate and ignorant, unable to even count properly.

Dr. R. interrupts him, in Arabic (visibly not to exclude the mother from the conversation, she doesn't understand French): "U nta 'arfti? [And you, can you do it?]," she asks. Reda is reluctant, annoyed by the obvious, finally says "forty-two" and insists that he shouldn't be in this hospital, that he requests a lawyer, he demands his rights: *Je demande un avocat, je demande mes droits!*"

"*Elle veut me rendre fou* [she wants to make me crazy], she forced me to consult with a *fqih* [Qur'anic healer] against my will." Reda insists on speaking French, ignoring the injunction of Arabic, the psychiatrist's refusal to reply in the language of his choice: the colonial language, language of the hospital files, but also, for him, language of his scientific studies and of his literary journeys, language his mother doesn't understand.[9] It is the only language in which he is able to articulate his request, his appeal to the Other, embodied in the room by this frail young woman sitting behind a desk.

"Why should I take medications?" "*Takhod dwa!* [Take your medications!]," (alluding to his mother), "I should instead take a lawyer because of the suffering she is inflicting to me. As for this language I am speaking [French] she [his mother] is illiterate and we are entering the twenty-first century." He repeats this in Arabic, perhaps to make his mother feel the humiliation: "*Makatfehemsh lfranse, maqariash.* She is illiterate, doesn't understand French, while I have a Troisième Cycle in Mathematics." (The mother signals to the psychiatrist that this corresponds to reality.)

I ask Reda about his education. "I have a university degree, a *maitrise* with equivalence in the French system, pure math, logic. I am a logician, only I disguise myself, and play instead my literary games [*je fais des jeux de littérature*]. I studied pure mathematics, pure logic, I have a degree in linear algebra, ʿ*arfti ashna hia la géometrie algèbrique?* [Do you know what linear algebra is?]" (violently to his mother).

"*Maʾarfa walu,* I don't know anything," submits the mother.

Reda turns to his mother aggressively and says in Arabic, "ʿ*alesh dditini ʿand llfqih* [why did you take me to the healer], against my will, and with the Fire Department? [The ambulance of the Protection Civile took him to the hospital that morning, but in his accusation the institutions overlap.] Why? To feed me herbs [ʿ*ashub*] and potions, nutmeg [*lgusa*] and fennel [*habt lhalawa*], to subjugate my will. I can still understand a girl who does that, she desires you and puts *twkkel* in your food, feeds you a couscous with magic to make you marry her. . . . But this woman?"

And then to the psychiatrist, and to me, in a mixture of Arabic and French: "They made me swallow meals of God only knows what, dog and cow brains . . . garbage [*les dechets*], cow dung they mix in with couscous, and much much more. In our region laboratory experiments are made with couscous!"

Insisting on using Arabic as the language of the interview, Dr. R. asks Reda whether he really thinks that his mother put magic in his food. Reda replies that he is suspicious, he doesn't trust her, her cooking, her food. Exasperated, the mother denies having put anything in the food, and Reda replies that in any case her cooking is poisoning him, and he makes once again an appeal to the mediation of the law, a law that might speak in his behalf—literally, to a lawyer: "I request a lawyer, for a lawyer who may defend my case, for all the suffering that I endured with this woman . . . [repeats in Arabic], because I have suffered so much . . ."

The scene in the emergency room becomes a trial in which Reda is at once plaintiff and defendant. It is a trial and a self-defense made possible by the summoning of the institutional code, calling subjects in the position of patients, protected by the recognition of their illness. Reda's passionate self-defense, and his request for mediation, are a testimony of his struggle for creating a "place," a space in which existence might begin. The absence of place, of horizon—in a physical and symbolic sense—is a poignant feature of Reda's claustrophobic speech, aimed at pushing back an aggression, distancing an invader, striving to protect the possibility of a vital movement threatened at his core.[10]

Reda is upset, the atmosphere is tense. I recall the anxiety and the way his voice affected me; I remember thinking that the psychiatrist must be affected as well—because the drama that was unfolding in his voice, and before our eyes, resonated as something larger than a personal or a family affair. It overflowed the specificity of his personal history and resonated for me (and how could it not for Dr. R.) as a historical and political affair. In that overflowing, the possibility of a personal history was reduced (or imprisoned, in the vocabulary of *daseinanalyse*) in what L. Binswanger (1958) calls the splitting off of experiential consistency into alternatives, into a rigid either-or. Reda, his voice, his body, became a rift where intersected and clashed the cleavages of Moroccan modernity, the ideology of modernity, the same cleavages by which his life was furrowed and that underpin the possibility of this hospital scene. Speaking in the name of that which was attacking him, the problematic of the subject was to push back the offensive, in the two opposed camps of magic-tradition and psychiatry-modernity. The psychiatrist, the mother, and I were at once spectators and characters on the scene of this recital. Reda was in it by his struggle, his search for an exit, most of all by way of his rage.

TWKKEL: Topography of the Unlivable

As I listen back to Reda's words in the transcript of that conversation, I attempt to follow the figures of his despair, analyze its images, as one follows the images of a dream.

He outlined the main themes at the outset, in a sort of poetic condensation. Poisoning and incorporation by ingestion, cannibalization, illiteracy, the theme of the Mother. She wants to make me crazy, she wants to kill me. And, *"we are entering the twenty-first century"*: exit and forward movement—science, mathematics, logic, and geometry, education by the intercession of the foreign tongue. Murderous persecution by "her cooking," her food and her magic, and by the intimate relationship his mother entertains with the *fqihs*, traditional healers and agents of traditional culture. The magic Reda refers to and specifically names is itself called *twkkel*, from the Arabic root *akal*, "to eat" (in this form of the verb, to be devoured, eaten away, destroyed). *Twkkel* is a technical term, the name of a magical operation and of a form of illness attack described in manuals of healing and magic, and it is a key notion in the vocabulary of affliction, in the discourse of healers as well as patients and their families. Unlike other conditions, more directly related to the jinns, complaints of *twkkel* are rarely censored in the illness narratives of patients in the psychiatric hospital, perhaps because of its perceived equivalence with psychiatric symptoms of persecution (by poisoning or, more culturally specific, in terms of a "delusion of sorcery"), or because of its more bodily, physical connotation. Intentionally harmful *twkkel* can be obtained by natural means (attempting to kill a person with poisonous plants or other toxic substances mixed in food or drink), but in its most dreaded form it is *sihar*, "witchcraft," a quest for power involving the intervention of the jinns in the realm of death and the manipulation of the forces of harm.

In the explication of a healer with whom I discussed this point, if *twkkel's* destructive force, as *sihar*, is channeled through magical operations that summon the malevolent intervention of a jinn, its origin, its source, is always in an envious passion, a devouring desire of the person to incorporate and/or annihilate the other. A desire and a rivalry, he added, that have become endemic in the current conditions of social injustice in Morocco and in the world, generalizing the model of *sihar* to a global struggle for power and destruction. (As we talked in the living room of his house, one of the rare concrete constructions alongside a shantytown in the outskirts of Rabat, this healer, who is also a preacher of Muslim revivalist orientation added, "Human beings exist in justice [*adami wajudi al-ʾadl*]. And justice is violated by coercion [*ikrah*].There is no justice in this world. . . . There are laws, but there are people who are *too* power-*ful*, and interfere with the law. How do the powerful prevent the exercise of the law? By pecuniary corruption (*maddian*), or by coercion and intimidation. In this situation the poor and powerless person turns to sorcery, because he or she has been offended and hurt. . . . ")

Unlike the healer I am citing, a real interlocutor and acute clinician and exegete, *fqihs* keep coming back as phantasmatic figures in the emergency room discussion with Reda and his mother. In Reda's account they are persecutory agents, pointing to a secret complicity between his mother, his cultural milieu, and the forces of tradition in the insatiable passion to subjugate others, him, and *enslave his free will*. In his mother's account instead, the mention of *fqihs* traces the secret map of a quest for healing in the home town, the neighboring region, and all the way to Rabat; a quest the mother cannot fully acknowledge in the psychiatric context, where that idiom of illness is invalid (and in a way couldn't fully acknowledge in general, for the realm of the jinns is ontologically elusive), and that she imputes to Reda himself. It is he, she says, who speaks of the jinns, who complains of being possessed, who seeks the cures of a fqih, although admitting later to have herself sought their intervention repeatedly, even without her son's approval or physical presence, as when she stood in line with her son's photograph in her hands at 5:00 A.M. at a healer's door—for the popularity of the young fqih was such that petitioners had to take a number to be received, as one did in the hospital. That healer told her that Reda was mqiws, "touched" by the jinns (tqas, "had been touched," registering the event of an initial demonic entanglement), and gave her an amulet she stitched in his pillow; yet another fqih diagnosed that he was struck by a jinniya, a she-demon, and prescribed the sacrifice of a ram. With great difficulty, she said, she gathered the money to buy the ram, and called the 'Issawa brotherhood to perform the trance dance, and brought in Reda with a stratagem (b-l-hila) so that he might be smeared with sacrificial blood, fall into a trance, and be healed. Reda danced all night to the rhythm of the music, but did not "fall" (ma tah-sh, that is, into a trance). In the end he got up and left and didn't come home for several days.

In Reda's account, the image of couscous is the condensation of his haunting, pregnant with what Freud called unheimlischkeit—the uncanny unfamiliarity of what is at once intimate and foreign. Drawn from the Maghribi repertory of magic, feminine magic in particular, couscous becomes for Reda a figure of the murderous forces of the Home that threaten his psychic and physical integrity. There are echoes in his words of well-known magical recipes aimed at destroying an enemy or subjugating another person's will, recipes mentioned in magical books, but even more in the anonymity and terrors of rumor: such as the secret practice of digging out a corpse in the cemetery and mixing the couscous with the hand of the dead, or seasoning it with excrement and other bodily scraps, before feeding it to the victim. Couscous is an emblem of the most familiar and intimate, the definition of the communal meal itself, prepared by the maternal hand on Friday and other holidays, offered as sadaqa (charity) to the poor, eaten in common at holy festivals in the space surrounding a sanctuary. In some legends, human settlements are said to have been founded around a gsa', a large wooden couscous plate, as in a mythical narrative from a region in the Moroccan south about a gsa' full of couscous that descended from the sky brought by the angels, in the midst of an open space in the palm groves; people gathered to eat the miraculous meal, and from that gathering a community was born.

But for Reda the communal meal becomes a mortal threat. This possibility was already inscribed within the affective ambivalence of the image of couscous, metonym of the identification with the group, which disclosed its destructive pole in the magical use. Yet the historical contingency of colonial and postcolonial expropriations in Reda's experience, and the way that contingency took a specific form in his life and rehearsed itself through him, painfully and madly, suggests that we should approach that image as something more than cultural psychology or as the inherent reversibility of symbols. To belong to the "we" of the cultural identification means to swallow that meal and to be killed.

Later in the course of the interview Reda came back to this theme. Dr. R. asked the mother whether she had in fact taken Reda to a healer, or were his accusations unfounded? And the mother replied that Reda went to the fqih on his own, because he felt he was "inhabited" (kan keygul fih jnun, rah ni mskun). Reda interrupted her angrily, beginning in Arabic but quickly turning to French (because the real interlocutor was Dr. R., to whom his appeal was addressed): "Nti lly dditina ʿand lfuqqaha f tiflet! [It is you, you took me (us) to the healers in Tiflet!] I never agreed to go. Je suis maladif [I am vulnerable and sickly], and you made me do unbelievable things . . . the fqih would order me to smoke his magical writing on the blue paper of the sugar loafs, to vomit and smoke my vomit, I don't know, this woman is going to kill me with her healers!"

"It was to cure you," says the mother.

In Arabic: "Cure me, she says! What cure, and what doctors? Why did you take me to the healer, to push me to my ruin? In French: Because I have eaten something, she fed me something, she'd grab me, she'd say eat, eat, eat! She said, go to the psychiatrists of our town, go to the healers!"

If eating and being fed/devoured imply the omnipotence of the Mother-Tradition, the illiteracy of the mother suggests impotence and amputation. It is an impotence that bears a sign of forbidden entrance, interrupted trajectory, lack of exit. Ignorance, paralysis, subordination to "tradition," blocked access to modernity, to language and critical thought: "elle est analphabète et on rentre dans le vingt et unième siècle [she's illiterate and we are entering the twenty-first century]."

The mother's illiteracy is the son's loss of voice, if he doesn't manage to get away, to distance himself, escaping their capture ("it was to elude the grip of these two analphabètes," he says later on in the interview, referring to his parents). The we of "we are entering the twenty-first century" indexes a desire of community, to rejoin those who "enter" the future, those who have access: to modernity, to language, to the self. Exit and forward movement: science, mathematics, logic, and geometry, education by the intercession of the foreign tongue. In this configuration "reading" understood as a form of resistance and an inalienable right holds a central place in what should be understood as Reda's *requisitoire,* at once a self-defense and an indictment.

In "the twenty-first century" Reda finds sanctuary against the persecution of the "home," which returns to attack him in the Real, from the outside, menacing and deadly—a threat of amputation by the hand and the speech of his mother. His reiterated request for a lawyer is an appeal to mediation—literally, insulation; the insulation of a "skin" that may draw his boundaries, the mediation of the law of the state by which he may declare his right to exit, and of the law of discourse, the possibility of an authorized speech. In the economy of his saying, the use of French is also this.

At stake is Reda's struggle against the annihilation of himself.[11] The theme of persecution and of his "suffering" (*cette souffrance*) in the hell of his experience are the negative and tragic dimension of this: imprisonment and paralysis, cannibalization, estrangement of the self and affirmation of a right to existence by refusal of identifications—with his mother, his language, his tradition. The theme of Exit—through education, science and reading, and later through literature and the Imagination—raises the question of freedom.

"KANHARAB B-LA LITTÉRATURE [I escape, save myself with literature]"

Dr. R. asks Reda whether he hears voices, "*Makatsma'sh aswat?* [Don't you hear voices?]," suggesting in her question that he might. It is a key question to establish the presence of psychosis and to possibly move toward a diagnosis of acute psychosis, paranoia, or schizophrenia. "Voices," auditory hallucinations, signal in psychiatric semiology the loss of connection with reality and of relation to other fellow beings that are characteristic of psychotic delusion. They are intrusive injunctions coming from the outside; they can be aggressive, injurious, give orders, or can provide an external commentary. In psychoanalytic terms, they witness a tear in the subject, a hole, filled by the work of delusion, that ultimate retreat.

The psychiatrist's question, asked routinely in clinical evaluations, marks a critical turn in the conversation, a metamorphosis in the scene of Reda's speech.

Makatsma'sh aswat? (Don't you hear voices?) is an ambiguous question in its Arabic formulation, albeit routinely asked in clinical interviews. Reda does not deny, he does indeed hear voices, attacks coming from the outside, just as this voice that is addressing him now. He assumes the place assigned to him by the institution and from there operates a displacement, wards off the threatening voice.

"At night," he replies to the psychiatrist, hinting that the invasive voices come at night, "*et alors je fais jouer les voix de Cervantes, comme si je faisais la comedie.*

Kanḥarrab b la littérature [and when that happens I rehearse Cervantes' voices, as if I was staging a play. I fight back with literature, I escape, and save myself with it—*kanharab b la littérature*]."

Then to his mother, in Arabic: "You don't know Cervantes, you don't know anything, this is suffering, you only know how to make couscous . . .

It is at that point that the anguish of persecution and imprisonment gives way to an imaginary experience of creation, a "flight" of the imagination, where Reda stages his characters in the open spaces of a literature in the foreign language.

We—his interlocutors—won't witness the immediacy of his flight. Reda presents his experience in the form of a reflection, offered in the distancing mode of commentary. Because for him what is at stake is a "retreat," an exit into another scene where the Self may be rescued and healed. Granting to it the status of a concept, Reda calls that other scene *le Stade Cervantes* (the Cervantes Stage). It is a "stage that exists in literature," he explains, but that sometimes he experiences in life. This "Stage" (a term he uses in the double sense of stage in the theater and human developmental stage) has the configuration of an intermediate world. I say this with a term of comparison in mind, one to which Reda would not have referred explicitly: *Al-Alam al-Mithal* (the World of the Imagination) in the thought of the thirteenth-century mystic-scholar Ibn al-ʿArabi.

The literary identification by which Reda says to "escape" and "fight back" (I will return to the double play of his expression) oscillates between the roles of Cervantes-the-author and Don Quixote-the-character—between a controlled staging of madness in a Baroque self-reflexive literature and the madness without return of the wandering knight, prisoner of his imaginary combats, suspended between the books and the life. Yet, for Reda, all this happens in solitude, because rare are those who, in his surroundings, in his small town as in the emergency room, are familiar with Cervantes, Don Quixote, and the story of the windmills. And this independent of the fact that Cervantes, the historical author, was in his time influenced by the reading of Arab texts, and in particular by the narrative strategies of the *Arabian Nights* as well as, perhaps, by the reflection on madness and healing the *Nights* represent.[12]

But first of all the voices.

In French to Dr. R. and increasingly to me, Reda says: "I wake up very early in the morning just to read, because with the crisis of the economy, there are no jobs, there is so much unemployment, and we live in Yacob El Mansour [an underprivileged neighborhood in Rabat], there is so much noise during the day, it is impossible to read!" (Reda had registered my reaction at his mention of Cervantes, and a connection was created between us, a connection through reading. Physically foreign, with a foreign accent in both Arabic and French, a "researcher," from his perspective analogous to him, I am perceived with complicity and included as a character in his tribunal.)

In this as other public hospitals, where the majority of the patients speak vernacular Arabic and are unfamiliar with medical and psychiatric concepts, the staff makes use of an intermediate vocabulary supposed rhetorically to be "that of the patient" (la langue du patient). It is a language of trade, in fact, loosely codified and deployed in the effort to make possible clinical interviews across experientially incommensurable conceptual worlds. It is a vocabulary based on the implicit assumption of the one-to-one translatability of symptoms or, more precisely, of the referential transparency of psychiatric symptomatology, which, whatever its symbolic expression, will necessarily translate into its true referent, that of a recognizable disease entity. Lwusuwas, for instance, that demonic haunting, maddening whispering in one's ear, temptation of unreason, which is a central figure of madness in the Qur'an as well as in everyday speech, becomes the equivalent of obsessive neurosis or, in the terminology of the fourth edition of the Diagnostic and Statistical Manual of Mental Disorders (DSM-IV), obsessive compulsive disorder. Hence to make a differential diagnosis the psychiatrist will attempt to isolate lwusuwas from the "voices" of schizophrenia.

Or when the presence of a jinn is at issue (in the complaints of the patient, never in the questions of the psychiatrists, unwittingly registering, by that reticence to enter the "patient's language," the vulnerability and risk of the "psychiatric operation,"[13] the task is to detect the symptom behind: the question becomes whether the entity, or voice, is internal or external to the subject and what the patient replies to that voice. As a senior psychiatrist put it at a staff meeting, discussing the case of a young man possessed by a jinn who, rather than speaking through him, never stopped talking to him: "From a purely psychiatric point of view what we want to isolate is the type of symptom, beyond the anecdotal figure of the jinn, which is drawn from our available cultural repertory and is not interesting in itself. We know that there is something embodied [incorporé], which causes the patient to do certain things, which gives orders to the person. It could just as well be a device implanted by the CIA in his body. From the semiological point of view in all these cases we have one and the same symptom, which we recognize as automatisme mentale." Such is the risk, and the violence, of concepts in translation, when translation no longer discloses the foreign nature of language, but becomes instead the apparatus of appropriation and reduction to the same.

Wash katsma' aswat f-udnik? (Do you hear voices in your ear?) Formulating the question in Arabic is not obvious, even though it is done all the time. Because in the larger sense indexed by the Arabic language and rooted in the specific way of experiencing subjectivity exemplified in the discourse of the jinns, as well as, at a more philosophical level, in the ecstatic dimension of religious experience, hearing voices is not equal to madness. Or at least a certain madness, a certain "exit" from the self, is foundational for the possibility of subjectivity and truth. The Qur'an was reveled in a visionary dream by the voice of an angel speaking in Muhammad's ear. Revelation, as argued by Fethi Benslama (1988) in his book on the Qur'an, is the result of a moment of radical ultimate existential risk, a passage through madness in which the Prophet might be lost, but that instead gives way to the interpretation of the voice as divine utterance—an interpretation made possible, and literally engendered, by the feminine intercession of Mohammed's wife, Khadija, on whose "lap" the divine's message becomes audible and can be received as a divine utterance.

Later in the interview the mother tells of an episode that illustrates the function of "exit" Reda imputes to reading, to the use of a foreign language, and to that experience of journeying he calls literature. One day, toward the beginning of his illness, he took off with his books in the wilderness: "Once, when he was first sick, during the time when he was praying a lot, he vanished for three weeks, went out into nature [kharj ll tabi'a], into the countryside [f-l-khala], into the wilderness of open empty spaces. He spent there his days and his nights, he took his books with him, said he was going to read his book to the land! Imagine, three weeks like that, he walked from Tiflet to El-Hajeb through the countryside, he slept outdoors and begged for food."

Reda opposes that all this is none of his mother's business. He turns to Dr. R, and to me, in French: "I searched and searched in the books, I was forced to hide the Italian language, because you realize, chez nous, in Tiflet, it's impossible to show it in public . . . because I love languages, I love reading, I love nature, it is my right, I request a lawyer immediately, it is my right to go out into nature and do what I wish, here in Morocco, it is my right! I respect the constitution of the king, and I demand a lawyer, a lawyer here and now!"

Kanharrab b la littérature: I save myself with literature. Kanharrab, a fleeing from an aggression, a dangerous situation, an attack or an invasion. A fleeing that is also a distancing, a departure that can save oneself. Kanharrab, I escape, resembles and in Reda's use rhymes with kanharrab, "I fight back, engage in a struggle," as in an armed counterattack, "I fight back with literature." In this sense, for Reda literature is a "counterdelirium" comparable to the counterdelirium of witchcraft, according to Favret-Saada (1977), as well as to the counterdelirium of literature for Deleuze (1998). But unlike the aggressive metaphor of witchcraft, the saving doesn't reestablish the Self as a presence, for what departs, in his image, what is no longer there, is precisely the self that is saved, that is both lost and saved. "I flee/fight back with literature," that is by way of literature, but also literally "with it," with the books on my back, for a life of wandering with "my" characters, the other voices, on the stage of "my" comedy, Cervantes' Stage, the mise-en-scène of the voices. Myself, Don Quixote, Cervantes' mad reader and wandering knight. The Cervantes Stage is "another scene" where all persecuting others have vanished, including himself as a narcissistic injury. It is an "open empty space," l-khala, where he can be alone and find sanctuary with his stories and his books. In this place Reda reads to nature: an empty listening, the only interlocutor that, he feels, doesn't reduce him to silence.

Later, after his hospitalization, in a room in the men's locked ward, I ask Reda about his encounter with literature. He tells me about the public library in his hometown, where people don't read, are illiterate, and don't speak other languages (they do speak Berber and Arabic!); he tells me about reading Voltaire and about his passion for Dostoevsky and Cervantes. He read *Crime and Punishment*, but it is *Don Quixote* that really had an impact on him. When I ask him why "literature," he explains that since he started having difficulties in concentrating (this is how he speaks of the "strangeness" of his condition), he had to abandon his scientific studies and began to read—to dig in literature (*fouiller dans la littérature*). And why Cervantes? I asked. He returned the question to me, do I know the story of Don Quixote? "Don Quixote has read all the books," he explains, "the books of world history, and he wanted to fight with the windmills, and for his love Dulcinea wanted to show to be a great knight, and this is why he took on traveling with his friend Sancho, but most often, in fact, with no one [he laughs]. He doesn't do any harm, to anyone, but the important thing, the important thing is that each time he creates a story for himself [*chaque fois il se crée une histoire*]."

TRANSLATIONS

According to the structure of the clinical interview, Dr. R. moves on to the mother. Dr. R. must collect information about family history and the early signs of the illness. There emerges, at this point, an important issue of translation, predicated on a play of reciprocal projections and on a certain complicity in misrecognition. To proceed, there must be a sense of common ground, a common ground that both parties assume is lacking. The psychiatrist must translate her diagnostic concepts in terms the mother can understand, in vernacular Arabic and in images borrowed from everyday language, without however surrendering to the presumed interpretative schemata of the mother, that of possession by the jinns; the mother must describe her son's condition in terms the psychiatrist can accept and validate, that is, she must objectify and translate her own experience of his state as if in a foreign language. This double translation produces important alterations that cannot be recognized by either party. Misrecognized also is the disquieting sentiment that, even when they seem to have reached an agreement on the representation used, saying for instance that "something is ringing in his head," each interlocutor situates this image in her own frame of reference, which is at odds with the that of the other. They know this, Dr. R. and Reda's mother, but can't acknowledge it and perhaps can't even formulate it. They can't, because the institution itself, its symbolic efficacy, requires that silence.

And things are even more complex if one considers that the psychiatrist, Dr. R., even though she is external (by choice, by chance, and by historical reason), is not at all foreign to the symbolic universe of Reda's mother, who could easily be her own mother. This fact raises the unresolved and in a way unspeakable question of cultural belonging as open injury and interrupted transmission. And, at the same time, one can consider that the mother came to the hospital to contain, control, and help her son, but also for a desire impossible to avow, to be able to speak her own rage.

Dr. R. turns then to the mother and asks in Arabic when her son's illness began. The mother relates how Reda started to change (keytghiyyer) two years earlier, when he suddenly embraced religion and took on assiduous praying—even the prayer of dawn, at the mosque, in the middle of winter. What's wrong with praying? Dr. R. opposes. Attempting to construct her case, the mother speaks of the old men's surprise at Reda's sudden religious turn (keytʾajbw), for he used to drink and to smoke. His prayer was not normal (keysalli sala mashi tabeʾya). What else was "strange"? asks Dr. R.

"Yes, strange [ghrib]!!!" The mother struggles to represent that strangeness: she speaks of her son's sleepless nights, his aggressive tone, the transformation of his bodily expression. "Mabqash kima kan [he was no longer himself]," she concludes.

The psychiatrist provides a vocabulary, "Did he look at himself in the mirror, did he notice a transformation in his image?" The mother says, "Yes, and he would talk to himself, at first he'd stop if we walked in the room, then didn't care anymore, would just go on speaking to himself in our presence." And he hit another boy with a knife, she adds. "When?" the psychiatrist asks. "Just a few months ago, and he spent two months in jail, that's what finished him up." The psychiatrist interrupts the mother to order, she wants a chronological account, "from beginning to end," and to ask whether Reda complained about his strangeness, whether he felt the world around him was becoming uncanny, ghrib.

"He complained that something was ringing in his head [katsonne lih shy hajja f-rras], that he was possessed, 'there is a jinn in me' [keygullik mskun, 'rah fiya shy jinn']."

Dr. R. makes a gesture of recognition, moving toward a possible diagnosis. The mother acknowledges her gesture in silence, with what I read as a sense of relief. Only later, after the psychiatrist left us alone in the room, she stated that those signs, "that juggling of the limbs and the speaking to himself, the ringing of something in his head," were signs of demonic possession, and they were not the reason she had come to the hospital. She had come because of Reda's drug habit, his hashish smoking, because she thought the hashish might have got to his head and, in that case, he would be treated with hospital drugs. In a way, she hoped so. Because in that case doctors could do something; Reda would take medications, and perhaps he'd be cured. But for a demonic possession, the hospital can provide no cure.

Afterward, as I listened to the tape recording of the interview, I asked myself if the truth of the mother was in that discreet revelation of her interpretive universe, which she had omitted in her conversation with Dr. R., or if it was instead in the story she was able to tell after her son's departure, and because of the active listening of the psychiatrist, in the foreign country of the psychiatric institution.

THE KNOT OF THE SOUL

Later, after her son was escorted to the men's locked ward, Reda's mother spoke differently. Her tone changed, and the anguish that froze her as a character, forced to speak the phantasm in the scene of her son's persecution, loosened into voice and made possible the enunciation of her own injury—the story of her own pain and the way that pain crystallized into the "knot" of her son's existence. Yet, as stories of suffering in situations of oppression are rarely innocent in their address and rhetorical scope, her story is an ambiguous one, where her pain is both revealed and reinvested in an ultimate appropriation.

It is Dr. R. who can receive her speech within the constraining space of the emergency room. And the mother speaks of a wound, a "knot of the soul," l-'aquda nefsyia, with an evocative expression by which she reckons the intertwining of her suffering with that of her son and laments his fate as an offspring of her own. He is "knotted," she says, maʾaqqad, with an evocative "intermediate" concept, a bridge between two worlds of interpretation—at once an image of bewitchment from the vocabulary of magic and a term for "complex" in that of modern psychology.

The knot of the soul is the hidden wound, physically expressed by the urinary incontinence that accompanied Reda through his adolescence; a wound hidden inside and suddenly exploded to the outside, into the other world of his illness. But the l-'aquda nefsyia is also the knot of her own soul: her unhappy marriage, alcoholic husband, the violence of her evenings, the sleeplessness of her nights, the tears. The husband, a policeman who beat her, and Reda, the little boy who watched the violence, who cried and later interceded for her with his father. The eldest of her children, he saw everything and was traumatized. She uses the technical term *sadama*, "shock" or "trauma," a term she learned from her children who accused them, the parents, of having traumatized them. Yet despite all this Reda was managing; despite the "knot," the knot remained hidden and he could succeed in school, the only one of the children to have had an education. But when he got his university degree and didn't find a job, when he found himself on the street, unemployed, a *chomeur*, all that came out in the open, like a blister, impossible to contain.

Now that the children have grown up, she decided to get a divorce. She was lucky because her husband did not oppose her request. She sought a divorce to try to give a chance to Reda, for the trajectory of his life is cut off. She knows, she says, that it is her own injury that implanted itself into the life of her son and is slowly destroying him. She suggests that I go to visit him in the ward; he will be glad to talk with me.

DON QUIXOTE AND THE CERVANTES STAGE

Sitting on his chair without moving, Reda has been listening in silence to his mother's description of his state. But when she mentions his experience of possession by a jinn he protests, in Arabic, that the jinns are also God's creatures, that they are found everywhere in the world, and that they are mentioned in the Qur'an. The mother opposes that she is just reporting things he said in the past. Reda explodes, in French: "I lied so that she gets away from me, that she leaves me alone, because she's illiterate, she and her friends are the enemies of science, the enemies of reading! [*J'ai menti, pour qu'elle s'éloigne de moi, parce qu'elle est analphabète, elle et ses copines, des ennemies de la science, des ennemies de la lecture*]."

The mother talks about his drug habit, his use of hashish, and the recent degeneration of his state. Not sleeping, wandering on the beach, talking about the jinns. Reda protests, "*C'est le Stade Cervantes dans la littérature* [it is the Cervantes Stage in literature]."

Irritated, Reda starts speaking a sort of Italian or Spanish (he had asked me where I was from), his own linguistic creation, in which can be recognized the name of Don Quixote. The mother explains that when he's feeling bad Reda starts speaking other languages, "French, English, Italian, and Berber . . . he's good with languages. . . .

Dr. R. is moving to a conclusion. The mother hesitates, "I feel I forgot something." And the psychiatrist asks her whether Reda ever claimed to be a prophet. The mother nods, "Imam 1-Mehdi," she says, "you're right, I forget some things, once he told me that a woman appeared to him in his sleep and told him, "You are the son of Myriam, you are l-Imam l-Mehdi, he said this to his father and myself. . . .

Reda protested in French, "This is Cervantes, I am telling you. . . .

The psychiatrist asks him directly, "Are you a prophet?"

"No! That's absurd," he protests, "it is a manner of speaking, like Cervantes [*c'est une façon de dire, comme Cervantes*]. It is manner of living, I do this, every once in a while, it is my way of going on living, time and again, I practice literature in life [*c'est ma façon de vivre, de temps en temps, je fais également de la littérature dans la vie*]. . . .What's wrong with practicing literature in life? I invent, create and recreate [*j'invente et je réinvente*]. . . .

"What is it that you invent?" asks Dr. R., interested, for the first time, in exploring Reda's site of flight, his recurrent recourse from the beginning of the interview.

"Stories such as those she's relating, stories with jinns. They say, for instance, back at home, that certain men have love affairs with she-demons. That's not true, can anyone really describe the procedure of nights [having sex with a jinn]? God created the jinns, and those jinns exist in religion as abstract terms of creature. But no one was ever married to a jinn. It the same thing that happens in literature, when it is applied to the practice of living, every once in a while I use terms such as jinn or jinniya, to live *le Stade Cervantes* in life. Just to get away from those illiterate ones."

"What is this that you call the 'Cervantes Stage'"? asks Dr. R., in Arabic this time, stressing the quotation marks as if not to validate Reda's concept as her own.

"In any case, this is what I call it. It means to make use of imaginary characters at certain times, to speak with the windmills, *tahuna* [mills]," Reda repeats in Arabic, aware that the audience might not be familiar with Don Quixote. "I as well, when I was speaking to myself, I was actually talking to the desk, *imagining it* as an enemy, as Don Quixote did. . . .

Dr. R. stops listening, asks the mother whether they ever took Reda to the hospital or to a fqih. At his mother's reply he becomes angry. Siding with Reda for the first time, Dr. R. addresses the mother in a reproachful tone. Dr R. is moved in her modernist sensibility closer to Reda, in fact, in her own experience: who are the healers her son is complaining about?

"They are well known in town," says the mother defensively. I ask her what was the healer's diagnosis: mqius, she says, "touched" (by the jinns), and starts talking about his excessive washing as evidence of possession (demons are said to like water). Reda opposes that it is his right to wash, to be clean, it is called hygiene.

A nurse comes in, and escorts Reda to the locked ward. Dr. R's quick notes, which will never become a formal patient file, mention psychotic symptoms, pointing to a psychotic personality and possibly an early onset of schizophrenia.

Later, at the ward, Reda is brought down by a nurse, who waits outside the door because the patient is "not cooperating" and opposes his hospitalization. Alone for the first time, we talk in a room by the main patio—about literature, Don Quixote, and what makes it difficult for him to concentrate. He asks me about my nationality, he already knew in fact, and starts speaking a sort of invented Italian that turns into Spanish and finally breaks into incomprehensible speech. Language hardens as a wall between us, and against this wall our conversation dissolves. When I come back to visit him the next morning, I learn that he has fled the hospital, climbing a high wall.

THE INTERMEDIATE WORLD

Aware of the risks of speculation (reducing Reda's suffering to my desire to understand), of that particular sort of appropriation that is anthropological interpretation, I attempt to reflect on the status of that other place, the Stage, where Reda retreats (*kanharrab*) and from which he fights back (*kanharrab*), in the rough moments of his illness as during the ER interview; the Stage to which he bestows the status of a theory, in which he is both a character and the director, and which is the site—rhetorical, existential, and physical—of his surrender to the Other and his desire for self.

I am encouraged in this reflection by the ambiguity of my position, a position I so often experienced as frustrating and even paralyzing, always external to the action, if also enmeshed in it (the anthropologist listening, asking questions, feeling directly concerned, affected, yet unable and unauthorized to "cure"), but which can be enabling of an oblique interpretative space, a space of "proximity," marginal to action and decision, a peripheral zone of speculation and critique. In attempting to inhabit this space, I am inspired by the strategy inaugurated by Reda himself, his "appropriation" of Don Quixote, which is also a dispossession of himself, and his multilayered use of characters and rhetorical figures by which, like the Spanish *hildago*, he labors at creating a multidimensional space where his uncanny experience of the world may find expression and elaboration. In this sense, his strategy can be called, as he calls it, literary.

Literature, writes Deleuze in one of his last essays, is the opposite of phantasms. Phantasms fix identities in place, personalize characters and seal possession, while literature is a process of dispossession, a becoming-other that dwells in a zone of proximity (*voisinage*), and is never saturated by an identity: "literature begins only when a third person is born in us that strips us of the power to say I" (Deleuze 1998: 3). In this sense, Deleuze says, literature is health—a vulnerable health (*une petite santé*) that almost choked in its experiences, but that gained in that process the capacity of becoming. It is born from within delirium, as a movement of straying, becoming foreign, from the mother tongue (from the Mother), from the madness of ideological identifications, and it transforms them from within, such an antidelirium; a becoming other that opens onto "visions," "ideas" that are not the projection of an Ego and that can become the singular-collective utterance of a people to come.

Reda has discovered his literary "procedure" in the work of Cervantes, where he encountered his own story in an exemplary form, translated into a foreign language. Thanks to this discovery, which coincided with his first realization of a feeling of strangeness in his experience of the world, he has taken on the practice of literature, which he intends from the point of view of the character as well as of that of the author. It is not by chance that in his literary search through Voltaire and Dostoevsky in the town library of Tiflet Reda settled on Don Quixote, the text that raises the ambiguity of character and author, ironical distancing and imaginary capture, life and fiction, to the principle of its narrative structure.

(Reaching back stenographically to the political questions raised earlier on in the discussion, it could be said that "literature," in Reda's use and as read through Deleuze, discloses an unforeseen possibility of *twkkel*, the murderous "us" of the collective identification. Literature opens for Reda the possibility of negotiating his debt to a failing cultural transmission in the form of a not-yet or no-longer us. While the objectifications of his modernity ideal are rigid, as the saturation of knowledge in a self-sufficient totality, the moving and multiple identifications of the *Stade Cervantes* are not.)

To phrase the question in terms closer to the clinical concerns of psychiatrists, it would be wrong to reduce Reda's procedure to the deployment of a delusion or to the commonly observed quest of patients at the onset of psychosis, trying to make sense and "rationalize" their experiences of growing strangeness in terms of a fantasy, which is then systematized into a delusion. That reduction would miss the dimension of struggle in Reda's experience, obliterating the sense in which his search is meaningful and his experience of otherness less unfamiliar than one may be willing to acknowledge. This was also the reaction of the psychiatrists at the hospital when we discussed a draft of this chapter: expressing the question in a diagnostic idiom, they said that if Reda had most likely a psychotic personality, he was however not fully psychotic, thanks to an element of creativity and to his ability to self-reflect.

First his symbolic geography. The Stage, as a topological elsewhere, is an effect of withdrawal, of breaking the ties with "home" (*chez soi*) in all its forms: the family, the home town, vernacular Arabic (the mother tongue), the space of the everyday, of social relations and tradition. It is the result of a radical disaffiliation of which Reda is at once the victim, the character, and the author. This "retreat" is a vital distancing from the mother, figure of the uninhabitable home, and from the magical logic of twkkel, the envious incorporation of the other. But the distancing is more than just a withdrawal. It is a departure, a journey, the metamorphosis of the self in a theater of imaginary forms, where the possibility of self-realization gambles with the risk of nonreturn.

On the one hand, le Stade Cervantes is for Reda the ironic moment of a coming of age, when the break with the forms of a fossilized tradition is consummated and "creation" becomes possible: "j'invente and je réinvente." The Cervantes Stage is the stage of "maturity" Reda reached in his evolution, inaccessible for his illiterate parents and from which are excluded all those who seek the reassurance of tradition. On the other hand, the "Stage," as Reda describes it, is also a scene of alienation, the fact of becoming a character in one's creation: "Je fais de temps en temps de la littérature dans la vie [time and again, I practice literature in life]." Reda becomes Don Quixote who, like himself, has read "all the books of history" and has given up all ties for a life of travel in the meadows of the imagination; Don Quixote who, like himself, lives at a time lag with his contemporaries, a temporal disjunction, speaks a "dead language" full of references they don't understand, because he himself has renounced their recognition. But Don Quixote is tricked by his imagination. Reda says this in full knowledge, as he looks at himself from the critical perspective of the author. He smiles and says that it happens to him too, sometimes, to fight against the windmills: he calls it living the Cervantes Stage in real life. Suspended between the author and the character, Reda doesn't seek a resolution: invention is something else than mastery, it is to practice literature in life, " to create stories for oneself." He claims for himself his j'invente as an exercise of self-fashioning, struggling to find balance on the line between delusion and creation.

Yet in his conception of the Stage there is the trace of a possible mediation. To the psychiatrist's question, "What do you invent?," Reda replies that he invents stories of jinns, jinns that he enacts in the mise-en-scène of voices to live the Cervantes Stage in real life; jinns that he glosses as "abstract terms of creatures" (in the Qur'an) and compares to figures of speech, styles of speaking, "manières de parler," when one practices literature in life. At once a space of language, where words materialize as images, and a mystical space, populated with jinns, le Stade Cervantes is an intermediate world, realm of the creative imagination: in Ibn al-'Arabi's Islamic metaphysics, Al-Alam al-Mithal. It becomes then the site of a possible mediation, a passageway between delusion and creation, where the rejected terms of cultural identification, the remains of an inaccessible tradition, are reencountered and can be symbolically transformed in that "foreign" space. For a moment the threatening otherness of the persecutory interpretation (the poisonous communal meal), becomes for Reda an ecstatic experience: "*inqui-etante familiarité*," *une fréquentation de "l'Autre"* (Certeau 1982: 20).

NOTES

I would like to thank the staff of the Hospital Arrazi in Salé, Morocco, and particularly Dr. Mehdi Paes, Jamaladdine Ktiouet, Selwa Kjiri, Jalal Toufiq, and Mustapha Laymani. Thanks also to Fouad Benchekroun, Abdellah Hammoudi, Mohammed Hamdouni Alami, Luca D'Isanto, Veena Das, M. Letizia Cravetto, Saba Mahmood, Lawrence Cohen, Eric Glassgold, Andrew Lakoff, Baber Johansen, M. Pia Di Bella, Byron Good, Mary-Jo DelVecchio Good, and Pete Skafish. Research on psychiatry in Morocco in 1998–99 was funded by a grant of the Social Science Research Council and in 2001–02 by a grant from the Sultan Committee, CMES, UC Berkeley.

1. See in this context Pandolfo (2006a, 2006b); on the history and predicament of colonial psychiatry, see Pandolfo (2000).

2. Article 11 reads, "L' hospitalisation dans un service publique ou un établissement privé de psychiatrie ne peut avoir lieu qu'au vu d'un certificat delivré par un médécin psychiatre qualifié mentionnant de façon detaillée et precise les anomalies du comportément du malade et concluant à la necessité de l'hospitalisation [Hospitalization in a public or a private psychiatric institution can exclusively take place at the production of a certificate issued by a qualified medical psychiatrist, describing in a detailed and precise manner the anomalies of the patient's behavior, and concluding to the need of hospitalization] (my translation).

3. The question remains open of how to understand this process from the point of view of psychic life, or what some psychoanalysts have called the institution and deinstitution of the subject. In a related context, psychoanalysts writing on exile and migration stress the crucial clinical dimension of "relating to the break," the trauma, as a recognition of radical discontinuity that is prior to the possibility of reinhabiting a space (cf. Deleuze 2001).

4. One of the prime consequences of the World Bank program of structural adjustment for Morocco in the 1980s has been the cutting of all forms of aid or subsidy for health care.

5. The French word *chomeur* means "unemployed" or "jobless person." In Morocco this is today a charged term, at once scornful and expressing a social and political discontent. Since 1990 there has existed a countrywide organized movement of "Chomeurs Diplomés," which has become symbolic of a generalized sense of distress and discontent among the youth. The senior psychiatrists commented at the staff meeting, "This patient's case helps us clarify the theme of *chomage.*"

6. Morocco has since had the experience of a truth commission, which concluded its proceedings in February 2006. L'Instance Equité et Reconciliation (IER; *Al-Insaf wa al-musalaha*) was created in April 2004 by royal decree, with the mandate to investigate and record human rights violations committed since national independence

and during the kingdom of the late king Hassan II (1956–99). The IER collected hundreds of testimonies of "victims" (al-dahia is the term officially used) or relatives of deceased victims and received over twenty thousand victims' requests of reparation. In spring 2005 public hearings were held by the IER in several cities, covered by the Moroccan and international media. The process stirred many hopes and a heated debate, with complex and unintended outcomes. Yet in the Moroccan situation the equation of witnessing, injury, and citizenship (based on human rights) is less obvious than in other international contexts. Among large unprivileged sectors of the Moroccan population, less conversant than the political elite with the international idiom of human rights, skepticism colored people's perception of the work of the IER, as well as the notion of accessing citizenship through witnessing.

7. I am referring here to the clinical-theoretical work on the *espace originaire*, or "primal space" (Aulagnier 1975), and the archaic experience of the body in psychosis and schizophrenia (Pancow 1969), as well as of recent contributions in cultural psychiatry (Jenkins and Barrett 2004, particularly J. Jenkins, chapter 1, "Schizophrenia as a Paradigm Case for Understanding Fundamental Human Processes," and E. Corin, chapter 4, "Living through a Staggering World: The Play of Signifiers in Early Psychosis in South India"). See also Corin (1990).

8. All names of persons in this essay, and specifically those of patients and psychiatrists, have been changed—unless reference is made to psychoanalysts or psychiatrists as authors of published texts.

9. The Moroccan university curriculum for the scientific disciplines, including mathematics (Faculté des Sciences), is entirely in French. The social sciences, as well as literature and philosophy, are instead taught in Arabic. At the Schools of Medicine, Architecture, and Engineering, instruction is in French.

10. The struggle for place, for horizon, for distance, is a central feature in the experience of youths with whom I spoke in poor neighborhoods. As I write about Reda, I think of a youth recounting to me his nights, sitting on top of a hill overlooking the freeway, in the silence in which one can breathe, following the movement of long-distance trucks with his binoculars, waiting for the truck in which he will hide, to risk his way beyond the Spanish border. See Pandolfo (2007).

11. In an essay on Schreber's *Memoir of My Nervous Illness*, Vincent Crapanzano (1988) describes a comparable struggle against annihilation, in which "space," "occupation," and "distance" play a fundamental role.

12. Abdelfattah Kilito, personal communication, February 2002.

13. See chapter 2, "The Historiographical Operation," in Certeau (1988).

REFERENCES

Agamben, G. 1998. *Homo Sacer: Sovereign Power and Bare Life*. Trans. D. Heller-Roazen. Stanford, CA: Stanford University Press. Originally published as *Homo Sacer: Il potere sovrano e la nuda vita* (Torino: Einaudi, 1995).

Arendt, H. 1971. *The Origins of Totalitarianism: Imperialism.* New York and London: Harcourt.

Asad, T. 2002. Interview by Nermeen Shaikh. *Asia Source,* December 16. www .asiasource.com/news/special_reports/asad.cfm.

Aulagnier, P. 1975. *La violence de l'interpretation.* Paris: PUF.

Benslama, F. 1988. *La nuit brisée: Muhammad et l'énonciation Islamique.* Paris: Ramsay.

———. 2000. épreuves de l'étranger. In "Clinique de l'exil," *Cahier Intersignes* 14/15:9–29.

———. 2002. *La psychanalyse à l'épreuve de l'Islam.* Paris: Aubier.

Berthelier, R. 1994. *L'homme maghrebin dans la littérature psychiatrique.* Paris: l'Harmattan.

Binswanger, L. 1958. The Case of Ellen West. In *Existence: A New Dimension in Psychiatry and Psychology,* ed. R. May, E. Angel, H. Ellenberg, 237–64. New York: Basic Books.

Borch-Jacobsen, M. 1993. *The Emotional Tie.* Trans. D. Brick. Stanford, CA: Stanford University Press. Originally published as *Le lien affectif* (Paris: Aubier, 1991).

Certeau, M. de 1982. *La fable mystique.* Paris: Gallimard.

———. 1988. *The Writing of History.* Trans. Tom Conley. New York: Columbia University Press. Originally published as *L'écriture de l'histoire,* (Paris: Gallimard, 1975).

Corin, E. 1990. Facts and Meaning in Psychiatry: An Anthropological Approach to the Lifeworld of Schizophrenics. In *Culture, Medicine and Psychiatry* 14:153–88.

Deleuze, G. 1998. *Critical and Clinical Essays.* Trans. D. Smith and M. Greco. Minneapolis: University of Minnesota Press. Originally published as *Critique et Clinique* (Paris: éditions de Minuit, 1993).

Crapanzano, V. 1998. Lacking Now is Only the Leading Idea, That Is—We, the Rays, Have No Thought: Interlocutory Collapse in Daniel Paul Schreber's *Memoirs of my Nervous Illness. Critical Inquiry* 24 (Spring): 737–67.

Fassin, D. 1999. Santé et immigration: Les verités politiques du corps. *Cahiers de URMIS* 5:69–76.

———. 2000. Politique du vivant et politique de la vie: Pour une anthropologie de la santé. *Anthropologie et Société,* 24 (1): 95–116.

———. 2001. The Biopolitics of Otherness: Undocumented Foreigners and Racial Discrimination in French Public Debate. *Anthropology Today* 17 (1): 3–7.

Favret-Saada, J. 1977. *Les mots, le mort, les sorts: La sorciellerie dans le bocage.* Paris: Gallimard.

Igert, M. 1955. Introduction à la psychopathologie marocaine. *Maroc Médical,* no. 360: 1309–32.

Jenkins, J., and R. Barrett, eds. 2004. *Schizophrenia, Culture, and Subjectivity.* Cambridge: Cambridge University Press.

Lacoue-Labarthe, P., and J.-L. Nancy. 1997. La panique politique. In *Retreating the Political*, 1–31. New York: Routledge.

Pancow, G. 1969. *L'homme et sa psychose*. Paris: Flammarion.

Pandolfo, S. 2000. The Thin Line of Modernity: Reflections on Some Moroccan Debates on Subjectivity. In *Questions of Modernity*, ed. T. Mitchell, 115–47. Minneapolis: University of Minnesota Press.

———. 2006a. Bghit nghanni hnaya (Je veux chanter ici): Voix et témoignage en marge d'une rencontre psychiatrique. *Arabica* 53 (2): 232–80.

———. 2006b. Nibtidi minin il-hikaya (Where Are We to Start the Tale): Violence, Intimacy, and Recollection. *Social Science Information* 45 (3): 349–71.

———. 2007. The Burning: The Theologico-Political Imagination of Illegal Migration. In "Transitional Transcendence," special issue, *Anthropological Theory* 7 (3).

Prakash, G. 1999. *Another Reason: Science and the Imagination of Modern India*. Princeton, NJ: Princeton University Press.

Roland, J. L. 1957. De quelques incidences psycho-pathologiques des phénomènes se surpopulation: Vue d'ensemble; Aspect propre du Maroc. *Maroc Médical*, no. 387 (Août).

Infant Death in the Postcolonial Time of Intervention

Sarah Pinto

NAMING DEATH

In considering languages of grief in relation to languages of certainty, there is a tension in the ways death can be thought of in connection to modern knowledge. On the one hand, we can consider death as that which underlies the possibility of knowledge, as that end point to the fostering or disallowing of life that stands for the modern configuration of power/knowledge (as Foucault [1978] had it). And on the other hand, we can imagine death as that which cannot be spoken in languages of modernity (as de Certeau [1986] suggested). Put differently, this is the distinction between death as the ultimate condition of biopower, the "absconding presence in the institution" (Chatterjee, Chattoo, and Das 1998: 189), and death as the final affront to the certitudes of knowledge-power, that which speaks the limits of human effort (de Certeau 1987). Yet, when death is spoken in a postcolonial site of poverty and intervention, when it is made to speak about the overwhelming quality of everyday life, death may dwell in both realms. This is especially true of infant death, which we might think of as posing a particular challenge to notions of normality, however imagined.

In rural areas of the north Indian state of Uttar Pradesh, part of the India representing the shadows of the "India shining" of call centers, technology, outsourcing, and shopping malls, infant death is at once a familiar part of life for many men and women and a key part of the way state and private institutions represent their own moral stances. In a region with some of the highest infant mortality rates in Asia, modes of subjectivity are on offer in relation to childbearing. This is so within health intervention schemes and amid the languages that circulate within and without them. This chapter asks how, in transnational structures of health intervention in the postcolonial world of the "developing country," ways of accounting for and recounting infant death give shape to as much as they describe conditions of suffering. For people who are defined through cross-cutting abstractions as those *for which* and *because of which* intervention exists—in this case rural poor women in north India—how does grief resonate with the political? Likewise, in the cosmopolitan spaces and socialities crafted by structures of health intervention, how does language about suffering bear the split-off, dissociated feel of melancholia?

Infant death plays a central role in women's everyday talk in rural north India, in the chitchat in which people establish the ground of intersubjectivity. In a setting in which women seldom exchange stories about pregnancy and birth, stories about infant and child death are common, shared within and between households, with greater and lesser detail, by way of introduction and after some intimacy is attained. Talk among women about past losses flows within and against a legacy of interventions that bears stamps of both colonialism and postcolonial politics. The stories of loss shared among the men and women with whom I lived in 2000–01 are part of an ongoing conversation about power and human action. Such talk shares with the universalizing languages of health momentary evasions of specificity that amount to a series of deferrals. Two interwoven ways of speaking of death, that refracting through structures of intervention and that reflecting on personal loss, converge in the way both involve the nonintegration of certain moments and memories into the flow of life and speech. These two forms of local discourse each, at the same time, speak *to* and *about* suffering. Both are modes of telling and creating the conditions of life and longing in which "the immediacy of the really real is promised by what appears in contrast to be the mere abstractions of structure, subjectivity, text, plan, or idea" (Mitchell 2000: xiii). Addressing the commonness of infant death in conditions of poverty and under the international gaze of intervention, they create and critique the "world-as-picture" that is modernity (Mitchell 2000: xiv), opening up spaces in which repressed meanings return as symptoms of social disarray. But recollections of loss can also diverge from prescriptive and diagnostic enunciations, even where they incorporate them. They do so both through what, specifically, is deferred and also through what, by extension, is allowed to reemerge as sign of a larger disorder.

In 2001, I was living in a small village about eighty kilometers from Lucknow, the capital of Uttar Pradesh. I was referred in my research wanderings by the regional supervisor of a state-NGO collaborative family planning program to one of the program's local health workers. She was an upper-caste Hindu woman who, prior to her involvement in the state program, had made herself a "ladies' doctor." In spite of a lack of certification or formal training, she taught herself about childbearing from books and experience and delivered babies in homes within the frame of education and rationality. Singled out for training and employment by this (now-defunct) program, she marketed and distributed contraceptives, gently suggested sterilization on the same rounds through the village in which she checked up on babies she had recently delivered, and noted local births, pregnancies, and contraceptive use in the program-supplied ledger. Her house was near the government health subcenter and an eight-kilometer journey to the primary health center. I passed the subcenter frequently on my visits. Though it was always shuttered and locked, when I asked whether the doctor had visited recently she was often vague. "Sometimes she comes. She might have been here yesterday, I don't really know." But this did not mean that other kinds of care were unavailable. In her village there were several compounders and a range of *kacca* (raw) doctors who, like her, practiced medicine without the benefit of training or certification. The monthly health camp that was part of the reproductive health program came through here as well.

To walk home from her house, it was better to leave the main road. In shortcuts through the fields, at times it was necessary to balance on the grassy *mer*, the raised ground between fields. To walk on the *mer* was to cross over burial places of children. Among most rural Hindus, children, unlike adults, are buried rather than cremated, having not reached the age of knowledge (*shayani*) in which sexuality, reproductive capacity, and rational worldliness converge. They are often put under these lines of demarcation between plots and crops, at the edges of fertility and sustenance. At the edges of celebration and auspiciousness, too, dwelt an embodied memory of these losses. At home in the village where I lived, women gathered in the house one afternoon to sing songs in honor of the maternal goddess Maia. The drum was passed to a woman who waved her hand to decline. "Since the death of my son, I do not sing," she said, to nods of recognition. In Sitapur, the loosening and tying of expression were part of the ways pain was shared.

At the same time, flowing and foreclosed speech made life accountable to the social and political worlds through which people moved. For rural men and women, this includes an extensive apparatus of "intervention" into childbearing, a social-political matrix that enters into and recedes from daily life in cyclical fashion, aiming to improve conditions for living while, in effect, mapping the limits of possibility. Reproductive health and family planning schemes—public and private, transnational and "grassroots"—come and go in tides of acronyms. Though formulas and models are often similar, institutions, names, and actors change repeatedly. The then-new collaborative family planning scheme active in 2001 ceased operation in 2006, while a new government rural health program began its early stages of design and implementation. The "dai trainings" (the term "dai" generally refers to traditional birth attendants, or TBAs) so often presented by NGOs and the government as part of "innovative" designs have been a familiar feature of intervention from the late nineteenth century, and the village health worker, with an ever-shifting set of responsibilities, has been a staple of postindependence health planning.

In the circulations of what Michel Foucault (2000) called "governmentality," morally laden messages and biomedical techniques flow across boundaries between institution and noninstitution, between real and ersatz doctors, clinics and households. Here, pedagogy is integral to caregiving; as everyday folks become practicing doctors by adopting techniques and ways of speaking, "training" is replicated through daily encounters. The us/them imaginary familiar to structures of development is repeated in Dumontian fashion up and down the hierarchies of development, establishing the distinction between who gives knowledge and who receives it in extra-institutional settings—in households, among "self-made" doctors—as well as in pakka (cooked, legitimate) clinics (Pinto 2004). Where bona fide health institutions are concerned, governance is made up of recurring, short-term schemes aimed overwhelmingly at limiting births, though many also intend to provide care, often in traveling "camps" and by way of local agents. Part of longstanding attention to population, such cyclical practices are part of the linear social agendas of development. Amid the cycling of schemes, things meant to be permanent—government health centers and hospitals—are at best unreliable, at worst empty shells, a set of inconsistencies and uncertainties in which poor infrastructure means not knowing when or for how long there will be electricity, when or if a bus will come, when or if there will be a doctor present at the health center, how much one will be expected to pay.

Uttar Pradesh is one of India's most populous states and bears many of its poorest indicators for health and development. While U.P.'s literacy and mortality rates are among the highest in India, so too is it among the world's worst in rates of polio and other communicable diseases. At the time that research for this chapter was conducted (2000–01), the infant mortality rate in U.P. (death under one year of age) was 86.7 (deaths per 1,000 births), ranking U.P. second highest in infant mortality in India (the highest rates were found in the northeast province of Meghalaya at 89.0; the lowest in southern Kerala at 16.3, and the overall rate for India was 67.6; GOI 1999). Across India, rates are significantly higher in rural (73.3) than urban areas (47.0) (GOI 1999). While the purpose of this chapter is not to delineate causes of infant death, in the small village in which I lived in the Sitapur District, about eighty kilometers north of U.P.'s capital city, Lucknow, I recorded deaths (during my stay and before it) from dehydration, diarrhea, dysentery, birth trauma, tetanus, accident, and "no reason at all." But causality is complex and layered in people's own accounts; deaths that "just happened," those that God hands out for reasons that cannot be known, and those for "no reason" cannot be separated from those preceded by warning signs or symptoms.

In the 1980s medical anthropologists writing about infant mortality described modernity as a condition in which "the dialectic between fertility and mortality has lost its edge" (Scheper-Hughes 1987: 1). Noting that childhood mortality was not considered a social problem in Europe prior to the twentieth century, Nancy Scheper-Hughes paralleled early modern mortality patterns in Europe, as described by Arthur Imhof (1985), in which deaths were concentrated in infancy with "old" patterns of reproduction, in which higher numbers of births and briefer intervals between them go along with uncertainty about child survival. Accompanying this uncertainty, Scheper-Hughes wrote, was a particular pattern of parental disinvestment, "allow[ing] parents a certain emotional distance that is psychologically protective" (1987: 11) (she clarified that this "old" pattern is hardly premodern, in that it is familiar in locales of intense poverty and limited resources characteristic of industrialized societies).

However, the "investment" and "strategy" model of childbearing, and by extension parental affect, may preclude a sense of the ways that not only conditions of modernity but histories of intervention and their attendant structures of meaning have rendered lack of affect or resignation a characteristic pathology of the subaltern woman. As moral, even soteriological, qualities of explanation enter into and give shape to the lives, memories, and interactions of the people in question, the notion of "fatalism" may leave less room for the varied languages of parental grief. Fatalism must be approached not just in itself, but as a founding moment of imagination upon which interventions are built. Even where it feels muted, the communication of grief in story, image, and action may speak to (rather than being cancelled out by) complexities of living and caregiving amid state and transnational structures that both insert into and recede from everyday life. Where for Scheper-Hughes, in her anguishing account of infant death in Brazil (1992), a quality of maternal detachment arises precisely from unbearable social and political conditions including the "averted gaze" of the state, in north India, it is under the gaze of the state that expressions of grief and causality speak to, as well as from, the politics of daily life.

As part of a larger discourse on fatalism, the pedagogical nature of postcolonial health interventions and their reliance on subject transformation make "awareness" a central construct in the framing of a healthy citizen. But in grappling with memories of loss, "knowledge" or "understanding" in the simple sense of "awareness" becomes an insufficient category. In rural India there are few firm divisions between subjects and objects of intervention beyond the moment of their performance, only imaginaries thereof. Thus, by disarticulating forms of speech from their camps, the historical and political genealogies of moral claims become more vivid. If we must deal with knowledge, let it be in the sense of these histories, of the biotechnical apparatus of intervention that gives shape to interactions in the rooms and courtyards where women gather to speak, sing, and labor. Here, at what some might consider the "margins" of the state, and others might imagine as its "center" (through either persistent fantasies about "the Indian village" or "target" metaphors of intervention), there is little purchase to the argument that a particular display of knowledge is a condition of consciousness.

THE DEPRESSING SPEECH OF INTERVENTION

On the third day of its life, a newborn baby girl died in the straw bed that had been made for her. As her mother stared quietly at the empty indentation, neighbors and relatives visited, discussing in soft voices what might have gone wrong. The baby had refused to drink. It was weak from the beginning, in spite of the efforts that had been made to invigorate it at the moment of its birth—warming the placenta, rubbing and massaging the baby. When I mentioned the death to the women in the upper-caste household where I was living, the younger daughter-in-law asked what happened.

"They said it did not drink."

"Those people never feed their babies right away," she said.

"It must have been born early." Uma, the elder daughter-in-law came over to hear about the death.

"No," I said, "It was born on time. They said it was weak from the beginning."

"Those people will never show a baby to the doctor. They never take their children to show the doctor," the younger said.

"Come off it," replied Uma, who had lost two babies herself. "Everything is in the big, big hands of God."

In assessments and recollections of death, it often feels that agency is under debate. Cause and human action continually encounter limits posed from out-side—God, doctors, ghosts, pathogens, fate. As it vacillates between these poles, the moral status of the mother remains ambivalent. Likewise, the relationship of the individual to kin group, caste group, class, and the broader world is under negotiation as a space of moral subjectivity. Charging these negotiations are fea-tures of expression characteristic of longstanding discourses on inaction and flawed affect. Replicable elements of intervention, especially those aimed at reproduction, involve patterns of speech and argumentation as much as they depend on material signs of authorization (identity and referral cards, delivery kits, shoulder bags, the ability to dispense drugs, injections, contraceptives, and so on). Phrases and ideas circulate from policy text to courtyard conversation through official and unofficial channels, in directly pedagogical encounters as well as in conversations less overtly aimed at education. Knowledge as a moral category infuses this system of unfolding hierarchy. But also present may be a splitting, repressive capacity not unlike that of melancholia, as Freud (1963) described it and Julia Kristeva (1989) later elaborated upon—dissociated, removed, nonspecific, and repetitive—emergent in colonial modes of uplift and reappearing in postcolonial and transnational institutions.

In early policy statements of the Safe Motherhood Initiative, a World Bank pro-gram, an approach to rural women's health was founded on what amounts to a theory of suffering. Central to this was the notion that a certain category of per-son—"poor women in Third World countries"—represented a premodern dislo-cation from universal knowledge, in this case, knowledge of how their condition was located on a scale of global norms. "Their" failure to be able to describe "their" conditions in a statistically oriented rationality, the "fact" that "they don't notice" such things as "high rates" of mortality or recognize "global standards" (Hertz and Meacham 1987: 1) provided pedagogical imperatives to intervention. Risks of pregnancy and childbirth, Safe Motherhood argued, "go almost unno-ticed" because "women have always died in childbirth" and because such risks are "overshadowed" by other "disadvantages" (Hertz and Meacham 1987: 1). As early Safe Motherhood documents asserted, not only do women not understand that repeated childbearing adversely affects health (their own and that of their children), "they" don't understand that ill health is bad (Hertz and Meacham 1987: 4). Such ignorance was described as a defining mode of existence of those targeted by interventions. Through the causal place given lack of historical vision, Safe Motherhood (not independently—other traditional birth attendant training programs demonstrated similar orientations) marked a path for intervention: "self-help programs" by which women would be instructed to "want help," understanding they would demonstrate by "demanding" services (Hertz and Meacham 1987: vii, 4).

Decades later, such etiologies remain vigorous in text and practice in India. A doctor who ran an NGO that trained rural midwives in Uttar Pradesh related a similar orientation at the same time that she professed admiration for rural women. As we spoke about her group's efforts to encourage women "that someone must be present at births," she said, "Otherwise, they see it as just a normal thing." The breadth of the "it" allowed a pathological "normality" to extend from birth to infant death: "They also consider it normal to lose a baby or two," she went on. "They are always surprised to hear that I gave birth to only two children, and to this day still have two children. They must be taught that [infant death] does not need to be normal." A failure to recognize "what is wrong" was the root of loss as blame for high rates of mortality rested primarily in a perceptive ability of the individual, blinded, in more sympathetic languages, both by and to her conditions.

In spite of being part of new endeavors, the authority of such statements may come from their familiarity. In South Asia, human (and especially female) emotion has long been understood in relation to the *purdah* of ignorance, a veil lifted through knowledge of universal modes of accounting. In the early twentieth century, Katherine Mayo's *Mother India*, a popular (and notoriously scathing) account of Indian women's lives, literalized the metaphoric association of veiling with lack of perspective. Mayo rendered conditions of poverty at once natural and traditional, and response to death epitomized by insufficient speech. In her writing, excessive (male) sexuality and a predatory nature were counterpoint to the rational world of enumeration, holding together the abject qualities of Indian life: "If a baby dies, the mother's wail trails down the darkness of a night or two. But if the village be near a river, the little body may just be tossed into the stream, without waste of a rag for a shroud. Kites and the turtles finish its brief history. And it is more than probable that no one in the village will think it worth-while to report either the birth or the death. Statistics as to babies must therefore be taken as at best approximate" (Mayo 1997 [1927]: 110).

If the abject, the part of the self that must be repressed for the subject to cohere (Kristeva 1982), bolsters discourses and interventions of imperialism, so too does it continue to circulate as both longstanding and local language of change. Where doctors and NGO workers are an on-again off-again presence in rural life, the languages they speak are more permanent, an integral part of rural women's interactions and reckonings of themselves in the world. Many caste-Hindu women in particular use bland languages of biological and technical explanation to account for the health and life outcomes of those around them (Dalit and Muslim women were, I felt, more ambivalent about these languages). They speak of low-caste and lower-class people with a language of hygiene and compliance with health institutions in which blame for over-reproduction and ill health is wrapped up in accountability for infant death. Exactly whom they describe may be vague, though social categorization is the same as in overtly caste-ist discourse. "Those people have too many babies." "They never get sterilized." "They never go to a doctor." "They live in filth."

Ashis Nandy describes the bifurcations by which "postcolonial structures of knowledge" are characterized by "a peculiar imperialism of categories" (2001: 61): "Within this form of imperialism, a conceptual domain is hegemonised by a concept produced and honed in the West, hegemonised so effectively that the original domain vanishes from awareness. Intellect and intelligence become IQ, oral cultures become the cultures of the non-literate or the uneducated, the oppressed become the proletariat, social change becomes development" (61).

Similarly, it seems that a transformation is occurring, or, in the phrasings of psychoanalysis, something is being swallowed whole in fragmented moments of intervention. In the individualizing causalities of Katherine Mayo and Safe Motherhood, grief may be absented from the experience of loss in the production of a new sign: the fatalistic rural woman, the uneducated peasant who is an essential figure in the myth of national development and, thus, national identity. As non-specific tropes of hygiene and inaction locate entire, if vaguely defined, groups on a grid of threat and value, Nandy's "peculiar imperialism of categories" involves new subject positions. The split-off, repressed specificities that make the language of population, hygiene, and compliance carry the same venom as languages of hate create out of infant death a discourse on the limited humanity of those yet-to-be-reached, as Arturo Escobar described for development broadly speaking (1994: 53). In what is seen as a fundamental misrecognition of death and its causes, lies an inability to count/account this lack of the same order as the lack of hygiene and noncompliance with institutions also referenced in accounts of rural women's lives. Embedded in intervention through training, then, is the idea that rural women must be taught to feel. With rationality comes affect.

In a postcolonial lineage of interventions, some bluntly coercive, memories of past interventions are dominated by the emergency of the late 1970s as the "time of *nazbandhi*," the time of sterilization. Where those most disenfranchised fear that, as one woman put it, "the state wants to eliminate the small people," or, as another described, hospital births may involve forced sterilizations or "poison in the needle," colonialism's "calm" and turbulent violences resonate in the dehumanizing structures of interventions in the name of humanism or populism. Such interventions come through a state (or its legitimating structures) whose motives are not always trusted, whose ability to care for its citizens is given little credence.

Amid such tangles of fear and longing, interventions' liberal humanist speech denies the presence of affect other than that demonstrating a universal knowledge. A sense of limited humanity takes shape in the conversion of grief into nongrief, in the swallowing whole of individual suffering in accounting for social pathology ("high rates," etc.). I argue elsewhere (Pinto 2006) that similar repression and mythologization, in slightly different terms, make "untouchability" integral to the moral structures of public health in India. As nonspecific signifiers ("those people") replace more specific terminology, forms of loathing based on pollution and consumption are no longer distinguishable from categories of hygiene and compliance. This process extends to all rural women through the "imperialism of categories" by which progress is posed through imaginaries of culpability and humanity—imaginaries in which objects must participate to forestall the deaths that are the crux of their modern condition.

CONSUMING GRIEF

But blame is always under negotiation. Death haunts all rural women. On a visit to the home of the ladies' doctor I was shown a photograph of her grandchild. "My oldest daughter . . . this is her baby. She is finished." When I asked how old she was, she said, "About seven months," though the child looked older than that. I asked what had happened, and she said the death was sudden—she just got sick and died, no one can say exactly what happened.

I looked again, realizing that the picture was not one of the child in life, but in death. "This is at that very time?" She nodded and turned the page. Another photograph, a close-up of the child, its head at an awkward angle against a male adult elbow. She turned the page again. The child in someone else's lap, a crowd of faces, mostly young ones—children, teenagers—surrounding her. Another picture. The baby's mother holding the dead child, her other children—four boys— around her, their faces wet with tears, her own expression unreachable. We both gazed at the pictures preserved behind plastic and talked about how this happened, about the unkindnesses of fate, until conversation turned to other topics.

Another day, she comes to see Amma, the elderly mother/mother-in-law of my household, to whom she was distantly related. As she and her sister were welcomed into the courtyard, relationships and hierarchies were established as all touched the feet of their elders in turn. The visitors discussed with Amma how they were related, enumerating households and kin networks, who was the wife of whom, how many children each had, who was grown, who was married. Kin mapping stopped when it was mentioned that Uma had only one living child.

"Only one? Why?"

"There were two others, but they died," Amma said.

Uma emerged with the tea. "Yes," she said, "One died when it was three months old and the other died immediately, meaning at that exact time [of its birth]." Amma repeated the information.

The visitors asked at the same time, their voices overlapping, "Did you give the babies the t.t. *tikka* [tetanus vaccine]?"

"Yes, we gave everything," Uma said.

"Did you give the *tikka* shots then, at that time?"

"Yes, we gave everything."

"And before, meaning when you were pregnant, did you get the *tikka* then?"

"Yes, everything. Both times. We gave all the *tikka*. But sometimes it just happens like this. That something is not right."

"Yes, yes. It's true."

Later, while Uma was rinsing dishes at the hand pump, her mother-in-law described the ill-fated delivery, speaking in a soft voice. "There was some kind of confusion. The water broke, but then the baby did not come right away. It didn't come for a long time."

One of the visitors whispered, "If all that water is there and the cord gets twisted the baby has to take in that dirty water, so it dies."

"What can it breathe? It has to take in all that dirty water," Amma said in a hushed voice. "Its eyes weren't even open." She glanced at Uma, "Sometimes this is what fate gives us."

The morning after the reproductive health program has put on a *navtanki* (a promotional performance in the idiom of "tradition"), I passed two men on the road and we got to talking. I was curious about a small grove of trees nearby where I had heard there was an old well, unused because, as someone once told me vaguely, something bad happened there. I asked about it and got a brief, dismissive answer, and then one of the men recognized me. "I remember you. You were at the *navtanki* about *larka-bacca* [children and babies]."

"That's right," I replied.

"I remember," he went on, then said half to me, half to his companion, "They were right. It's good to have only two children."

A third man stopped on the road and got off his bike to join our conversation. "Two or three is good. Three is good too." There was a pause. Then his voice rose, "But look, they say 'have two children, have two children,' but I had two children and they both died."

The other men looked at him, "Really?"

"What happened?" I asked, and another man asked the same thing. "Were they sick?"

"No, no illness, nothing. Sometimes it is like this. The first one was born and then three days later he died. Then the younger one was born and he lived a few hours but died the very same day."

"Oh ho," said one of the men. "Were they born here in this village?"

"Yes."

"So sad," we all agreed.

The first man said, "Did you do anything?"

The man on the bike snapped back, "Like what? This is all given by the one above. It is out of our control, isn't it?"

In contrast to the inadequate grief described by languages of intervention, stories of infant and child death are in abundance in rural life, part of everyday interaction. A particular sense of what normality means is put forward in their sheer presence. Where pregnancy (or other forms of grief and trauma) is seldom spoken of beyond whispers and euphemism, these stories are traded regularly. They can be part of introductions when women first meet, as they tell about their families, their children, how many they gave birth to, how many remain. Deaths are invoked to explain a present way of being or moving through the world, a sense of constant limitation—as with the woman who no longer sings—or a sense of constant reckoning with unknown forces. They mark a space of intersubjectivity on the basis of what many refer to as a shared sadness and in a context in which sisters-in-law share households, labor, and, in effect, children. Mothers and mothers-in-law, sisters and sisters-in-law, daughters and daughters-in-law tell their own and each other's stories, reiterating familial ties tightened through grief, that one person's loss is also another's, also a household's loss. As neighbors visit a bereaved mother, they share their own stories to, as one woman put it, say, "This too happened to me," to ameliorate, momentarily, a pain that "does not go away."

Some stories are briefly eloquent, encompassing broad reaches of causality in a paucity of detail. Speaking with two sisters-in-law one afternoon as their collective crowd of children played around us, I was told by one woman about her daughter who had died: "She was this big," she said, holding out her hand to show the height of a child about three years old. When I asked what happened, she said, "Who knows? She just died. Sometimes it is like that." She waved her hand. "She was this big, and I don't know what happened. She was sick—"

Her sister-in-law cut in, "She was this tall. Her *mundan* had already happened. No one knows why she died." They pointed to the place in the fields where she was buried. Later, the first woman told me about the other woman's son. I would hear about him many times. He had died of tetanus when he was "this big"—about four or five. Together the two of them told the story, each interrupting the other, nodding while the other one spoke.

At times stories erupt into the apparently seamless realities offered by health programs. While I was speaking with two local birth specialists a neighbor woman and her daughter came onto the veranda where we sat. The daughter was wearing a nightgown and wrapped in a shawl, her head bent to the ground. "Her baby was born one month ago," the mother said, with little pre-amble. "There was so much pain and still the baby did not come." The daughter was taken to the nearest private hospital in a hired van. There was no doctor initially, though after some time she arrived. The baby was born by "operation" after "many people laid their hands." The newborn was weak, though they had difficulty convincing the doctor of this. "I told them, I said, 'Can't you do something?' But there was nothing, they did nothing. They said to us that sometimes a baby is born like this. What else?" She nods toward her daughter and says, "She did not want to live without the child. She said this to me, 'My life is trickling out.'"

After some time living in Uma's home, she related to me the story of the other death. "You cannot hear it without crying," she began. Her baby was sick with diarrhea and fever for several days, and after visiting several doctors, and giving it several kinds of prescribed medicine, she took the baby to a small city several hours away where there was a "big doctor," a pediatric specialist. He gave the baby more medicine and that night she slept for the first time in days. When she woke in the night the baby's skin beneath her hand was cold to the touch. She ran into the other room to call her aunt, and women of the house rushed in. As she waited in the outer room, she heard them say, "Poor bride, the baby is dead and she doesn't even know it." She must take the baby home on the train, they told her, wrapping it in a blanket and acting as though it were alive. When she finally arrived home, she collapsed. "It was like the breath was gone from the inside."

Stories share common refrains, embedded within, capping the end. Causalities may be listed—involving living conditions, interactions with health institutions, and failed attempts to get care ("we gave it this doctor's medicine and that doctor's medicine and nothing helped"), trips to nearby cities, chaotic unfoldings, the involutions within institutions. Explanations evoking biomedical frameworks may overlap with references to ghostly cravings, spirits of women dead in childbirth who "grab" the newborn and newly delivered. Even in the case of stories where "nothing happened, the baby just died," repeated narratives of infant death remind us that "everything is in the hands of God." "Sometimes babies just die like this." "Sometimes this is what fate hands us."

Rather than taking fatalism at face value, let us locate in it a quality of move-ment. Writing on women's sadness in India has focused on a tension between internal and external suffering—what is told and what is withheld. In her account of women's grief in the wake of the violence of Partition, Veena Das describes the interiority of women's suffering, using womblike metaphors and describing grief as "articulated through the body" and formed through "transactions" with meaning (1997: 68). Enunciations in the wake of subject-shattering violence, Das says, speak of "healing as a kind of relationship with death" (78), a sustained rather than absolved relationship to social and physical death. At the same time, expressions of grief may be collective, vitally gendered and embodied in the female as "the one that will carry this pain within forever" (80). In constituting a subject through grief, the very presence of those who have suffered is a continuing commentary on political realities, at the heart of the existence of the nation, even as suffering may be normalized into the flow of life. Where in lamentation the "inner state" is "finally given a home in language," making the world livable again (68), such mitigated strangeness signifies the ever-unfinished project of healing.

Infant mortality is a different social crisis than rape or brutal violence, a different rent in the fabric of normality, and poses different challenges to the future of self, kin, and nation. The ability to speak or not speak violence may constitute a different dilemma than that posed by speech—or constraints on it—in the context of infant death. For one thing, the latter aims less at nationalized politics than at transnational, indeed, denationalized structures of biotechnique put in the service of national progress but never reducible to it. But in its description of the shape of grief's ability to be sustained as commentary on political conditions, Das's account gives us material for understanding grief not just in but *as* a relationship to power. It demands we juxtapose it to the very languages meant to intervene at the site of loss. In particular, we can emphasize the "work," in Das's terms, that runs eloquently against the grain of healing.

As moments of suspended resolution, suspended healing, stories of infant death speak to violence more akin to the structural violence described by Scheper-Hughes (1992) but involving an emotional ground and semiotic framework that speaks to the ever-reiterated presence of state and transnational attention. Infant death's symbolic place in the apparatus of public health and development, the structures of governance and symbolic hierarchies in which infant and child death become meaningful (particularly as a "Third World" problem), and, most importantly, the distinctly diffuse causalities of infant mortality mean that in repeated stories of loss, while certain things are being made—or kept—visible, other things are continually obscured, rendering them part of social life in a different, symptomatic way. Perhaps unlike laments, rather than transforming the strangeness of death into something more comfortable, women's stories obscure links of certainty in which medical practice and biotechnical moralities and "embraces" (Good 2001) are supposed to exist. They speak to an aspect of the postcolonial Indian nation understood through idioms of "progress" and the technoscientific rationalities of health-related development, genealogically connected to structures and meanings that emerged under British rule and dependent on notions of "internal others."

If stories of infant death become instances of suspended grief, running counter to processes of integration as well as, perhaps, to those moments in which awareness of human suffering is repressed, then engulfing grief frames a continuous deferral. What *was* spoken—causality, the social—is deferred, replaced by singular, encompassing Causality. For Freud (1963), the melancholic overidentifies with the lost object, remaining entangled in a longing turned upon itself that creates an experience of self-negation and despair. Narratives of infant death, even those that rage at entangled causalities, often end with a gulp of all-consuming causation—the hands of God, the gifts of fate. These moments swallow, in a powerful moment, the locatedness of death that, in many cases, has just been elaborated. But rather than abrogating causality, they express a broader sense of contingency. Overwhelming causation emerges in the symptom of repetition from what the narrative swallows whole, through the grief consumed and the consuming grief.

For many critics who have commented on melancholia, depressed speech has the capacity to "devitalize" structures of language and power—through what is repressed and what returns as symptom. As such, saying *less* amid repeated iterations amounts to "an impossibility to give up the object" that *maintains* a relationship to Law, rendering it weak and invalid (Kristeva 1989: 45, 47). In Kristeva's words, "the depressed subject has remained prisoner of the non-lost object (the Thing)" (47). Where the "depressed subject" is, in this case, dispersed across a social landscape, all may be imprisoned.

When Michel de Certeau (1984) says that death is not named, he refers to the speech of the dying person in the space of biomedicine and European narratives of progress, for which death is an unspeakable affront to the given conditions of reality. Within such contexts, he says, "death is an elsewhere," and when repressed as such returns as a "wound on reason" (192). For the rural poor in and at the edges of the machinery of intervention, the ghost in the machine is the certainty of knowledge/causality, of what brings death. The realities of life for the rural poor put lived causality at odds with the rational-technical language of certainty. As much as pain exists here as a transaction and healing "relationship with death" (Das 1997: 78), speaking death may also be a mode of devalorizing, a way of eviscerating certainty, transforming causality into symptom, part of a particular condition of modern subjectivity. Pain puts death within and in opposition to the maps of causality that are meant to locate persons as political subjects. In being left unresolved the dead child and the child's death are indices of the overwhelming conditions of everyday life. Rather than normalizing loss, it is as though they say, "Look at what is normal."

SYMPTOM

"It was as though the breath was gone from the inside." Uma's embodied grief was also a challenge to her body's ability to speak, but one that found, finally, its space of expression. Her reminder to her sister-in-law that "everything is in the big, big hands of God" posed an epistemological impasse at the site of explanation—explanation that, under the circumstances, may never be capable of being anything other than reductive. To these moments, notions of failed affect and flawed perception eclipse complex expressive, bodily, and intersubjective processes. Denoting a particular postcolonial order that is at the same time a quiet state of disorder, rural women's grief keeps loss in conversation with the discourses that aim to observe, categorize, and evaluate it. Such memories share a common reality with authoritative speech—a quality of vagueness and obfuscation, the weight of things not spoken. Two things are held in suspended ambiguity in efforts to speak to and about the dead: the political domain, and a particular kind of postcolonial female subject—the latter is flooded with a moral urgency, in the sense identified by Arthur Kleinman, in which "experience is moral" because it is "the medium of engagement in everyday life in which things are at stake and in which ordinary people are deeply engaged stake-holders who have important things to lose, to gain, and to preserve" (1999: 362).

At this intersection of moralities is the threat—and critical power—of the return. We can think of this symptom in terms of the haunting quality of a not-quite-forgotten other, historically and in contemporary flows of subjectivity. Narratives of otherness in terms of sex, race, and the primitive that were integral to colonialism and nineteenth-century sciences that buttressed it amounted, Ranjana Khanna (2003) suggests, to a web of techniques of knowledge and therapy. A key way such techniques functioned, Khanna argues, involved processes of literalization similar to those of melancholia. Such demetaphorization, the literal engagement with ideas, was akin, Khanna says, to those disavowals by which colonialism performed its "calm violence" on the other (even as it enacted violences that were not so calm). As melancholia carries the threat of the return, in the form of the symptom, the melancholic structure of colonial forms of appellation left for the postcolonial nation-state a "specter of colonialism (and indeed its counter—the specter of justice)" (Khanna 2003: 25).

Let us retrieve Khanna's specter of justice from its parenthetical location. At the same time that the "rural woman" haunts the forward motion of progress, the symptomatic quality of restitution emerges in the melancholic language droning on through postcolonial interventions. This may be especially so of efforts to enter those spaces in which present is linked to future: the household, female and infant bodies, sexuality and reproduction, and the affects that bind them. So, as the quiet catastrophe of infant death hollows out the very certainties that aim to contain it, notions of flawed humanity and their countermemories write death into the discourse of living (pace de Certeau); if, as Giorgio Agamben says, we must question "the status of violence as the cipher of human action" (2005: 59), then we must also question the status of infant death as the cipher of human inaction. In what infant death says about the limits of human action—caregiving, care getting, fostering life—and what it is made to say about certain people as representatives of human inaction, speaking about it destabilizes languages of justice, health, and cure. In stories where past deaths are kept in the discourse of the present, the big, big hands of God may be the only things capable of holding in one place the complex and unbearable contingencies of living.

NOTE

Research for this chapter was conducted with an International Dissertation Field Research grant from the Social Science Research Council and was written with the support of an NIMH Postdoctoral Research Fellowship at Harvard Medical School, under the valuable guidance of Mary-Jo DelVecchio Good, Byron Good, and Arthur Kleinman. In framing and formulating the ideas in this chapter I have also been fortunate to be in conversation with Chris Dole, Sarah Horton, Everett Zhang, Cesar Abadia, and João Biehl. Any errors or missteps are, of course, my own.

REFERENCES

Agamben, Giorgio. 2005. *States of Exception*. Chicago: University of Chicago Press.

————. 1986. *Heterologies: Discourse on the Other*. Trans. Brian Massami. Minneapolis: University of Minnesota Press.

Chatterjee, Roma, Sangeeta Chattoo, and Veena Das. 1998. The Death of the Clinic?: Normality and Pathology in Recrafting Aging Bodies. In *Vital Signs: Feminist Reconfigurations of the Bio/logical Body*, ed. Margaret Shildrick and Janet Price, 171–96. Edinburgh: Edinburgh University Press.

Das, Veena. 1997. Language and Body: Transactions in the Construction of Pain. In *Social Suffering*, ed. Arthur Kleinman, Veena Das, and Margaret Lock, 67–91. Berkeley: University of California Press.

de Certeau, Michel. 1984. *The Practice of Everyday Life*. Berkeley: University of California Press.

Escobar, Arturo. 1994. *Encountering Development: The Making and Unmaking of the Third World*. Princeton, NJ: Princeton University Press.

Foucault, Michel. 1978. *The History of Sexuality*. Vol. 1, *An Introduction*. Trans. Robert Hurley. New York: Random House.

——. 2000. Governmentality. In *Power: Essential Works of Foucault 1954–1984*, vol. 3, ed. James Faubion, trans. Robert Hurley et al., 201–22. New York: The New Press.

Freud, Sigmund. 1963. Mourning and Melancholia. In *General Psychological Theory*. New York: Touchstone Press.

Good, Mary-Jo DelVecchio. 2001. The Biotechnical Embrace. In *Culture, Medicine and Psychiatry* 25:395–410.

Government of India (GOI). 2001. *National Family Health Survey*. New Delhi: Government of India.

Hertz, Barbara, and Anthony Meacham. 1987. *The Safe Motherhood Initiative: Proposal for Action*. Washington, D.C.: The World Bank.

Imhof, Arthur E. 1985. From the Old Mortality Pattern to the New: Implications of a Radical [Change] from the Sixteenth to the Twentieth Century. *Bulletin of the History of Medicine* 59:1–29.

Khanna, Ranjana. 2003. *Dark Continents: Psychoanalysis and Colonialism*. Durham, NC: Duke University Press.

Kleinman, Arthur. 1999. *Experience and Its Moral Modes: Culture, Human Conditions, and Disorder*. The Tanner Lectures on Human Values. Salt Lake City: University of Utah Press.

Kristeva, Julia. 1982. *Powers of Horror: An Essay on Abjection*. Trans. Leon S. Roudiez. New York: Columbia University Press.

——. 1989. *Black Sun: Depression and Melancholia*. Trans. Leon S. Roudiez. New York: Columbia University Press.

Mayo, Katherine. 1997 [1927]. *Mother India*. Delhi: Low-Price Publications.

Mitchell, Timothy. 2000. Introduction to *Questions of Modernity*, ed. Timothy Mitchell, xi–xxvii. Minneapolis: University of Minnesota Press.

Nandy, Ashis. 2001. *Time Warps: The Insistent Politics of Silent and Evasive Pasts*. Delhi: Permanent Black.

Pinto, Sarah. 2004. Development without Institutions: Ersatz Medicine and the Politics of Everyday Life in Rural North India. *Cultural Anthropology* 19 (3): 337–64.

——. 2006. Globalizing Untouchability: Grief and the Politics of Depressing Speech. *Social Text* 86 (Spring): 81–102.

————. Forthcoming. *Global Untouchabilities: Tales of Birth and Death in Rural India.* Oxford: Berghan Books.

Scheper-Hughes, Nancy. 1987. Introduction: The Cultural Politics of Child Survival. In *Child Survival: Anthropological Perspectives on the Treatment and Maltreatment of Children*, ed. Nancy Scheper-Hughes, 1–32. Boston: D. Reidel Publishing Co.

————. 1992. *Death without Weeping: The Violence of Everyday Life in Brazil.* Berkeley: University of California Press.

Stewart, Kathleen. 1996. *A Space on the Side of the Road: Cultural Politics in an "Other" America.* Princeton, NJ: Princeton University Press.

POSTCOLONIALITY AS
THE AFTERMATH OF TERROR
AMONG VIETNAMESE REFUGEES

Janis H. Jenkins and Michael Hollifield

In this chapter we examine the problem of subjectivity as a transformation of lived experience in the wake of civil warfare and formation of the postcolonial nation-state. The specific terms of subjective alteration—collectively imprinted as a clash of political ethos[1] and personally imprinted as a shattering of identity and sentiment—are considered in relation to a culturally produced anguish in the aftermath of a conflict. Our ethnographic illustration of this process is the well-known case of the Socialist Republic of Vietnam.[2] Prior to this political formation in 1975, multiparty warfare was waged throughout a fractured nation, as anticommunist armies comprising "South" Vietnamese, Americans, and holdover loyalists to French colonialists collided with anticolonial and communist armies of "North" Vietnamese, the Viet Minh or Viet Cong. The suffering wrought by the defeat of South Vietnamese forces provides the primary reference point for this chapter.

This defeat of South Vietnam was, from the perspective of North Vietnam, a defeat of colonial intruders under the banner of authentic Vietnamese nationalism in the aftermath of renewed French colonial incursions in 1859 that only apparently ended following occupation at Dien Bien Phu in 1954. This in turn led to a further and different invasion of U.S. military advisors and troops through 1973. The eventual expulsion of a great many decades of colonial forces by the Viet Cong produced as much disintegration as resolution, however, and the aftermath of these successive conflicts produced a multilayered shattering of economy, community, and family in postcolonial Vietnam.

In his discussions of hermeneutics and narrative analysis, Paul Ricoeur has observed that both the telling and the hearing of a story require that one be able to "extract a configuration from a succession" (1981 : 278). In what follows we extract a configuration of cultural and personal meaning from narratives of often traumatic, disjointed successions of events experienced by refugees who fled the violence of war and detention in Vietnam during the late 1980s and '90s, ending up in the culturally alien and ambiguously welcoming urban environment of Albuquerque, New Mexico.[3] Our intention is to show how experiential themes of alterity, trauma, and memory are wedged in the political divides that make up the longstanding colonial and postcolonial conflict within Vietnam.

Broadly speaking, we are pressed to understand the effects of warfare in postcolonial settings as a matter of global public health and human rights. While pathbreaking work has been undertaken on the state production of dysphoric affect, mental disorder, and social suffering (Good, Good, and Moradi 1985; Kleinman 1986, 1995), the human and medical sciences have yet to flesh out fully the particular dimensions of such experience as the occasion for bodily and psychic marring, on the one hand, and remarkable resilience, on the other (Jenkins 1991). This chapter is an effort to extend contemporary thinking on these transformations of lived experience as reciprocally produced within the nation-state and body-self.

POSTCOLONIAL REGIMES AND BODY-SELVES

Understanding the direct parallels between a postcolonial regime and the body-self productively shifts the discourse from the political and economic impacts of postcolonial transformations to the experiential impact of these developments. Shelley Wright advances this issue with her argument that "(1) colonialism involves the deep cultural and psychological penetration of both colonizers and colonized as well as profound economic, political and legal changes; and (2) decolonization must therefore go well beyond the creation of new nation-states or even the reformation of neo-colonial economic structures. It must also involve the decolonization of our minds and bodies" (2001: 58).

Thinking about "the violence within" in reference to Kay Warren's (1993) phrase for violence within a national political entity would then come to incorporate the notion of what we can consider an intrapsychic and intrasomatic violence. The question becomes how to conceive at once the collective incorporation of public violence and the tormented inner conflict of a fragmented self. The mode of analysis we invoke plays on this kind of dual sensibility wherein the meaning of violence is ambiguously constituted, but with quite specific consequences in defining the lives of people and the emotional atmosphere they inhabit.

CONUNDRUMS OF SUBJECTIVITY: ALTERITY, TRAUMA, AND MEMORY

In a recent volume by Janis Jenkins and Robert Barrett (2004), the rise of anthropological thinking about subjective experience is traced in relation to current ideas in culture theory, which include (1) the primacy of lived experience over analytic categories imposed by anthropological theory; (2) the active engagement of subjects in processes of cultural construction; and (3) the irrepressibility of subjectivity as embedded in intersubjectively created realms of meaning and significance. The authors argue that the notion of intersubjectivity provides an important bridge to a more precise understanding of the interactions among cultural representations, collective processes, and subjectivity.

Below we explore the specific ambiguities that guide our analysis of political culture and subjectivity in Vietnamese exile narratives, developed in part on the basis of previous anthropological and psychiatric work on political violence (Jenkins 1996; Hollifield et al. 2002). Three much contested domains of subjectivity are identified as central to an analysis of the lived experience of warfare and political violence: alterity, trauma, and memory. In this chapter, we can only briefly sketch the ways in which attention to the interpenetration of these subjective domains helps to illumine transformations of lived experience produced reciprocally by and within political and personal bodies.

The postcolonial problem of alterity—marking the threshold of "otherness"—is the crossroads or site wherein subjectivities are transacted in relation to geography, religion, and political affiliation. Personal and collective trauma is embedded within these deeply disputed sites, particularly with respect to the expulsion of "foreigners" and "invaders." While issues of alterity have long been central in psychoanalytic studies, their anthropological integration into postcolonial studies of subjective processes have been cautious in relation to misgivings surrounding the traditionally narrow social scope of this line of thinking. Nevertheless, Paul Antze and Michael Lambek (1996) underscore the anthropological value of Freud's formulation of trauma and memory as inexorably linked to repetitive, patterned productions of the self embedded within a social field.

In a treatment of subjectivity and alterity in postcolonial settings, Leela Gandhi (1998) argues that narratives of the aftermath of warfare and violence often reveal an ambivalent and symbiotic relationship between colonizer and colonized. Thus "the battles between native and invader are also replicated within native and invader. . . . The crisis produced by this self-division is at least as psychologically significant as those which attend the more visible contestations of the colonizer and the colonized" (1998: 11–12). Gandhi (1998: 11) invokes Albert Memmi's classic text (1968) to argue that the "perverse mutuality between oppressor and oppressed" is nothing less than an attempt (successful or otherwise) to shed light on why subaltern groups revisit rather than flee entirely the scene of oppression.

A sense of self in relation to traumatic memory entered European thinking at a time when doubts about colonial projects (for colonizers and colonized alike) had come to the foreground. With the 1889 publication of *Psychological Automatism*, Pierre Janet helped to specify how traumas produce their disintegrating effects in proportion to their intensity, duration, and repetition. The initial response combines what he termed "vehement emotion" and a cognitive interpretation resulting in dissociation of memory or identity processes and attachment to the trauma such that the person has difficulty proceeding with her life (see Jenkins 1991).

Summarizing models for the analysis of memory and trauma, Ruth Leys (2000: 8–9) argues for the theoretical value of hypnotic imitation or identification (mimesis) as opposed to neurobiological models that otherwise dispose of what she calls "narrative or implicit memory" in favor of neurological imprinting in response to external trauma that leads to plastic changes in neural pathways of the brain. This view of trauma, as deployed in contemporary psychiatry, radically removes the role of agency and moral meanings (Young 1995; Freyd 1996). Drawing on Janet's work, trauma can be better understood within an analytic tradition summarized by Leys as "imitation, identification, or mimesis" (2000: 8). Clearly this locates subjective experience within the realm of historical and social processes.

Thus the study of remembering and forgetting of the colonial past in the postcolonial present hinges largely on formulations of ways in which the mind extends beyond the individual while at the same time collective experience informs individual consciousness. Jennifer Cole's *Forget Colonialism? Sacrifice and the Art of Memory in Madagascar* (2001) is an ethnographic account of this process that approaches the question through a focus on "the social and cultural practices through which individual and social memory are woven together" that "affords a way out of the dichotomy that sees memory as either locked inside people's heads or available only in collective representations and embodied practices and ritual" (2). She implicitly identifies the existential common ground of this reciprocity between individual and social memory by acknowledging that "many traces of the past may be incorporated into the sociocultural environment so that they are not consciously remembered" (2).

A more explicit political formulation of social processes of trauma and memory in relation to alterity is found in the work of Ignació Martín-Baró (1988,

1989), who maintained that individualized accounts of trauma and illness are insufficient in the context of warfare. Although the trauma and suffering are manifest in personal psychic suffering, it is more useful to think in terms of psychosocial trauma or "the traumatic crystallization in persons and groups of inhuman social relations" (1988: 138). Trauma and suffering become manifest in psychic suffering, dysphoric affects, and a variety of forms of psychopathology. This psychosocial crystallization of trauma is particularly evident in the collective experience of anxiety, terror, and, above all, denial of reality. Moreover, this process affects all members of a society, either directly or indirectly. No one remains untouched, or unchanged, by civil warfare and its aftermath.

THE CONTEXT: WHAT POSTCOLONIAL PERIOD?

In Vietnam, a longstanding ambiguity of national identity was only intensified by the French takeover in 1882–83 in the wake of political and civil unrest between the north and the south. In response to this internal crisis, the "Vietnamese" ruling elite sought to incorporate some elements of the "other," considering parts of the West equal or superior to Sino-Vietnamese civilization (Duiker 1995: 29; McLeod 1991). They considered hybridization of identities as an avenue to other goals, including political, educational, and economic development. William Duiker (1995: 29) frames this desire for national survival as a concern on the part of many Vietnamese intellectuals that the fate of their nation hinged on a willingness to articulate with and even incorporate elements of European political and cultural organization. Over the course of the next thirty-five years, the imagined advantage of such alterations did little to improve the lot of Vietnamese peoples. Further, the internal structure of what had been "Vietnam" was being as much dis-integrated as identified. Chinese characters were replaced in official circles with the Roman alphabet (a process begun in the seventeenth century under French missionary incursion). Older leaders could no longer lead because their Confucian teachings and literacy were now at odds with the (French colonial) administrative culture. Land and economic wealth were not distributed as well as hoped, and only a minority of children (about 10 percent) received European-based education, leaving the majority at cultural odds with their own political structure (Duiker 1995: 29–33).

This colonial failure, and the building perception by the Vietnamese that the French could not and would not help with their collective toil, led to new construction and resistance against the colonial "other." Ironically, it was in part from the new Franco-Vietnamese group that grew the resistance movements that worked toward expulsion of the French colonial invaders. Ho Chi Minh, the founder of the Indochinese Communist Party (ICP) in 1935, led the movement that culminated in the military defeat of the French at Dien Bien Phu in April 1954. However, in efforts to recruit young Vietnamese to the struggle, Minh placed rhetorical emphasis on nationalism. The notion of nationalism was itself ambiguously layered, with many Catholic and Buddhist Vietnamese secretly fighting with the French and against the antireligious ICP (McLeod 1991; SarDesai 1992).

This period was followed by years of political struggle (involvement in World War II, Japanese occupation of Vietnam from 1941 to the end of the war in 1945, and the long postponement of independence following a well-planned revolution by the IPC in August 1945). Following World War II, independence was narrowly defeated by forces of resistance from other national and external anticommunist interests. This postponement again served to create internal strife and disagreement about what was self and what was other, and about what was vital to and for Vietnam. While the termination of nineteenth-century French colonial rule of Vietnam formally took place in 1945 with Ho Chi Minh's declaration of independence for the Democratic Republic of Vietnam (DRV), a nine-year guerilla war ensued between communist Viet Minh and the French and the Viet Minh's antireligious allies (Marr 1995). Following this perpetuation of colonial conflict, a 1954 Geneva agreement provided for a temporary north-south division of Vietnam until elections could bring the two provisional territories into a united government.

The Geneva Convention of 1954 only formalized what had been going on for decades, even centuries, providing for two zones, splitting north and south at the Ben Hai River on the seventeenth parallel, with the north dominated by the Viet Minh and the south dominated by the Bao Dai puppet government of the French. General elections were to be held in both zones by July 1956 to ascertain the future will of the Vietnamese. The fact that this did not happen only underscored the ongoing crisis in national identity for the Vietnamese. Indeed, 1954 was not the first time the "Vietnamese" garnered their independence from a foreign invader.[4] This second retaking was an issue of "nationalism." The South Vietnamese refusal to accept this arrangement resulted in their counterdeclaration in 1955 as the Republic of Vietnam.

The suffering that arose from this ongoing crisis was fueled by persistent confusion about the parameters of identity. In the north resided ethnically diverse Vietnamese, whose leaders were intellectuals not necessarily aligned with religious groups. In time, the DRV became increasingly less tolerant of religious practice generally. Hundreds of thousands of people of traditional Confucian, Buddhist, and Catholic persuasion fled to the south to join the burgeoning group of ethnic Vietnamese mixed with French who at once tolerated and advocated religion. Both the north and the south attempted to tolerate and to incorporate the ethnic Chinese, who over time became a focus of contempt. Non-Vietnamese ethnic groups who resided in the western and central mountains were provided cultural autonomy but were controlled politically by the DRV, who saw the central highlands as the route to final control of the cities in the south. Thus entering this postcolonial period, it remained uncertain what the Vietnamese "self" was constructed of, what the "other" consisted of, who were distinctly "we," and who were unambiguously "they." This confusion was carried into the next period and through the second Indochinese war, that of the Viet Cong against the South Vietnamese and the United States.

Subsequent American invasion by military advisors and regular troops (escalating to 534,000 by 1969) to support the noncommunist southern forces failed in its effort to overthrow Viet Cong and the northern forces. While there was a withdrawal of U.S. troops following the Paris Accords of 1973, other military personnel remained through 1975. Following reunification of the Democratic Republic of Vietnam (north) and the former Republic of Vietnam (south) in 1975, hundreds of thousands of former South Vietnamese government and military officials, as well as intellectuals and private citizens suspected as anticommunists, were subjected to the newly victorious governmental campaign of retribution through systematic imprisonment, toil, and torture within now-infamous socialist "reeducation" camps. While it is unknown how many perished (through torture, starvation, overwork, or suicide) in these camps, several thousand survived and were ultimately released to return (under surveillance and drastically reduced circumstances) to the community. After their release from prison, many (some over the course of a decade) managed to borrow or save the approximately $150 necessary to process their application for emigration to the United States. The particular vantage point for this chapter is the subjective experience of South Vietnamese who survived and ultimately fled following long-term imprisonment and torture subsequent to the fall of Saigon.

Being expelled from one's country was followed by a long and frequently dangerous migration often coupled with a randomness of relocation site. Attempts at reidentification of self took place in this subjectively chaotic context. Refugees left Vietnam in three main waves: a mass exodus with the Americans in 1975, escape during the years 1975 to 1989, and the joint government-sponsored Orderly Departure Program beginning in 1989.

A former U.S. Air Force officer residing in Albuquerque sought to locate friends he had fought with in Vietnam and to that end traveled to each of the four refugee camps established in the United States to process the mass exodus in 1975. This he did in tandem with helping to establish the first Vietnamese refugee resettlement program in New Mexico. By the end of 1975, this program included over three thousand in population. Over the years there has been much secondary migration. In 2000, approximately five thousand Vietnamese resided in Albuquerque, 80 percent of whom were Catholic while most of the rest were Buddhist. Until 1990, the majority lived in the southeast heights area, where the majority of earlier established Vietnamese shops still exist. Currently, social and economic mobility within the population has led to a diffused expansion of Vietnamese who now work in a variety of jobs and utilize the health care systems widely.

CASE STUDIES

The narratives of the Vietnamese refugees with whom we worked are distinguished by experiential themes of alterity, trauma, and memory located in the political cleavages of colonial and postcolonial conflict. We bring into play four principal signifiers in terms of which these themes are narratively grounded: (1) contestations of regional borderlands; (2) religious and godless combatants; (3) political party affiliations; and (4) human compassion and cruelty. Grafted into our psychopolitical analysis of the Vietnamese case is the substantial confusion in identifying who constitutes self and who constitutes other. This experiential conundrum is central to the genesis of trauma, repetition compulsion seeking out the oppressor, and creative strategies for the formation of temporally fluid selves, at once articulating with the social past and present.

We draw from two case studies to shed light on the transformation of subjectivity under conditions of civil warfare and formation of the postcolonial nation-state. The cases selected from the larger study sample of Vietnamese refugees are those of elder males. While obviously each individual is distinct, we consider that the two cases selected for presentation are representative of a certain segment of politically active and militarily involved men who bore the brunt of reprisals following the defeat of the south. Both men held relatively prominent positions within the South Vietnamese military forces prior to their detention in "reeducation" camps in 1975. Thus the narratives are gender-specific insofar as the particular terms of analysis apply to men whose political commitment to their version of the nation-state was forged in opposition to the antireligious, communist north. Women's experience in the south following the fall of Saigon was generally different, with many left to care for their families under drastically reduced economic and sociopolitical circumstances.

Informed consent and Institutional Review Board approvals for the use of these narratives were obtained from each person and through the University of New Mexico as part of the New Mexico Refugee Project. In addition, the cases discussed here have some detail alteration to assure anonymity. However, both men were nevertheless clear about their willingness and even desire to have their identity known, which, from the authors' viewpoint, appeared to indicate a desire to tell their story as part of personal projects to re-create self-experience intersubjectively.

Mr. H: "It was the biggest and most terrible shock in my life"

Mr. H. was born in Nihn Thuan Province in December 1936 and was raised in a Catholic village with strong anticommunist sentiment. He joined the secret police as an undercover agent in 1954, following the activities of the Viet Cong. In 1957, at the age of twenty-one, he was offered better training and better pay and over the next decade worked in various locales. In 1969 he was promoted to the chief of police back in his home province, where he remained until 1975. In a battle with communist forces, he was captured and imprisoned on March 18, 1975, for what was to be a period of seven weeks as a prisoner— "reeducation detainee." Mr. H remained in the camp until 1983, conducting hard and mostly useless labor.

After having severe back pain over a period of eighteen months, he was provided medical attention, and it was determined that he needed surgery to repair a herniated disc. He was returned to prison for three months after the surgery, only to be released when it was determined that he could no longer perform hard labor. Back at home, he was forced to report to the police station and write reports on his activities every week. Along with his wife, he remained under near-constant watch of the communist authorities. Reporting to this police station operated by young Viet Cong with virtually no police training or education—from the site where he had once supervised the entire province—was no small source of anger and humiliation. In addition, Mr. H suffered from medical inattention to the aftereffects of his back injury: chronic bowel and urination problems, erectile dysfunction, and constant pain. In 1984 the authorities allowed him to travel out of town to work for six-month periods, during which, in spite of his back injury, he worked on road construction and cultivated rice on the 0.15 acre of the 2 acres of family land that the government returned to him after having confiscated it. He continued doing this until 1995 in order to feed himself and his family, all the while his back becoming progressively worse. Ten years passed before he was able to save $150 to pay the requisite fees to come to the United States.

Throughout narration of these trials, he notes that his mood is better now that he has been in the United States for a few years and that he has received treatment for his multiple medical problems. He is also concerned, however, that at some point he might not have access to medical care and that American doctors give him medicines for pain relief but not cure. As a means of preventing anxiety, he notes that he tries to think of happy things, although while saying this his mind wanders to another time and he comments, "I have no doubt in my mind that I would have killed myself [in prison] if I were not a Catholic." He saddens, developing halting almost dissociative speech, recalling coprisoners and friends who killed themselves while in prison; he is certain that at least two hundred of the some eighteen hundred detainees in his camp committed suicide. Telling this, tears stream and he literally chokes them back, spewing out a few words, holding his chest, asking to stop for a few minutes. Five minutes later, he wants to continue:

> At first, individual guards would say, "I would kill all of you but the government won't let us." They made camp such that people wanted to kill themselves. This reminded me of friends who would kill themselves by hanging by their own clothing, and the communists began to not let us wear any clothes—we were so cold. Then, others would kill themselves by biting their tongue off and bleeding to death, or by hitting their head on the wall, or by running into the wall with their tongue in between their teeth. We were made to bury our own fellows, and were made to promise to never speak about it.

In his narrative of rebellion against the Viet Minh, Mr. H provides the cultural rationale that undergirded the construction of the enemy as alien other against whom he and his comrades must fight:

> From the beginning, since we were colonized by the French, they [the French] would protect the villages that had a lot of religion. The French protected the Catholics although they would also protect the Buddhists. Therefore Catholics and even Buddhists would be the more likely to follow the French because they would get protection. It doesn't mean they wanted the French, or that they followed them politically, but it was the best option for many people, for the Catholics and Buddhists.

His opposition includes both explicitly and implicitly the four narrative signifiers we have identified as central to issues of alterity: north-south regionalism; religious orientation; political affiliation; and human cruelty:

> There were three reasons we were so much against the communists. The first was because of their involvement with the countries of China and Russia so we knew who their leaders were. The second thing is that they were against any religion in the world. Anybody with religion, it didn't matter whether

they were Catholic or Buddhist, they would kill them and they didn't believe in religion. The third thing was that they were very cruel. If others did not follow them or believe them, they would be willing to kill them. They would often kill people by burying them alive, by cutting their necks, and other horrible means. It's really kind of simple: the communists were very much against human nature. We learned to forgive many people and many things that happened, but not the communists because they were so much against human beings and human nature.

This apparently clear-cut schema for constructing the enemy other was inadequate, however, to the everyday flow of one's assumptive social world. Sorting religious and political groups was a source of considerable anxiety and proved shadowy at best:

> There were so many doubts and mistrusts among people, even between Buddhists and most Catholics and Buddhists. . . . You could no longer automatically trust some of your older Buddhist friends. I became more distrustful of even long-time friends [whether] they were with the communists or not. Everybody seemed to divide by religion. Even in my job, I couldn't tell whether my bosses or my commanders were followers or if they were kind of followers and not leaders.

The confusion over leadership turned to insufferable grief and rage with the assassination of President Diem in 1963. Mr. H specifies the type of postcolonial problem with alterity this posed as a kind of sociologically failed autoimmunological response to recognize the self:

> I was very shocked and it was the biggest and most terrible shock in my life. I had followed him since I was young. I had a good position in his cabinet and so it was a big shock to me. [Choked up, crying:] I was so certain that Diem would fight to win and beat the communists, but then the conflict with the religion rose and made everybody distrustful of each other and that was part of the problem with the fall of Diem. To me, the assassination of President Diem was very brutal and unforgivable. The way I looked at him is he was just like our family.

Mr. H continued his narration by saying that not only was he angry at the time at what transpired: a group of generals, with General Minh as ringleader, assassinated President Diem in what he and his associates considered a coup d'état. Still, today, he finds this event to be unbearably painful and indeed became tearful and choked up at the time of this narrative (March 2003). He explained the pain in the following way. Despite alternating assistance and interference on the part of the American government, this was fundamentally a Vietnamese problem and a Vietnamese betrayal. Following the assassination of President Diem, he says that he sent his family away for their safety but also because he simply wanted to be alone and that he became "very mentally isolated," angry, anxious, had nightmares, headaches, poor concentration, and near anorexia. During the course of the interview, Mr. H. became so "choked up" while holding his chest at times that the interviewer (Michael Hollifield) was concerned about his immediate health.

Mr. H stated that what he felt most angry about was that the future of the country was in peril:

> We could never beat the communists with the current leaders. And besides, we now had no one really who was competent to follow or trust. I started having constant headaches at that time and it was hard for me to focus on conversations. I was very distractible and could not concentrate well. And I also could not eat very well because I would choke up easily. After 1965 I knew for sure we would lose Vietnam.

Narrating these times was particularly difficult for Mr. H, who noted that he really has a hard time ever thinking about this time in the past because it hurts his head so much. He says he knows that even now most Vietnamese in the country are still miserable and poor. He is convinced that this was the result of all the corruption and lack of leadership.

It is clear that Mr. H's lengthy imprisonment hardened his categorical distinctions between those social groups with whom he identified and those whom he reviled. In prison, he was placed in a special unit because "to them I am very, very bad. I was in a special group that they took revenge on. They always made me write and rewrite things in the past that I did and if anything happened in the outside [political or social events] they would interrogate me about my knowledge about what that was or what was happening." He noted that prior to prison, communists could be friends and were primarily simply Vietnamese with "different mindsets," but certainly not people he hated. However, the prison experience "made me see that they were different and they were my enemy. We knew the communists would maybe keep us until we were old or until we died so I didn't have any feeling of belonging or being possessed by anything or anyone." Even after his release from prison, he noted that his experience was quite similar in that he was still required to write reports and could not talk or go freely: "It really didn't matter when I was in prison versus when I was not in prison, I was still miserable, and I was not free and I was having the anxiety and the nightmares and all those other symptoms. The feelings of belonging when I came to the United States were much different than the time in prison or out of prison in Vietnam."

Mr. T: "There was political confusion and I felt confused"

Mr. T was born December 1921 in the central highland town of Qui Nhon. He was educated through college and later in the army commander general staff college in Kansas in 1959–60. He worked on his family farm for much of his adolescence and joined the military (mandatory) in 1940 at the age of nineteen, on active combat duty, but soon after fought as a company guerilla commander in a "revolution to fight French domination." But by the end of 1945 the French "took us back and we collapsed." Following French return, he was arrested and imprisoned as a Viet Minh guerilla commander. Since he was Catholic and fluent in French, he was recruited to collaborate and in fact became a double agent working in clandestine relation with Viet Minh. At that time, he reports feeling quite torn, since he remained loyal to the Viet Minh cause of nationalism and was willing to subvert the French goals to this end. Things became entirely disorienting for him by 1950 when the Viet Minh became increasingly intolerant of Catholicism and oriented more toward communist discourse from the Soviet Union. This was experienced as a betrayal and was so threatening that he defected at the time under Emperor Bao Dai and went to the Da Lat military academy, graduating as a first lieutenant. Thus his nationalist loyalties remained intact although the reference group for pursuing those goals had shifted dramatically. Even so, no dramatic affect appeared to accompany this changeover, which he reported as "just business." The dividing line for him was "religious versus antireligious," which he reported as likewise affecting Buddhists within the country.

In the mid- and late 1950s, Mr. T was director of military instruction for the reserve officers school, in charge of demonstrating American training for the Vietnamese military. It was during this time that he traveled to the United States for advanced military training. He later joined the South Vietnamese military and, following the assassination of President Diem, was transferred in 1964 to the police force in Saigon. He recalled that "at that time there was political confusion and at that time I felt confused about the situation . . . and I can say exactly, it [the assassination] was by rebel generals, it was Minh, and now everybody knows that this general organized this coup d'état . . . supported by Americans." He reported feeling very confused and sad, yet he came to feel that Americans did not understand what Vietnam needed, citing (Robert) McNamara in recognizing with him that "America was wrong . . . very wrong for doing so."

Following the death of President Diem, Mr. T decided to quit the army and to stay home. However, a colleague from the U.S. embassy came to his home and asked him to collaborate on a rural development program, which he did for three months. He then determined to quit all things he associated with the state and politics due to increasing personal conflict about what causes were morally worthy. Mr. T and a group of friends began to privately invest to construct an amusement park for children, which Mr. T was relieved to undertake since he was "tired with government and these political matters, with everything, so we went to spend time with the children." He had lost his interest and will to continue to try to build Vietnam along the lines he had previously pursued and was sickened by the corruption of the new administration. He worked toward this new project (actually constructed in 1970) with a sense of relief and pleasure.

When Saigon fell in 1975, he remained near Saigon, but soon after was captured and put into a reeducation camp, where he stayed for five years, six months, and twenty-four days. The Viet Cong (VC) ordered him to write about his life and family and to confess to being an enemy of the state. He reported that the VC would look for inconsistencies in the writing, which they could then take to mean that the prisoner was lying, which would bring beatings, torture, and perhaps death. People who resisted or who even talked back were tortured. Mr. T knows approximately thirty people who were killed while he was a prisoner, sometimes for inconsistencies of story, but most often for trying to escape. Multiple disappearances occurred, perhaps fifteen to twenty-five people. He reported humiliation insofar as "we were made to be totally dependent on having to be a certain way for food and for life." His survival strategy was to "stay indifferent" and to not take actions against the guards, waiting for the "orderly departure program" under negotiation with the new government and American intervention.

Mr. T recalls that following his internment in 1975 at the age of fifty-four, he rapidly developed episodes where his mind would go away, where he would not even notice the present, and that the duration of these periods could be short or last a long time. He developed nightmares and daytime flashbacks of some of his war experiences and prison experiences. As he had more intrusions about the past and present, he developed more fear about the future. Panic attacks and worry in the context of these fears developed, and he began to "live like a machine," going through the motions of the reeducation camp without any interest in life. He was always "on guard," not knowing what might happen. Over the years, he felt more and more "like an automaton," and the experience of depression and trauma remained with him after his release. Following his release, he noted his sense that although he was home, he was not at home. Two children had been killed and his wife was dead. There was no work, and the authorities had taken all of his possessions. He was watched by police, and his movements were monitored. For thirteen more years his life was spent in this way: moving motionless, thinking thoughtless, and being nothing.

This way of being in the world began to change after moving to the United States as a refugee. Mr. T was granted refugee status and arrived in the United States with a surviving daughter in December 1995. He worked in the Southwest in a factory and was able to engage in routine daily activities, though persistent jaw pain—from a physical attack while in prison—prevents him from doing heavy work for lengthy periods. Even so, he had never wanted to leave Vietnam: "I wanted to stay. Because I was an old man, I wanted to stay and die in my country. But I was always disturbed by the police, they would always come to me and ask me why you didn't leave the country, start the paperwork with the ODP program. . . . If I stay, maybe I have some clandestine project against them." He claims to have become inured to the harassment and to always being an "outsider."

An author of poetry and songs, Mr. T anticipated having a book completed within a few months, entitled Gone with the Waves. His national identity is not that of a "United States person" but instead "always Vietnamese . . . mentally I am Vietnamese. Now, I can only dream of patriotic change in Vietnam. The best I can do now is to leave knowledge to the young people."

AFTERMATH

As narrative elements, the themes of region, religion, political affiliation, and human cruelty signify not only categories of social organization and action, but also domains of subjectivity. The fragmentation and realignment of the nation by north and south has its parallel in the psychogeographical sense of displacement and forced migration in the context of flight from warfare: Where is my home? Where is my 'north?'" Similar points can be made about the layered religious terrain with successive strata of Confucianism, later Hinduism and Buddhism, and later still Islam and Catholicism, and the political terrain marked by colonialist and communist identifications.

We suggest that it is this displacement that links the three subjective themes of alterity, trauma, and memory with which we have been concerned and places them in relation to the social and collective. The subjective displacement in this instance is not only the psychoanalytic transference of emotion from one object to another, but a psychic diaspora that began long before the physical diaspora that made refugees of these Vietnamese. The displacement of trauma is to be found in the enduring residue of chronic pain.[5] The displacement of memory is that of constricted temporal horizons. And the displacement of alterity is that of experiencing oneself as automaton, as well as that of no longer being able to distinguish self and nonself with respect to who is on one's side and to be trusted—the Buddhists but then no longer, the communists who once could be friends but then no longer. Alterity as an otherizing tendency is quite literally present in the discourse of Vietnamese, with reference to the source of evil, danger, or violence as the others. During the war, violent acts were simply attributed to others or "them," both because one feared to identify attackers and because one never knew for sure whether the perpetrators belonged to the government or to the Viet Cong.

Yet if the displacement we are discussing is not primarily that of psychoanalysis, it might be said that the South Vietnamese engaged in repetition-compulsion insofar as the past trauma of politicoreligious tension was played out by those, many of them Catholic, who fled the communist north asking yet another paternal authority—the United States rather than France—to take on the role of the "good father." Not only were the South Vietnamese primed for this paternally complex relationship (by the previous one with the French), but the United States was primed for the role of "guilty father" out of its abject fear of failure in the self-perceived (and psychopolitically distorted) obligation of "taking care" of the world. With the burgeoning fear of communism in Russia and China, the United States became the willing, then abusive, father, but because its motive was pathologized by guilt it could not live up to the goal of "freeing" the Vietnamese.

As a result of its own trauma, and very much like South Vietnam and its leadership, the United States itself became a "fragmented state," fraught with internal disagreement about identity and alterity and how to proceed with war and peace. If this analysis has merit, then it leads to the further question of the psychic dynamic of those who are now refugees in "the house of the father," particularly as postcolonial Catholics surrounded by a patriarchal aura that is both political and theological. The majority, perhaps as much as 85 percent, of the refugees were Catholic. Indeed, some of the refugees expressed elements of retraumatization during our study when a wave of insecurity and xenophobia swept the United States following the September 11, 2001, attacks on New York and Washington.

Over twenty-four centuries ago, Hippocrates taught his students that disease is not only suffering (*pathos*) but also toil (*ponos*) to repair. While there is an invader causing disease and suffering, there is also the fight of the body to restore itself. This *vis medicatrix naturae*, the healing force of nature, was imagined to be a resilience that cures from within. Groups of people are analogous to individual persons in this respect: a collection of elements that can either act to be harmful to the whole or to be healing to the whole. The fight of an individual body or a group to heal itself necessitates that the elements of the body or group first recognize each other as "self." Even when an element is enclosed in the body, that element, when recognized as "other," will be "attacked" by yet other elements, with the hopes of expulsion. Where that element is erroneously recognized as other when it is really an important element of self, damage to the collective body or group occurs. It is this confusion of recognizing self versus other that is the basis for some inflammatory and autoimmune diseases, and it is this same confusion that is responsible for the harm done to individuals and their *ponos*, their attempt via resilience to restore themselves to health. In a group, if an individual continues to be viewed as other, then it will be more difficult for restorative functions to be successful.

Colonialization of societies by foreign invaders, like colonization of individuals by pathogens, demands a response of recognizing self from other and mobilizing forces to expel the other and retain and heal the self. The health of individuals in postcolonial societies parallels the process of identifying self, other, and mechanisms of toil toward health. In Vietnam, invaders and healers had come and gone for over two centuries. The confusion about self and other gave rise to the parallel confusion in bodies, minds, and interrelationships that characterized the role of war and trauma in postcolonial Vietnam.

NOTES

1. The term "political ethos" has been defined by Janis Jenkins as "the culturally standardized organization of feeling and sentiment pertaining to the social domains of power and interest" (1991: 140).

2. The historical complexity of the colonial encounter in Vietnam is beyond the scope of this chapter, but includes forays on the part of the Chinese, French, Japanese, and Americans. In addition, Vietnam has also engineered forays of its own, including in 1471 the Champa Kingdom (now central Vietnam) and more recently Cambodia (1978–89).

3. The ethnographic case materials for the present chapter are taken from a much larger study called the New Mexico Refugee Project. This research studies trauma, torture, and health among Vietnamese and Kurdish refugees relocated in North America. Dr. Michael Hollifield, professor of psychiatry and family and community medicine at the University of New Mexico, is principal investigator for this NIMH-funded study, "Epidemiology of Torture and Trauma in Two Refugee Groups," MH 59574–01. Dr. Janis Jenkins, professor of anthropology and psychiatry at Case Western Reserve University, has served as anthropological consultant to the study.

4. It was the second time that the French were expelled, the first being the removal of French missionaries in the 1700s wherein conflict over religion was salient.

Prior to the 1700s, the Vietnamese had fought other invaders based on notions of "ethnicity" and "geography" (Duiker 1995; SarDesai 1992).

5. See the collected volume of Mary-Jo DelVecchio Good and colleagues (1992) for an ethnographic array of analyses of chronic pain.

REFERENCES

Antze, Paul, and Lambek, Michael, eds. 1996. *Tense Past: Cultural Essays in Trauma and Memory.* New York: Routledge.

Cole, Jennifer. 2001. *Forget Colonialism? Sacrifice and the Art of Memory in Madagascar.* Berkeley: University of California Press.

Duiker, William J. 1995. *Vietnam: Revolution in Transition.* Boulder, CO: Westview Press.

Freyd, Jennifer J. 1996. *Betrayal Trauma: The Logic of Forgetting Childhood Abuse.* Cambridge, MA: Harvard University Press.

Gandhi, Leela. 1996. *Postcolonial Theory: A Critical Introduction.* New York: Columbia University Press.

Good, Mary-Jo DelVecchio, Paul E. Brodwin, Byron J. Good, and Arthur Klienman, eds. 1992. *Pain as Human Experience: An Anthropological Perspective.* Berkeley: University of California Press.

Good, Mary-Jo DelVecchio, Byron Good, and Robert Moradi. 1985. The Interpretation of Iranian Depressive Illness and Dysphoric Affect. In *Culture and Depression,* ed. Arthur Kleinman and Byron Good, 369–428. Berkeley: University of California Press.

Hollifield, Michael, Valerie Eckert, Teddy Warner, Janis H. Jenkins, James Ruiz, and Joseph Westermeyer. 2005. Development of an Inventory for Measuring War-Related Events in Refugees. *Comprehensive Psychiatry* 46 (1): 67–80.

Hollifield, Michael A., Teddy Warner, Ntyamo Lian, Barry Krakow, Janis Jenkins, James Kesler, Jayne Stevenson, and Joseph Westermeyer. 2002. Measuring Trauma and Health Status in Refugees: A Critical Review. *Journal of the American Medical Association* 288 (5): 611–21.

Janet, Pierre. 1889. *L'automatisme psychologique: Essai de psychologie expérimentale sur les formes inférieures de l'activité humaine.* Paris: Alcan.

Jenkins, Janis H. 1991. The State Construction of Affect: Political Ethos and Mental Health among Salvadoran Refugees. *Culture, Medicine and Psychiatry* 15: 139–65.

———. 1996. The Impress of Extremity: Women's Experience of Trauma and Political Violence. In *Gender and Health: An International Perspective,* ed. Carolyn F. Sargent and Caroline B. Brettel, 278–91. Upper Saddle River, NJ: Prentice Hall.

Jenkins, Janis H., and Robert J. Barrett, eds. 2004. *Schizophrenia and Subjectivity: The Edge of Experience*. Cambridge: Cambridge University Press.

Kleinman, Arthur. 1986. *Social Origins of Distress and Disease. Depression, Neurasthenia, and Pain in Modern China*. New Haven, CT: Yale University Press.

———. 1995. *Writing at the Margin: Discourse between Anthropology and Medicine*. Berkeley: University of California Press.

Leys, Ruth. 2000. *Trauma: A Genealogy*. Chicago: University of Chicago Press.

Marr, David G. 1995. *Vietnam 1945: The Quest for Power*. Berkeley: University of California Press.

Martín-Baró, Ignació. 1988. La violencia política y la guerra como causas del trauma psícosocial en El Salvador. *Revista de Psícología de El Salvador* 7: 123–41.

———. 1989. Psícologia política del trabajo en America Latina. *Revista de Psícología de El Salvador* 31: 109–22.

McLeod, Mark W. 1991. *The Vietnamese Response to French Intervention, 1862–1874*. New York: Praeger.

Memmi, Albert. 1968. *Dominated Man: Notes toward a Portrait*. London: Orion Press.

Ricoeur, Paul. 1981. *Hermeneutics and the Human Sciences*. Ed. and trans. John B. Thompson. Cambridge: Cambridge University Press.

SarDesai, D. R. 1992. *Vietnam: The Struggle for National Identity*. Boulder, CO: Westview Press.

Warren, Kay B., ed. 1993. *The Violence Within: Cultural and Political Opposition in Divided Nations*. Boulder, CO: Westview Press.

Wright, Shelley. 2001. Witches, Slaves, and Savages. In *International Human Rights, Decolonisation and Globalization*, 36–61. London and New York: Routledge.

Young, Allan. 1995. *The Harmony of Illusions: Inventing Post-Traumatic Stress Disorder*. Princeton, NJ: Princeton University Press.

CROSS-CULTURAL PSYCHIATRY IN MEDICAL-LEGAL DOCUMENTATION OF SUFFERING

Human Rights Abuses Involving Transnational Corporations and the Yadana Pipeline Project in Burma

Kathleen Allden

This chapter describes the suffering and hardship of several villagers from Burma who are now refugees in Thailand. Their life experiences reflect the large population of villagers whose families were forced to leave their homes and villages to make way for the construction of a natural gas pipeline in the Tenasserim region of Burma by US and French transnational oil companies in collaboration with the Burmese military government (*EarthRights News* 1996b). The villagers, mostly ethnic Karen people, were subjected to forced labor, torture, rape, death of family members, and other severe human rights abuses. The consequences of the atrocities committed during the construction of the pipeline continue to have far-reaching effects on the lives of the villagers. They live as "illegal migrants" in rural villages or as "displaced persons" in refugee camps in Thailand. As such, they are not allowed to work legally, which makes it extremely hard to support and feed their families and has resulted in poverty and desperation.

In a precedent-setting human rights legal case, eleven villagers are suing the Unocal Corporation for the damage done to them. The plaintiffs in the suit against Unocal are using the Alien Tort Claims Act to prosecute the corporation for human rights abuses that it allegedly colluded in and/or committed in Burma. The Alien Tort Claims Act states: "The district courts shall have original jurisdiction of any civil action by an alien for a tort only, committed in violation of the law of nations or a treaty of the United States" (Alien Tort Claims Act 2000). The attorneys representing the plaintiffs asked the author to perform psychiatric/psychological evaluations on each plaintiff to help document the pain and suffering they endured. The information will be used for expert testimony in the case against Unocal.

Since the early 1980s, medical and psychiatric experts have increasingly been involved in the legal investigation of human rights abuses. The purposes of medical and psychiatric evaluations and expert testimony include reports of assessments of individuals who allege torture and ill treatment to judiciary bodies such as war crimes tribunals; human rights investigations monitoring; assessment of individuals seeking political asylum; defense of individuals who "confess" to crimes during torture; and assessment of needs for clinical care of torture victims and other victims of human rights abuse. The psychiatrist is conferred the special job of ascertaining an individual's credibility and of qualitatively documenting his or her suffering.

In performing these tasks, the psychiatrist who works with victims of human rights abuses must be sensitive to particular historical, social, and political contexts, as well as to the specific cultural, interpersonal, psychological, and even biological contexts unique to each individual (Kleinman 1986). Multiple layers of analysis are required to capture and understand the complexity of meanings of the events to the individual, as well as the meanings of symptomatic reactions and the events' consequences to the individual (Engelhardt 1975; Westermeyer 1985). Because this work is usually performed by psychiatrists from different cultures and countries than the victims, psychiatrists have to deal with the tension between what is universal in a victim's experience and what is culturally specific (Friedman and Jaranson 1994).

Additionally, these tasks present the psychiatrist with a complexity of roles. As caregivers, psychiatrists are concerned with easing the pain of the victims, but during the investigation and documentation of human rights abuses, psychiatrists are also intervening as political actors, criminal investigators, and scholars. As a political actor, the psychiatrist can be viewed as an activist, a player in a worldwide campaign to raise human rights standards and prevent human rights abuses. As a criminal investigator, the psychiatrist gathers evidence in interviews that can be used to prosecute torturers, war criminals, and those who perpetrate or authorize torture and human rights abuse. As a scholar, the psychiatrist may also strive to expand his or her profession's collective knowledge of how the human mind works and how human beings respond and heal after traumatic assaults and atrocities. Arguably, rather than conflict or detract from one another, these roles complement, enrich, and augment each other.

This chapter briefly reviews how the author and other medical, psychiatric, and forensic experts developed international guidelines for medical-legal investigation of torture and severe human rights abuses, and it introduces the reader to the new United Nations document, "Manual on Effective Investigation and Documentation of Torture and Other Cruel, Inhuman or Degrading Treatment or Punishment," also known as the Istanbul Protocol (IP) (Iacopino, Özkalipçi, and Schlar 1999). Then the chapter describes how the IP was used in the case against Unocal. These topics allow for a discussion of the active role for medicine and psychiatry in the struggle against human rights abuses in the context of corporate globalization and the new global economy.

THE ISTANBUL PROTOCOL

In 1984, the United Nations adopted the Convention against Torture. Torture is defined as "any act by which severe pain or suffering, whether physical or mental, is intentionally inflicted on a person for such purposes as obtaining from him or a third person information or a confession, punishing him for an act he or a third person has committed or is suspected of having committed, or intimidating or coercing him or a third person for any reason based on discrimination of any kind, when such pain or suffering is inflicted by or at the instigation of or with the consent or acquiescence of a public official or other person acting in an official capacity" (UN General Assembly 1987). The World Medical Association, in the Declaration of Tokyo, interprets torture more broadly. In this declaration, torture is defined as "the deliberate, systematic or wanton infliction of physical or mental suffering by one or more persons acting alone or on the orders of any authority, to force another person to yield information, to make a confession, or for any other reason" (Declaration of Tokyo 1975). Since World War II, there has been much scientific investigation concerning the consequences of severe psychological trauma. Nevertheless, until recently there have been no international guidelines for documenting the consequences of torture and other cruel, inhuman, or degrading treatment. The IP is the first comprehensive set of guidelines for this purpose.

The IP is the result of three years of analysis, research, and drafting by more than seventy-five forensic doctors, physicians, psychologists, human rights monitors, and lawyers who represent forty organizations and institutions from fifteen countries. The IP was first conceptualized in March 1996 after an international symposium held by the Turkish Medical Association, called "Medicine and Human Rights," held at the Department of Forensic Medicine, Cukurova University Medical Faculty in Adana, Turkey. The drafting process culminated at a meeting in Istanbul in March 1999. The author cochaired the subcommittee on psychological evidence and was one of the leading editors of the IP.

On April 20, 2000, the UN Office of the High Commissioner for Human Rights unanimously annexed the principles included in the IP to resolutions E/CN.4/RES/2000/32 and E/CN.4/2000/43; the UN General Assembly passed the resolutions in late 2000 (UNHCHR 2000). In 2001, the UN Office of the High Commissioner for Human Rights published the IP as an official UN document in all five official UN languages.

The IP contents include information on the following relevant material:

International legal standards such as international humanitarian law, UN legal obligations to prevent torture, UN bodies and mechanisms such as the Committee against Torture, Human Rights Committee, Commission on Human Rights, Special Rapporteur on Torture, Special Rapporteur on Violence against Women.

Regional organizations including the Inter-American Commission on Human Rights and Inter-American Court on Human Rights, European Commission on Human Rights, European Convention for the Prevention of Torture and Inhuman or Degrading Treatment, African Commission on Human and People's Rights.

The International Criminal Court.

Relevant ethical codes such as Ethics of the Legal Profession, Health Care Ethics, UN Statements Relevant to Health Professionals, statements from international professional bodies, national codes of medical ethics.

A section discussing principles for health professionals with dual obligations.

A model protocol for legal investigations of torture and cruel, inhuman, and degrading treatment with procedures for determining an appropriate investigative body, interviewing alleged victims and witnesses, obtaining consent, safety concerns, use of interpreters, securing physical evidence, developing a commission of inquiry, choosing experts, performing the physical and psychological exam, interpretation of findings and recommended content, and format of final reports.

THE ROOTS OF POSTCOLONIAL CONFLICT IN BURMA

Burma (now called Myanmar) is geographically divided into lowlands surrounded by a ring of mountains. The dominant majority group, the Burman, lived in the lowlands along with minority groups such as the Karen, Mon, and Arakanese. The surrounding mountainous area is inhabited by many other minority groups such as the Chin, Kachin, Karenni, Nga, Pa-o, Palaung Wa, and others. Large populations of Karen also live along the Thailand-Burma border.

The Shan, who live in the northeast hills, traditionally paid tribute to the former Burmese kings but were never directly administered by them. "Burmese" refers to the language spoken by Burmans and to all citizens of Burma. Many of the non-Burman groups converted to Christianity. Burmans and Shan remain largely Buddhist (Fink 2001).

British merchants entered Burma in 1600, but it was during the mid- to late 1880s that the British established their rule. As the United Kingdom drew up the country's boundaries, parts of the highland and hill populations who were never controlled by the Burmese kings became part of Burma while other segments of the hill-tribe population found themselves living within the newly drawn boundaries of neighboring countries (Fink 2001).

When the Japanese invaded Burma in World War II, many nationalist Burmese viewed them as liberators. Although disillusionment with the Japanese quickly followed, after the war when the British tried to reinstate their rule, the Burmese nationalists insisted on independence. Burma won its independence in 1948. Ethnic minority leaders, some of whom had fought on the side of the British during the war, however, were reluctant to join the union of Burma. Since shortly after World War II, the Karen, Shan, Mon, Karenni, and others have been fighting for independence from Burma.

"Karen" refers to a group of indigenous people who live in the hills and plains on both sides of the Thai-Burma border. Historically, they have resisted the efforts of the more powerful lowland states to assert authority over them (Hinton 1989). The combined Karen population in Southeast Asia is approximately 3.5 million (Hovermyr 1989). The Karen are swidden farmers whose language has a Sino-Tibetan origin (Stern 1968). A small minority of Karen have assimilated into the mainstream culture in both countries. The major subgroups of the Karen are Sgaw, Pgo, Bghe, Pa-O. The Karenni, meaning Red Karen, has its own insurgency against the government and refuses to be associated with the major Karen subgroups (Hayami and Darlington 2000).

Burma attempted to form a democracy between 1947 and 1958. In 1958, the military took over the government. Since then, the ruling military junta has waged a bloody offensive against ethnic minorities. Documented government atrocities include looting and burning of villages, rape, torture, forced labor, arbitrary detention, and summary execution. It is estimated that millions have been internally displaced during this struggle and that there are between five hundred thousand and one million Burmese living in Thailand illegally (Fink 2001).

In response to severe economic decline, political oppression and human rights abuse, in 1988 university and high-school students, joined by monks and many others, led a popular prodemocracy movement. The prodemocracy movement was brutally suppressed by the government. In 1990, the citizens of

Burma overwhelmingly elected Aung San Suu Kyi and her party, the National League for Democracy, to lead their government. Aung San Suu Kyi is the daughter of General Aung San, the man who facilitated Burma's independence from Britain. (His assassination in the 1960s led to the military takeover of the government.) Following the elections, the Burmese government immediately placed Aung San Suu Kyi under house arrest; many of her associates, the new democratically elected officials, were killed, imprisoned, and tortured. Her leadership and commitment to nonviolent change won her the Nobel Peace Prize in 1991 (Fink 2001).

THE YADANA NATURAL GAS PIPELINE IN BURMA AND TRANSNATIONAL CORPORATIONS

In 1982, large natural gas deposits were discovered in the Andaman Sea off the coast of Burma. In the early 1990s the Unocal Corporation conducted oil and gas exploration in central Burma. Several companies including Unocal began negotiating with the State Law and Order Restoration Council (SLORC) for oil and gas exploration rights. Unocal hired a consulting firm to evaluate the risks involved with investing in Burma. The report stated that "Burma and the government habitually makes use of forced labor to construct roads. In Karen and Mon states, the army is forcing villagers to move to more secure sites. . . . The local community is terrorized; it will regard outsiders apparently backed by the army with extreme suspicion" (*EarthRights News* 1997).

Despite the consulting firm's cautionary recommendations, Unocal bid on a contract to produce and sell oil and gas products. They lost the bid to the French oil company, Total. Later in 1992, Total negotiated an assignment of a portion of Total's interest in the project to Unocal. Unocal then incorporated Unocal Myanmar Offshore Company. Total and Unocal, together with the government of Myanmar/Burma, planned to construct a pipeline from the Andaman Sea, through the Tenasserim region of Burma, to the Thai border. The Thai government signed a thirty-year contract with Myanmar Oil and Gas Enterprise to purchase the gas.

Human rights investigators in Burma uncovered disturbing findings about the project. Reports found that the oil companies ignored local peoples' calls for a moratorium on international investment in Burma. The companies contracted with the Burmese military to provide security for the pipeline project. In providing security, Burmese military abuses of the local population were alleged to include extrajudicial killings, torture, rape, and extortion. A second category of abuses by the Burmese military is alleged to involve construction of the pipeline itself, including forced portering of materials and ammunition by local villagers and forced labor for constructing barracks, a railway, and other pipeline infrastructure necessities. With increased presence of the military in the region, residents reported that in addition to forced labor, forced relocation, rape, and summary executions, civilians were seized by the military and forced to work without pay or food on roads and the construction projects related to the pipeline. The only way for villagers to avoid forced labor was to pay a tax or "porter's fee" (*EarthRights News* 1996a).

In 1996, a historic lawsuit was filed in US federal court. Victims of rape, forced labor, forced relocations, assaults, and death of family members sued Unocal and other corporations as well as Unocal executives John Imle and Roger Beach individually for their complicity in the pipeline project and the abuses surrounding it. The plaintiffs filing the suit are villagers from Burma who are currently refugees in Thailand. Most are from the Karen ethnic minority group (*EarthRights News* 1997). In a landmark decision in 1997, the judge ruled that transnational corporations could be held responsible for violations of international human rights law in foreign countries and that US courts have the authority to adjudicate such claims. This sets a groundbreaking precedent in the field of international law. The court rejected Unocal's argument that only "governments" violate international law and that corporations are shielded from suit (*John Doe I et al., Plaintiffs, v. Unocal Corp. et al., Defendants* 1997).

In 2000, the court made a summary judgment on Unocal's motion to dismiss the charges. In its decision to grant Unocal's motion to dismiss the case, the court wrote,

> Plaintiffs present evidence that before joining the (pipeline) project, Unocal knew that the military had a record of committing human rights abuses; that the project hired the military to provide security for the project, a military that forced villagers to work and entire villages to relocate for the benefit of the project; that the military, while forcing villagers to work and relocate, committed numerous acts of violence; and that Unocal knew or should have known that the military did commit, was committing, and would continue to commit these tortuous acts. . . . Unocal and (the Burmese military) shared the goal of a profitable project. However . . . this goal does not establish joint action. Plaintiffs present no evidence that Unocal "participated in or influenced" the military's unlawful conduct; nor do plaintiffs present evidence that Unocal "conspired" with the military to commit the challenged conduct. (*Doe v. Unocal* 2000)

The plaintiffs appealed to the Federal District Court of Appeals. A parallel case was filed in the California court system. On June 11, 2002, the California Superior Court rejected Unocal's argument to dismiss the case and agreed to move the case to trial. In preparation for deposition and testimony, the author traveled to Thailand to reevaluate the plaintiffs during August 2002.

PSYCHOLOGICAL/PSYCHIATRIC EVALUATION OF PLAINTIFFS

The author performed psychological/psychiatric evaluations on the plaintiffs in 1999 and follow-up evaluations in 2002. All plaintiffs live in refugee camps or rural ethnic Karen villages on the Thai side of the Thai-Burma border. They came to Bangkok in October 1999 to give their depositions to Unocal attorneys. During that period, the author met and interviewed each plaintiff twice. A total of eleven people (three woman and eight men) were evaluated. Their ages ranged from twenty-three to fifty-eight. Most were ethnic Karen people, but one was Tavoyan and one was ethnic Burman. All were from the Tenasserim region of Burma. In August 2002, the author traveled to the Thai-Burma border region to meet with the plaintiffs again. The following two case vignettes illustrate the types of trauma and suffering that the plaintiffs experienced and the consequences that the violence has had on their lives since the events took place.

Case Vignette: Jane Doe I

Jane Doe I is a thirty-three-year-old Karen woman. She is a Christian and is married. She has four living children and five dead children. She was living in a refugee camp at the time of the 1999 interviews but had moved with her husband to a Thai-Karen village by the time of the 2002 reevaluation.

Jane Doe grew up in a Karen village in Burma. She lived with her mother, father, four sisters, and two brothers. She did not attend school because the family could not afford to send her. She learned how to raise animals and cultivate plants and trees. She married at age nineteen. Her husband is Tavoyan and grew up in a nearby Tavoyan village. She met him when he came to Jane Doe's family's farm to provide paid labor. Her parents gave them land where they built their own house, raised animals, and farmed. She said that in those days they had no worries until 1991.

In 1991, the Burmese military began to make demands on Jane Doe's village. The military demanded forced labor and portering and took whatever food and material they wanted from the village. In 1992, the military ordered the entire village to relocate. The forced relocation was part of the plan to clear the pipeline route and to provide a ready pool of forced labor for the pipeline project. Out of fear of forced labor and paying fees to avoid forced labor and portering, Jane Doe and her husband decided to go into hiding. The family moved to a secluded jungle area near a stream where wild vegetables were plentiful.

They remained there until 1994. One day in 1994, Burmese soldiers came to her hut when Jane Doe was alone there with their children—her husband was away fishing. The soldiers demanded that the family move to the designated location. A soldier kicked Jane Doe and pushed her down the stairs of their hut. Another soldier took an ax and destroyed the family's rice storage room. Jane Doe was nursing her new infant when the soldier kicked her; she and the baby fell into the fire pit. Jane Doe fell unconscious briefly. Jane's arm was burned and the baby's head was very badly burned. As soon as the soldiers left, the family fled to the Thai border. The trip took several days. The baby died from burns and infection within two days of their arrival in Thailand.

In 1999, Jane Doe said she thought about the death of her baby nearly all of the time. When she thought of the baby's death she felt pain in her heart, head, and neck. She tried to distract herself and avoid thinking of the baby by keeping busy or singing, but this did not help. She felt depressed and hopeless and frequently thought of taking poison to kill herself. She didn't tell her husband about these thoughts because if and when she tries to kill herself she said that she wants to be successful and does not want him to interfere. She said that only the thought of her living children prevented her from committing suicide. She said there is nothing on earth like a mother's love so she cannot deprive them of that.

Additionally, she said she could not sleep at night and that she lies awake most of the night thinking about all she has lost and worries about what kind of future her children will have. She said she felt that she and her family are like "beggars" because they were trapped in a refugee camp and had to depend on others to give them food and supplies. She wished they could work and care for themselves.

She reported having no appetite. She said she felt weak and tired throughout the day. She described having several episodes of shortness of breath, palpitations, and anxiety every day. She has intrusive memories and nightmares of her traumatic experiences. She also dreams about her previous life and the dead baby. She worried that she was losing her mind because she was easily distracted; sometimes she left her house and then discovered that she had walked to the wrong destination, or she had forgotten her wallet at the market, or to light the fire when she was trying to cook. She worried that some day she would wander off and not return. She denied hearing voices or seeing things.

By the time of the reevaluation in 2002, Jane Doe had become psychotic and her husband had left her. She reported that all of her previous symptoms were worse. She described frequent prolonged episodes of dissociation. She also described auditory hallucinations such as hearing the crying of her dead baby and the voices of the soldiers who attacked her. Four months before the reevaluation, she gave birth to another child. Shortly afterward her husband left the family. Jane Doe said that they had argued constantly about money and that she believed he had another woman somewhere. She criticized her husband for not being able to find enough day labor to buy food and necessities for the children. When he was able to find work, which was approximately two to three times per week, he was paid no more than the equivalent of US$2 per day, amounting to US$6 per week for a family of six. With her husband gone, Jane felt overwhelmed with despair and did not know how she would manage. She earned a small amount of money by foraging for wild vegetables and selling them in the village. Her mother is blind and lives in a refugee camp two hours (by foot) from the village. Jane considered going to the camp, but she and her children missed the official camp registration in 2001, so even if she went to live with her mother, she would not be an official camp resident and would not qualify for food distribution.

Case Vignette: John Doe

John Doe is a forty-nine-year-old Karen man. He is married and has seven children. He is Christian. He and his family live illegally in Thailand in a Thai Karen village. John Doe grew up in a Karen village in Burma. After his father died when he was a young child, he and his mother and sister lived with his grandparents. He left his grandparents' home when he got married at age nineteen. He said that he and his wife led a happy village life. They were given land on which to farm and raise animals. John Doe said everything was peaceful until after the birth of their third child in 1992. Things began to change at that time. The Burmese military demanded that the villagers relocate to a new village. When they heard the order to relocate, John Doe said they didn't believe they would actually have to move. They built huts close to a "car road," which they had been instructed was the site of the new village. He said that they never really lived in the huts. The villagers believed they would be able to negotiate with the military. A second order came from the military that the village must comply with the relocation within ten to fifteen days, and if they were found in the old village after that time they would be arrested and shot. At that time, John Doe said that he and the other villagers finally realized they risked being killed and their property destroyed if they didn't follow the order. The move was done with haste and was very difficult, especially for those villagers who didn't have bullock carts.

Life in the new village was not good. The land was flat and dry. Their pigs and chickens could live there without problems, but the cows and buffaloes wandered back to the old village where they could find grass to eat. In order to go to the old village, villagers needed to obtain a pass. They were told they would be shot if they were found in the old village without a pass. Everyone in the village began to feel very depressed and desperate about their situation.

Once they were in the new village, the villagers were frequently called upon to provide forced labor and portering for the military. They had to supply building materials such as wood, leaves for roofing, and bamboo. In addition to portering, they were forced to build military buildings and work on the construction of a railroad. The amount of labor demanded of them was very great. The forced labor made it nearly impossible for John Doe and the others to do their own farm work and support their families. He said, "I felt like I didn't own myself" because he had no free time at all for his own work.

During one particularly horrible episode, he recalled that he was at his farm when the military arrested him and forced him to porter. As the group was walking, they encountered fighting. There was an explosion and he was wounded on the right shoulder and back. He walked back to his village where the headman helped him. He received no medical attention. Two days later he learned that the military had burned down his hut and barn and all of the family's food that was stored there. They had nothing to eat. At that time, he said he considered killing himself and his entire family by giving everyone poison. He said that this was the worst he has felt in his entire life. He told his wife about these thoughts. She comforted him and told him that their children are young so they must be patient.

John Doe said that when the pipeline survey and subsequent construction began there were even more demands for labor. Soldiers stole the villagers' possessions and took their animals and ate them. John Doe said that he and his family became so poor that the situation eventually became intolerable. He feared that if they stayed any longer, they would die. John Doe said he felt like his "mind was burning." He didn't know what to do for his family. He couldn't sleep or eat. He worried all the time about how to feed and clothe his children. In 1996, he and his wife decided to leave the village. They escaped at night carrying very little with them. They had to carry their children so they couldn't take many possessions. The escape was very dangerous. They had to sneak out without being seen. He knew they would be shot if the military spotted them. They traveled through the jungle along a river. They had to climb over mountains until they reached a region of Burma controlled by the Mon. They were safe in the Mon area and they stayed there for about one month. Eventually they made their way to Thailand. They currently live in a Thai Karen village.

At the time of the 1999 interviews, John Doe said he felt very depressed. He said that his sleep and appetite were poor. He felt tired and weak all the time. He reported constantly worrying about this children and thinking about everything they lost. He said there is little hope for his future or for his family. He was very discouraged but he said he did not think of killing himself anymore. He said he had to go on living because his children depend on him and that life would be much worse for them if he killed himself.

At the time of the reevaluation in 2002, John Doe and his family were still living in the Thai Karen village. He said that he supported the family by providing paid labor for Thai Karen farmers. His older children also worked, but his wife's health was bad so she could not help. He said that every day was a struggle to get enough food to feed his family. In 2001, a Thai man came to the village and offered a job to John Doe's fourteen-year-old daughter and her cousin. Due to the family's extreme poverty, he agreed to let his daughter go. He believed that his older children were needed at home to do harder labor such as farming. The Thai man said the girls would be helping to wrap bread and cakes in plastic wrappers and doing cleaning. According to John Doe, the girls were taken to a location where they were "sold" to a business and forced to work. They were not given any wages or money for their necessities. They reportedly had to work all day and long into the night and were not allowed out of the business compound. The gates were kept locked to prevent them from running away. Finally, the cousin, who speaks Thai and can read and write (John Doe's daughter is illiterate), was able to sneak a phone call to a public phone in the Thai Karen village where the families are living and to write them a letter. She informed the families of their plight and gave them the address. The parents were very upset. They were afraid they couldn't get the girls back and that the girls would be taken and "sold" to another location to work, possibly as prostitutes. The parents contacted a friendly Thai man in their region. He agreed to try to locate the man who originally took the girls away, but he was not able to find him. Next, they contacted the business where the girls were being held. The business owners said that they had given the girls' wages to the Thai man who brought the girls there and that they would not release the girls until the families reimbursed the 10,000 baht (US$240). This amount of money was frighteningly high for the families. They borrowed money and asked the church for assistance to get the girls out. Finally, after four months, the girls were released. This incident was extremely upsetting for John Doe and his wife. He said that his wife could not eat or sleep until the girls were safe. Now, she keeps the daughter close to home all the time. The child was extremely upset upon her return and is gradually recovering from this incident.

Also in 2001, John Doe had another frightening experience. He was hired by a Thai person to clear some land. As he was clearing the land when he was arrested by the Thai Ministry of Forestry. They put him in jail. He remained in jail for one month until his family could pay 10,000 baht to get him out. His wife and relatives had to work very hard to earn the money; they also borrowed some money from the church.

John Doe said that he felt more depressed and worried in 2002 than in 1999. He worried about not getting enough food to feed his family. He said he was becoming increasingly discouraged as he found himself getting older. He found he couldn't work hard enough for his family and that living in a foreign country where they were not legal had become increasingly difficult. He didn't see how things would improve. He said that his sleep, appetite, and concentration were poor and he was forgetful.

He described having frequent intrusive memories of forced labor, especially of the time when he was wounded while portering. He reported having nightmares of people trying to kill him. He described having a heightened startle response. In the past he thought of committing suicide, but in 2002 he said that things were a little more stable so he didn't want to kill himself. He said that his responsibility for his children helped him cope with his difficult life in that he had to function for their sakes.

John Doe also reported that his physical health had been poor between 1999 and 2002. He described having had ten episodes of total body paralysis. The episodes lasted for about one week. He was not able to consult a physician because he is undocumented and didn't dare travel outside of the village to go to a doctor.

SUMMARY OF PSYCHIATRIC/PSYCHOLOGICAL EVALUATION RESULTS

For many that have survived severe trauma, the experience can cause variable effects (Eisenbruch 1992; Weine et al. 1995; Wilson and Raphael 1993) at a deeply personal level that can persist and fluctuate for many years (Keller, Eisenman, and Saul 1997; Goldfeld et al. 1988). Some forms of severe trauma, such as torture, are thought to be powerful enough on their own to produce mental and emotional consequences, regardless of the individual's pretrauma psychological status (Iacopino, Allden, and Keller 2001). Psychological consequences develop in the context of personal meaning and personality development, and reactions are shaped by cultural, social, political, interpersonal, biological, and intrapsychic factors that are unique for each individual. Although one should not assume that all forms of trauma have the same outcome, since the early 1980s much has been learned about psychological, biological, and neuropsychiatric responses to extreme stress, and clusters of typical symptoms have emerged that are recognized across cultures (Friedman and Jaranson 1994). This appears to be true despite the fact that these symptoms may not be the chief concerns of the individual (Sartorius 1987).

The utility of diagnostic categories such as major depression and post-traumatic stress disorder (PTSD) from the fourth edition of the *Diagnostic and Statistical Manual of Mental Disorders* (DSM-IV) (APA 1994) in non-Western cultural groups has not been clearly established. Nevertheless, evidence suggests that the symptoms and signs of severe trauma across cultures have become increasingly clear (Marsella, Friedman, and Spain 1992, 1993). Additionally, high rates of depression and PTSD have been documented among traumatized refugee populations from multiple different ethnic and cultural backgrounds (Mollica, Donelan et al. 1993; Kinsie et al. 1990: Allden et al. 1996; Lopes et al. 2000; Mollica, McInnes et al. 1999). Therefore, the clinician's inquiry should include the individual's beliefs about their experiences and the meanings of their symptoms, as well as an evaluation of the presence or absence of symptoms of trauma-related mental disorders (Allden 2002). For these reasons, the evaluations of the plaintiffs included an assessment for symptoms of major depression, PTSD, and other psychiatric disorders as defined by the DSM-IV.

To make the diagnosis of PTSD, the DSM-IV requires that the individual have "experienced, witnessed, or [have been] confronted with an event or events that involved actual or threatened death or serious injury, or a threat to the physical integrity of self or others" (Marsella, Friedman, and Spain 1992). Several trauma events in Burma were reported repeatedly during the interviews. The following list summarizes the plaintiffs' reports of trauma in Burma, before fleeing to Thailand:

Forced relocation	11
Forced to be a porter for military (self or spouse)	8
Forced to perform labor (self or spouse)	7
Military stole possessions	7
Couldn't support family due to demands for labor	7
Forced to pay porter fees	6
Witnessed violence to others	6
Life threatened	5
Beaten/tortured/raped	4
Captured, imprisoned	4
Family member killed	3

The following is a summary of the frequency of common trauma-related psychiatric symptoms that were reported by the plaintiffs:

SYMPTOM	1999 (N = 11)	2002 (N = 10)
Depressed mood	7	7
Sleep disturbance	7	7
Nightmares	7	6
Constant thoughts of losses	7	9
Intrusive memories	7	8
Fatigue	4	4
Forgetfulness/poor concentration	4	7
Poor appetite	4	4
Hopelessness	4	5
Pain	4	4
Headache	4	5
Irritability	3	3
Weakness	3	3
Suicidal thoughts	2	3

In 1999, all but one of the plaintiffs had symptoms of major depression and PTSD. Seven had symptoms sufficient to diagnose major depression. Four had symptoms of PTSD sufficient to make a diagnosis. Of those with major depression or PTSD, four were comorbid for both disorders. For those without a symptom level sufficient to make a diagnosis, all still had some symptoms, such as sleep disturbance, depressed mood, and nightmares. Nearly all spontaneously reported that they constantly thought of all that they had lost. In particular they spoke of the loss of their homes, their farms, and their way of life in their home villages.

In 2002, only ten of the eleven plaintiffs were available to be reinterviewed. Of the ten who were reinterviewed, six plaintiffs met diagnostic criteria for major depression and five met criteria for PTSD. One plaintiff (Jane Doe I) had developed psychotic symptoms. Four plaintiffs were comorbid for both disorders. All those who did not meet diagnostic criteria for these disorders reported some symptoms of each disorder. In general, the plaintiffs were more depressed and symptomatic in 2002.

MAJOR THEMES FROM 1999 INTERVIEWS

Several common themes emerged over the course of the 1999 interviews. The first dominant theme was that all plaintiffs expressed a sense of deep hopelessness about their future and that of their families. They spoke at length of missing their old way of life in their villages and the loss of their ancestral land. Their actual homes and villages were burned and have disappeared into the jungle; they have no homes or villages to return to. Nevertheless, most plaintiffs expressed the dream of one day returning to their home region inside Burma. A second major theme the plaintiffs expressed in common was the way they said they coped with their losses and difficult lives. They all expressed that the only thing that helped them survive was faith in God or Buddha and prayer. (All of the plaintiffs are Christian except for one who is Buddhist.)

Regarding their lives in Thailand, in 1999, all but two were living in refugee camps on the Thai side of the Burma border. They spoke of the misery of the camps where they had no freedom, there was no work, and they had to depend on "hand-outs" from humanitarian agencies. The plaintiffs used phrases such as "living in a cage," "feeling like dogs," and "feeling like beggars" to describe life in the camps.

Regarding their participation in the law suit against Unocal, the plaintiffs each individually voiced the belief that if they communicated with Unocal and its directors, and if Unocal and its directors knew about and understood the violence and human rights abuses and degree of misery and suffering that were committed during the construction of the pipeline, that Unocal would stop the abuses and prevent further abuses from taking place. Additionally, plaintiffs expressed the altruistic motivation of informing the world through the lawsuit about the suffering in Burma and that somehow their efforts in the long run would benefit others who had suffered and were still suffering as a result of the pipeline project and from Burmese military repression and violence.

MAJOR THEMES FROM UPDATED EVALUATIONS IN 2002

New themes emerged during the 2002 interviews with the plaintiffs. In 2002, only three of the eleven plaintiffs were still living in refugee camps. Most had moved to live in Thai ethnic Karen villages. Those who remained in the camps all reported that life was far worse. The Thai government had moved the camp locations and consolidated a number of camps. Each family had less space so there was no longer any room for even small garden plots. The camps were guarded by Thai military to prevent movement out of the camps. This meant that refugees could no longer go out of the camps to find day labor. Without the opportunity to make any money and without small garden plots, the plaintiffs said that they only had food from the food distribution program. There were no vegetables or meats. The diet consisted of rice, fish paste, oil, and occasional beans. They all worried about feeding their families. Quantity of food was reported as insufficient and there was no diversity in the diet. Also, they had no means of providing any material goods such as clothing to their families.

Those plaintiffs who lived in Thai Karen villages reported that life as illegal migrants in Thailand was dangerous and miserable. They said that they were not legally allowed to work or own land. They had to depend on the Thai Karen to allow them to stay temporarily on their land. As illegal migrants, the plaintiffs did not have freedom of travel and so risked arrest, and detention and deportation if they were arrested. For these reasons, they rarely left the villages, even for necessary medical care. Unlike the camps, there was no food distribution for plaintiffs in Karen villages. They had to find day labor or grow food in hidden mountain plots in order to provide food for their families. All plaintiffs complained of chronically not having enough food for their families. Hopelessness was a pervading theme for all plaintiffs and three said that they considered suicide. Those who thought of suicide said that it is only their responsibility for their children that prevents them from acting on their suicidal thoughts.

In addition to hopelessness, the second major theme that emerged in the 2002 interviews was fear. Fear took many forms. The plaintiffs expressed fear of returning to Burma and facing further forced labor. They expressed fear of reprisals for participating in the Unocal lawsuit. All feared that the Burmese military would arrest, torture, and kill them if they found the plaintiffs and identified them as lawsuit participants. Two expressed fear of Unocal itself and said they worried that Unocal could hire Thai people or members of the Burmese military to disguise themselves and sneak into the refugee camps or villages to torture, harm, or kill the plaintiffs. No plaintiff wanted their neighbors to know of their participation out of fear that the neighbor might inform the Burmese government.

There was a shift or evolution of the plaintiffs' perceptions or beliefs about Unocal's knowledge about forced labor and human rights abuses. In 1999, most plaintiffs expressed a desire to inform Unocal about the abuses and believed that if Unocal and its directors understood the suffering that the pipeline construction was causing, the company would come to their assistance and prevent future exploitation of Burmese villagers. In 2002, however, most plaintiffs said they believed that Unocal knew about the abuses and forced labor but "pretended" not to know. A number of plaintiffs said that Unocal pretended not to know so they could continue to profit from the pipeline and avoid paying compensation to the plaintiffs. They said that Unocal must know because they had given them so much information in their depositions. Additionally, one plaintiff said that when Unocal staff visited the villages, some villagers such as school teachers who spoke English would certainly have secretly informed the Unocal staff of what was occurring. Only one plaintiff still believed that once Unocal learned about the abuses they would come to the villagers' assistance and prevent future harm. This particular plaintiff said, "They are educated business men with a lot of money. They would certainly protect the villagers from the military."

All but one of the plaintiffs reported that his or her health was failing. Again, as in 1999, all of the plaintiffs pointed to their religious faith, prayer, and meditation as the chief factor that helped them survive their past and current difficult circumstances.

CONCLUSION

This case study in human rights abuses by a transnational corporation draws attention to the long-range consequences of human rights abuses on the lives of those who endure the abuse. Clearly, it is not only the human rights abuse "events" that cause suffering; nor is it simply the psychological symptoms induced by the events, but the accumulation of trauma, symptomatic psychological responses, and the spiraling social consequences that unfold over years. There is a layering and synergistic interaction between events, symptoms, and social consequences that determines the impact on the individual, the family, and community over time.

The Unocal case also draws attention to the mental health and psychosocial problems among refugees and internally displaced persons in general and the need for social and political solutions as well as clinical and programmatic interventions. In its *World Health Report* 2001, the World Health Organization (WHO) stressed the mental health needs of refugees and internally displaced persons (WHO 2001a). The report also gave the discouraging news that of the 185 WHO member states, only 28.3 percent had any programs to address mental health needs of refugees (WHO 2001b). Clearly, there are no comprehensive solutions on the horizon, despite the increasing attention to these issues.

From this case study of the Unocal pipeline project, we see how psychiatry can be drawn into the debate on the excesses and abuses of transnational corporations that operate in the context of the new global market economy. This is a curious juncture for psychiatry, given the past three decades of intense focus on neurobiology, psychopharmacology, and quantitative analysis, and a simultaneous declining emphasis on, if not neglect of, the social, cultural, and political factors that shape and determine an individual's (or population's) health, well-being, and sense of purpose and meaning. Over the same time period, the social sciences have enriched their exploration of the complexities of psychological, sociopolitical, and sociocultural layers of human experience through critical analysis. The gap between rich and poor around the world is expanding. Suspiciousness and distrust of the "outsider," specifically asylum seekers, immigrants, and refugees, is growing. Psychiatry and medicine can play a role in giving a voice to those among the most marginalized.

NOTE

Addendum: In 2005, the plaintiffs agreed to a settlement with Unocal for an undisclosed but sizable sum. The plaintiffs and their legal team view the settlement as a historic victory for the human rights and corporate accountability movement. In addition to compensation for their personal suffering, the plaintiffs have substantial funds to develop programs to improve living conditions, health care, and education for the people from the pipeline region.

REFERENCES

Alien Tort Claims Act. 2000. *U.S. Code* 28 § 1350.

Allden, K. 2002. The Psychological Consequences of Torture. In *The Medical Documentation of Torture*, ed. M. Peel and V. Iacopino. London: Greenwich Medical Media Limited.

Allden, K., C. Poole, S. Chantavanich, K. Ohmar, N. N. Aung, and R. F. Mollica. 1996. Burmese Political Dissidents in Thailand: Trauma and Survival among Young Adults in Exile. *American Journal of Public Health* 86 (1): 561–69.

American Psychiatric Association (APA). 1994. *Diagnostic and Statistical Manual of Mental Disorders*. 4th ed. Washington, DC: APA.

Doe v. Unocal. 2000. 110 F. Supp. 2d 1294, 1310 (C.D. Cal.).

EarthRights International. 2005. Historic Advance for Universal Human Rights: Unocal to Compensate Burmese Villagers. EarthRights International, Saturday, April 2. www.earthrights.org/legalfeature/historic_advance_for_universal_human_rights_unocal_to_compensate_burmese_villagers.html.

EarthRights News. 1996a. John Doe et al. v SLORC, Unocal and Total. *EarthRights News* 1 (4).

———. 1996b. Total Denial. *EarthRights News* 1 (3).

———. 1997. Historic Ruling in John Doe I et al. v. Unocal et al. *EarthRights News* 2 (2).

Eisenbruch M. 1992. Commentary: Toward a Culturally Sensitive DSM; Cultural Bereavement in Cambodian Refugees and the Traditional Healer as Taxonomist. *Journal of Nervous and Mental Disease* 180:8–10.

Engelhardt H.T. 1975. The Concepts of Health and Disease. In *Evaluation and Explanation in the Biomedical Sciences*, ed. H.T. Engelhardt and S. F. Spicker, 125–41. Holland: D. Reidel Publishing Co.

Fink, C. 2001. *Living Silence: Burma under Military Rule*. London: Zed Books.

Friedman, M., and J. Jaranson. 1994. The Applicability of the Post-Traumatic Concept to Refugees. In *Amidst Peril and Pain: The Mental Health and Well-Being of the World's Refugees*, ed. T. Marsella et al., 207–27. Washington, DC: American Psychological Association Press.

Goldfeld A. E., R. F. Mollica, B. H. Pesavento, and S. V. Faraone. 1988. The Physical and Psychological Consequences of Torture. *Journal of the American Medical Association* 259:2725–29.

Hayami, Yoko, and Darlington, Susan. 2000. Endangered Peoples: The Karen of Burma and Thailand. In *Endangered Peoples: East and Southeast Asia*, ed. L. E. Sponsel. Greenwood Publishing.

Hinton, P. 1989. The Karen, Millennialism, and the Politics of Accommodation to Lowland States. In *Ethnic Adaptation and Identity: The Karen on the Thai frontier with Burma*. Philadelphia: Institute for the Study of Human Issues.

Hovermyr, A. 1989. *In Search of the Karen King*. Upsala: Studia Missionalia Upsaliensia XLIX.

Iacopino, V., K. Allden, and A. Keller. 2001. *Health Professionals Guide to Assisting Asylum Seekers: Medical and Psychological Evaluation of Torture*. Cambridge, MA: Physicians for Human Rights.

Iacopino V., Ö. Özkalipçi, and C. Schlar. 1999. The Istanbul Protocol: International Standards for the Effective Investigation and Documentation of Torture and Ill Treatment. *Lancet* 354 (9184).

John Doe I et al., Plaintiffs, v. Unocal Corp. et al., Defendants. 1997. 963 F. Supp. 880 (C.D. Cal.).

Keller A. S., D. P. Eisenman, and J. Saul. 1997. Evaluating and Treating the Psychological Consequences of Torture. *Journal of General Internal Medicine* 12 (suppl. 1).

Kinsie J. D., J. K. Boehnlein, P. K. Leung, L. J. Moore, C. Riley, and D. Smith. 1990. The Prevalence of Post-traumatic Stress Disorder and Its Clinical Significance among Southeast Asian Refugees. *American Journal of Psychiatry* 147 (7): 913–17.

Kleinman, A. 1986. Anthropology and Psychiatry: The Role of Culture in Crosscultural Research on Illness and Care. Paper delivered at World Psychiatric Association regional symposium, Psychiatry and its Related Disciplines.

Lopes Cardozo, B., A. Vergara, F. Agani, and C. Gotway. 2000. Mental Health, Social Functioning, and Attitudes of Kosovar Albanians Following the War in Kosovo. *Journal of the American Medical Association* 284 (5): 569–77.

Marsella, A. J., M. Friedman, and H. Spain. 1992. A Selective Review of the Literature on Ethnocultural Aspects of PTSD. *PTSD Research Quarterly* 3:1–7.

————. 1993. Ethnocultural Aspects of PTSD: An Overview of Issues, Research and Directions. In *Review of Psychiatry*, ed. J. Oldham, A. Tasman, and M. Riba. Washington, DC: American Psychiatric Press.

Mollica R. F., K. Donelan, S. Tor, J. Lavelle, C. Elias, M. Frankel., and R. J. Blendon. 1993. The Effect of Trauma and Confinement on the Functional Health and Mental Health Status of Cambodians Living in Thailand-Cambodia Border Camps. *Journal of the American Medical Association* 270:581–86.

Mollica R. F., K. McInnes, N. Sarajlić, J. Lavelle, I. Sarajlić, and M. Massagli. 1999. Disability Associated with Psychiatric Comorbidity and Health Status in Bosnian Refugees Living in Croatia. *Journal of the American Medical Association* 282 (5): 433–39.

Sartorius, N. 1987. Cross-cultural Research on Depression. *Psychopathology* 19 (2): 6–11.

Stern, T. 1968. Ariya and the Golden Book: A Millenarian Buddhist Sect Among the Karen. *Journal of Asian Studies* 27 (2): 297–328.

UN General Assembly. 1987. General Assembly Resolution 39/46, Annex, 39 UN GAOR Supp. (No. 51) at 197, UN Doc. A/39/51 (1984), entered into force June 26, 1987.

UN Office of the High Commissioner for Human Rights (UNHCHR). 2000. UNHCHR Resolution E/CN.4/RES/2000/32, Human Rights and Forensic Science.

Weine S. M., D. F. Becker, T. H. McGlashan, D. Laub, S. Lazrove, D. Vojvoda, and L. Hyman. 1995. Psychiatric Consequences of "Ethnic Cleansing": Clinical Assessments and Trauma Testimonies of Newly Resettled Bosnian Refugees. *American Journal of Psychiatry* 152:536–42.

Westermeyer, J. 1985. Psychiatric Diagnosis across Cultural Boundaries. *American Journal of Psychiatry* 142 (7): 798–805.

Wilson J. P., B. Raphael. 1993. *International Handbook of Traumatic Stress Syndromes*. New York: Plenum Press.

World Health Organization (WHO). 2001a. *The World Health Report 2001: Mental Health; New Understanding, New Hope*. Geneva: WHO.

————. 2001b. *The World Health Report 2001: Atlas; Mental Health Resources in the World*. Geneva: WHO.

World Medical Association (WMA). 1975. *Declaration of Tokyo*. Tokyo: WMA.

CONTRIBUTORS

KATHLEEN ALLDEN, an expert on refugee trauma and psychological consequences of torture and human rights abuse, coauthored the UN protocol
on medical-legal investigation of torture. She provides consultation to
international NGOs, government, and academic institutions. She is on the
faculty of Dartmouth medical school.

BEGOÑA ARETXAGA (1960–2002) was educated in Spain and the United
States, receiving a BA in psychology and anthropology in 1983 and an MA
in anthropology in 1985 from the University of the Basque Country. She
received her PhD in anthropology at Princeton in 1992, where she was a
lecturer. She joined Harvard University's Department of Anthropology,
where she taught from 1993 to 1999, becoming the John L. Loeb Associate
Professor of the Social Sciences in 1997. In 1999, Bego joined the anthropology faculty at the University of Texas at Austin. Her publications include
Shattering Silence: Women, Nationalism, and Political Subjectivity in Northern Ireland
(Princeton University Press, 1997); *Los Funerales en al Nacionalismo Radical Vasco*
(San Sebastian, 1987); "Maddening States," *Annual Review of Anthropology* 32
(2003): 393–410; *Empire and Terror: Nationalism/Postnationalism in the New Millen-
nium*, Center for Basque Studies Conference Papers Series edited with Den-
nis Dworkin, Joseba Gablondo, and Joseba Zulaika (University of Nevada
Press, 2005); and *States of Terror: Begoña Aretxaga's Essays*, edited by Joseba Zulaika
(Center for Basque Studies, 2005).

JOÃO BIEHL is associate professor of anthropology at Princeton University.
He is the author of *Vita: Life in a Zone of Social Abandonment* (University of

California Press, 2005) and *Will to Live: AIDS Therapies and the Politics of Survival* (Princeton University Press, 2007). He has coedited *Subjectivity: Ethnographic Investigations* (University of California Press, 2006).

DAVID EATON is assistant professor of anthropology at the California State University, Chico. He received his MPH in international population and family health from the University of California, Los Angeles, and a PhD in medical anthropology from the University of California, Berkeley. His research on AIDS outreach, awareness, and prevention has focused on men's lives in Rwanda, the Republic of Congo, the former Zaire (now Democratic Republic of Congo), and Cameroon.

MICHAEL M. J. FISCHER is professor of anthropology and science and technology studies at the Massachusetts Institute of Technology. He is the author of two books on anthropological theory and method, *Anthropology as Cultural Critique: An Experimental Moment in the Human Sciences*, with George E. Marcus (University of Chicago Press, 1999); *Emergent Forms of Life and the Anthropological Voice* (Duke University Press, 2003); and three books on Iran, *Iran: From Religious Dispute to Revolution* (University of Wisconsin Press, 2003); *Debating Muslims: Cultural Dialogues in Postmodernity and Tradition*, with Mehdi Abedi (University of Wisconsin Press, 1990); and *Mute Dreams, Blind Owls, and Dispersed Knowledges: Persian Poesis in the Transnational Circuitry* (Duke University Press, 2004).

BYRON J. GOOD is professor of medical anthropology, in the Department of Social Medicine at Harvard Medical School and in the Department of Anthropology at Harvard University. He is the author of *Medicine, Rationality and Experience: An Anthropological Perspective* (Cambridge University Press, 1994), which is based on the Louis Henry Morgan Lectures and has been translated into French, Italian, Japanese, Spanish, and is forthcoming in Chinese. Among his edited works with colleagues are *Clifford Geertz by His Colleagues*, with Richard Shweder (University of Chicago Press, 2005); *Subjectivity: Ethnographic Investigations*, with João Biehl and Arthur Kleinman (University of California Press, 2007); *Culture and Depression*, with Arthur Kleinman (University of California Press, 1985); *Pain as Human Experience*, with Mary-Jo DelVecchio Good, Paul Brodwin, and Arthur Kleinman (University of California Press, 1994); and a forthcoming work on panic disorder, with Devon Hinton. He was an editor in chief of *Culture, Medicine and Psychiatry*, 1986–2005, and chair of the Department of Social Medicine at Harvard Medical School, 1999–2006. Byron's field research and collaborations in Indonesia began when he was a Fulbright Senior Scholar in 1996 and have led to research on psychosis in Java and chronic trauma and conflict in Aceh. Since 1984 he has been the codirector of the NIMH postdoctoral program in Culture and Mental Health Services Research at Harvard.

MARY-JO DELVECCHIO GOOD is professor of social medicine at Harvard Medical School and in the Department of Sociology at Harvard University. She is the author of *American Medicine, the Quest for Competence* (University of California Press 1995, 1998); and *Pain as Human Experience*, with Paul Brodwin, Byron Good, and Arthur Kleinman (University of California Press, 1994). She has published over one hundred essays and journal articles, including in *Social Inequalities* (2005, ed. Mary Romero and E. Margolis) and in *Subjectivity: Ethnographic Investigations* (2006, ed. J. Biehl, B. Good, A. Kleinman). She was an editor in chief of *Culture, Medicine and Psychiatry*, 1992–2005, where she began as deputy to the associate editor (1983–85) and then associate editor (1986–92). Since 1984, she has been core faculty and director of research training for the NIMH postdoctoral program in Culture and Mental Health Services Research. She was a Russell Sage Visiting Scholar (2002–03) and launched two projects on the culture of medicine and disparities in psychiatric and medical care in the United States, funded by the Russell Sage Foundation (2002–08). Mary-Jo began her work in Indonesia as a scientific advisor to young medical faculty researchers in Aceh on child survival projects in 1988–92. She subsequently was a Fulbright Senior Scholar at the University of Gadjah Mada in Indonesia in 1996 and 1997, and she continues collaborative research there on the culture of medicine and bioethics. In 2005, she returned to Aceh as an advisor to the International Organization for Migration on mental health programs for the communities affected by the tsunami. She and Byron continue working on mental health programs for conflict-affected communities in Aceh. In 1999, Mary-Jo began her current study of political subjectivity of Indonesian artists.

MICHAEL HOLLIFIELD is associate professor of psychiatry and family medicine at the University of Louisville School of Medicine, and director of the Anxiety Disorders program. He is particularly interested in the effects of trauma on health outcomes and in behavioral medicine. Dr. Hollifield's work to improve assessment of traumatic experiences in refugees of war has resulted in the development of culturally sensitive measures that capture the experiences of soldiers and civilians, men and women, and young and old people. He and his colleagues have also completed the first study to demonstrate the effects of acupuncture on posttraumatic stress disorder. He is a board member of the Society for the Study of Psychiatry and Culture, the Academy of Cognitive Therapy, APA, AFP, and AOA.

SANDRA TERESA HYDE is assistant professor in the Departments of Anthropology and Social Studies of Medicine at McGill University in Montreal. In addition to being a coeditor of this volume, she is the author of *Eating Spring Rice: The Cultural Politics of AIDS in Southwest China* (University of California Press, 2007), which is based on ten years of research on HIV/AIDS in China. She began her work on AIDS in the late 1980s as an activist and as part of completing her masters in public health at the University of Hawaii. She is currently working on a new research project on injection drug use and how it is experienced, prevented, and treated in the border zones in southern China, and research in North America on how scientists and physicians reconfigure gender through the surgical treatment of intersexed infants.

ERICA CAPLE JAMES is assistant professor of anthropology at the Massachusetts Institute of Technology. A former SSRC-MacArthur Foundation Fellow on International Peace and Security, her research interests include violence, human rights, and justice; democratization, postconflict reconstruction, and the politics of humanitarian assistance; gender, race, and trauma; and religion and healing. She is currently researching two projects: the first focuses on the experience of Haitian refugees in the United States; the second explores the politics of complementary and alternative medicine in the United States. She is finishing a manuscript entitled *Democratic Insecurities: The Ethics of Intervention in Haiti*.

JANIS H. JENKINS is professor of anthropology at the University of California, San Diego. She was an NIMH Research Fellow at Harvard Medical School (1986–90). In 1990 she received the American Anthropological Association's Stirling Prize for Contributions in Psychological Anthropology and joined Case Western University as professor of anthropology and psychiatry. She was a visiting scholar at the Russell Sage Foundation in New York (1996–97), and the coeditor in chief of *Ethos, the Journal of the Society of Psychological Anthropology* (1997–2000). In 2002, Professor Jenkins was visiting professor at the Institute of Social Medicine in Rio de Janeiro. Her research interests include culture and mental illness, diaspora, violence, trauma and subjective experience, and the globalization of psychopharmacology. Her publications include numerous articles along with a coedited volume, *Schizophrenia, Culture, and Subjectivity: The Edge of Experience* (Cambridge University Press, 2004).

JOHAN LINDQUIST is assistant professor of social anthropology at Stockholm University in Sweden. He is currently completing a book entitled *Anxious Mobility: Development, Migration, and Tourism in the Indonesian Borderlands* and is conducting further research on transnational migration from the Indonesian island of Lombok to Malaysia. He is also the codirector and producer of the documentary film *B.A.T.A.M.*, which follows the lives of migrants on the Indonesian island of Batam, a free-trade zone located just off the coast of Singapore. The film won an award of excellence at the 2005 Society for Visual Anthropology film festival at the Annual Meeting of the American Anthropological Association. It is available from Documentary Educational Resources (www.der.org).

JOHN M. MACDOUGALL received his doctorate in anthropology from Princeton University, and for the past ten years has focused his research on religious movements and militias in Bali, Lombok, and Jakarta. Since Suharto's fall in 1998, John's research interests have shifted to study the way that organized crime and radicalized religion have decentralized identity and security among Indonesia's urban poor. John has worked for several NGOs in Indonesia and East Timor. Recently he studied organized crime and regional militias for the International Crisis Group in Jakarta (2002–04) and is currently working on the political-economy of trafficking networks for the International Organization for Migration in Jakarta.

MARIELLA PANDOLFI is professor of anthropology at the Université de Montréal. She has a PhD in anthropology from école des Hautes études en Sciences Sociales in Paris. As general secretary of Società Italiana di Psichiatria Transculturale and vice president of Società Italiana di Antropologia Medica (SIAM), her previous research on the anthropology of the body established a dialogue between psychoanalytic and phenomenological approaches to ethnopsychiatry. For the past decade her work has sought to penetrate a new field examining postcommunist Balkan territories that are marked by the breakdown of states, the explosion of violence, and the implementation of massive humanitarian and military-humanitarian interventions. She has published several books and has edited special issues on the body, suffering, traumatic events, and military-humanitarian interventions. She is currently on the editorial board of *Cultural Anthropology, Culture, Medicine and Psychiatry, Anthropology and Medicine*, and *AM Rivista della Società Italiana di Antropologia Medica*. She was a consultant for the United Nations in Vienna (1999) and for the International Organization for Migration in Kosovo (2000–01). In 2004, she received the Women of Distinction Award in Montreal for the field of education.

STEFANIA PANDOLFO is associate professor of anthropology at the University of California, Berkeley. She was educated in Italy and the United States and has lived an extended part of her life in the Maghreb. Her work has centered on cultural hermeneutics, subjectivity, memory, and the interface of political and psychic processes, with a focus on Arab civilization and Islam and the question of postcoloniality. More recently she has focused on transnational migration, youth, and the return of theological vocabularies. She is the author of *Impasse of the Angels: Scenes from a Moroccan Space of Memory* (University of Chicago Press, 1997) and is currently completing several publications, including a book entitled *The Knot of the Soul: Madness, Psychiatry, Islam*, based on research at a Moroccan psychiatric hospital.

SARAH PINTO is assistant professor in the Department of Anthropology at Tufts University. Her dissertation received the Sardar Patel Award in 2004 for best dissertation on modern India. Her book based on this research is *Where There Is No Midwife: Birth and Loss in Rural India* (Berghahn Books, 2007). Her interests include intersections between gender, caste, and medicine; and reproduction and mental health. She is also studying shifts in relationships between families and psychiatric institutions, and the lives of female long-term patients in in-patient psychiatric wards in India.

A. JAMIE SARIS is senior lecturer in the Department of Anthropology at the National University of Ireland, Maynooth. He has published extensively on how a large mental hospital in the west of Ireland effected certain historical changes at particular localities and how it was, in turn, partially domesticated by local forces.

INDEX

Abdurrahman Wahid (Gus Dur), 84,
100n1, 114, 115
Abélès, Marc, 160, 161
Abraham, Nicholas, 17, 49
Aceh, 62, 69, 83, 101n2, 103n13. See
also Indonesia; reformation
art/artists in Indonesia
acquired immune deficiency syndrome
(AIDS), 24, 196, 211–12n1, 252.
See also everyday AIDS practices; specific countries
activists: advokasi (community-based
activism), 112; and HIV statistics in
China, 196; theory-minded
activism, 114, 123, 127n6; and
victim as sociopolitical category of
activism, 152n5
advokasi (community-based activism),
112
Affandi (artist), 70
AFOR (Albania Force), 169, 179n3,
180n11, 181n18n, 181–82n20
Africa. See specific cities; specific countries
Agamben, Giorgio, 16, 159, 179n6,
333, 375
Agier, Michel, 161

Agus Yuliantara Yulikodo (Yuli). See
Yulikodo
AIDS (acquired immune deficiency syndrome), 24, 196, 211–12n1, 252.
See also everyday AIDS practices; specific countries
AIDS Law Project (ALP), 252
Al-Alam al-Mithal (the World of the Imagination) (Ibn al'Arabi), 354
al-Aqsa Intifada (the second Intifada),
263, 270
Albania: and Berisha sympathizers,
164–65; and "complex emergencies," 170; and geography of occupied spaces, 163, 164–66; and
global media, 173; history of,
161–62, 165, 179–80n9; and
humanitarian intervention, 169,
170, 181n16; and international
hotels as reflection of postcommunist transition, 165–66; and
Kosovo Albanians, 162, 170; and
Tirana, 163–66, 169. See also the
Balkans
Albania Force (AFOR), 169, 179n3,
180n11, 181n18n, 181–82n20

425

Alien Tort Claims Act, 397
Allden, Kathleen, 409, 410
Allied Harbour operation, 169, 179n3,
181–82n20
ALP (AIDS Law Project), 252
alterity: and Mucker cult, 282, 291,
303n12; and Vietnamese refugees,
28, 379, 380–81, 385, 387, 388,
392, 393. See also the "other"
Amado, Janaína, 292, 293
Amarapibal, Amorntip, 192
American Psychiatric Association (APA),
410
Amphibi militia, 116, 117–18, 119,
120, 128n10
Amok (amuk), 20, 29n2, 64, 83–88, 93
Anagnost, Ann, 212n3
ancestors/divine spirits (Iwa), 144,
145, 146
Anderson, Mary, 270
Andersson, E., 254n9
animating force of body (nanm), 145
anthropology. See ethnographic studies
anticrime campaigns (yanda yundong) in
China, 189, 209
anticrime militia (pamswakarsa) in
Indonesia, 111, 115, 126–27n1,
127–28n8
antiretroviral treatment (ART), 196,
252. See also AZT
Antze, Paul, 153n15, 380
Anzaldúa, Gloria, 192
APA (American Psychiatric Association),
410
Appadurai, Arjun, 161, 163, 189
Arendt, Hannah, 333
Arensberg, Conrad, 319
Aretxaga, Begoña, 6, 16, 17, 18,
19–20, 64
Ariès, Philippe, 248
Aristide, Jean-Bertrand, 133, 135, 136,
152n3
Arkinstall, William, 149, 248, 249
armed civilian gangs (zenglendo), 137–38,
152–53n8
Armstrong, David, 247
Arnold, David, 190

ART (antiretroviral treatment), 196,
252. See also AZT
Art Institute of Indonesia in Yogyakarta
(ISI-Institut Seni Indonesia), 63,
64–68, 65, 69, 101n5, 102n10. See
also specific artists; specific artworks
Asad, Talal., 336
Ashforth, A., 246, 251
Asia: and krismon (Asian monetary
crisis), 24, 65, 102n12, 221, 224;
and New Asia concept, 222. See also
the Growth Triangle; specific cities;
specific countries
Assu, Jacare, 285
Auftrag 1874, 283
Aujourd'hui (newspaper), 241, 254n6
Aulagnier, P., 356n7
Aung San Suu Kyi, 402
Australia, 128n10, 130–31n16, 200,
205, 211, 303n12
autonomy-control narrative: and
HIV/AIDS epidemic, 247
AZT: and drug trials in China, 198. See
also ART

Badie, Bertrand, 167, 175
BaKongo peoples, 243, 248–49
Balinese Hindus, 110
Balkanization, 56, 162, 178–79n2
the Balkans: and Balkanization, 162; and
biopolitical landscape, 157; and
biopolitics, 157, 159, 179n6;
defined, 161–62, 179–80n7; his-
tory of, 178–79n2; and humanitar-
ian intervention, 161–63;
International Commission on the
Balkans, 162; and international
community, 162; and No Man's Land
(Ničija Zemlja) (film), 260, 272n1;
and OSCE, 158, 177, 179n3,
180n11, 181n19; postcommunist
collapsed states of, 18
BaManianga peoples, 249
Bandung art, 101n3
Baroud, Ramzy, 266, 273n4, 273n6
Barrett, Robert, 356n7, 380
Basoglu, Metin, 139

Borchard, Günther, 289
Borchert, Thomas, 194
Borch-Jacobsen, M., 337
Borden, Anthony, 176
borderlands: and biopower, 22; and colonial ideas about minorities in China, 190, 193, 204, 210; and contradictions in everyday AIDS practices in China, 191, 192, 197, 204, 205–6, 210; and control by China, 193; and cross-border migrations in China, 189; and dis-ordering effects of HIV disease in China, 190, 192–93; and ethnic minorities in China, 23; and glob-alization, 22–23; and governmen-tality, 22; and HIV among minority populations in China, 22, 23, 24, 195, 196; and imagined percep-tions in China, 191; individual negotiation in China of, 192, 210; and intersubjectivities, 22–25, 192; and minority gender relations in China, 191, 194, 200, 202, 210, 212n7; and moral politics in China, 22, 199–200; and nation-states, 22; and outsiders in Asia, 230, 243; and policies for HIV dis-ease in China, 191, 210; and pros-titution industry in China, 194, 202; and role of borders, 232n11; and self-identity, 192; and state boundaries in China, 191–92. See also the Growth Triangle; Palestine/Israel borderland
Bosnia, 161–62, 179–80n9, 273–74n7. See also the Balkans
Bourdieu, Pierre, 190
Boyle, Paul J., 228
Brauman, Rony, 167
brave: in Indonesia, 67, 128n9
Brazil: and assemblages for construction of colonialism, 7; and Brummer settlers, 285–86; and Catholic Church, 280, 287, 289, 293, 294; and competition for immigrants, 285, 303n5; and economic resources, 280, 302n3; and fratri-cidal war, 26; and German Kultur, 26, 284, 285–87, 289–90, 296, 301; and immigrants' status, 280, 302n3; and Lutheran Church, 280, 288, 289, 291, 293, 303n7; and migrant violence, 280; and Porto Alegre, 280, 282, 286, 296; and religiosity, 289. See also Mucker cult; São Leopoldo, Brazil

Brazzaville, Congo: and blood donations tests for HIV, 245; and claims of source for AIDS epidemic, 243; and counseling for persons with HIV/AIDS, 245, 246; and effects of clinical disclosure of persons with HIV/AIDS, 239, 245; and healers' treatments for persons with HIV/AIDS, 241; and HIV testing, 244–45; and National Blood Bank, 246, 250; and Occupational Care Center, 250; and Outpatient Care Center, 245; political history of, 239; and public disclosure of per-sons with HIV/AIDS, 244; and public discourse about AIDS epi-demic, 242, 243; and seropositive identities, 246; and speech con-texts about HIV/AIDS epidemic, 248; statistics about HIV/AIDS epi-demic, 253n1

Brown, Karen, 144, 145, 146, 153n14
Brummer settlers, 285–86
Buddhism, Sasak, 110
Bu Mega. See Megawati Sukarnoputri
Bunyole, Uganda: and HIV/AIDS epi-demic, 243
Burma: and Aung San Suu Kyi, 402; and border with China, 189, 192, 193, 208, 209, 212n6; and Burmese military, 397, 402–3, 404–7, 412, 413; and Myanmar Oil and Gas Enterprise, 402; and postcolonial conflicts, 400–402; and SLORC, 402; and Tavoyan people, 404; and Tenasserim region, 397, 402, 404; and Total (French oil company),

China (*continued*)
and ethnic groups at risk for HIV
disease, 190, 195; and ethnic
tourism, 194, 200, 208; and geographic affects of HIV disease, 196,
200, 210; and geopolitical space,
192; and global intervention in HIV
crisis, 23, 210; and *gui* (ghost) as
metaphor for addiction, 213n10;
and harm reduction projects in
China, 200, 201, 202, 206–7, 210,
213n9; and Henan Province HIV
disease, 195–96; and hierarchical
relationship of the Tai peoples to
Han interior central government,
23; and HIV testing, 197–99, 200,
201, 205–6, 210; and homosexual
community, 196, 198; and
hybridization of NGOs with state
government, 191, 207, 211; and
IEC materials, 197, 199; and illegal
blood banks, 195–96; and imagined perceptions of HIV disease,
191; and knowledge about transmission of HIV disease, 194–95,
198, 200, 203; and Kunming HIV
epidemic, 193, 201, 202, 203,
210, 212n5; Lao Yan and the Security Drug Center narrative, 206–7;
and late-socialism, 190–91, 199,
200; and local intervention in HIV
crisis, 23, 210; and Mao period,
199, 205–6, 209, 210; and medicalization of marital arts and spiritual practices, 191; and Menglian
narrative, 200–206; and Ministry of
Health, 196, 197, 200, 201, 204,
205, 213n11; and minority gender
relations, 191, 194, 195, 200, 202,
210, 212n7; and moral stance on
people with HIV, 199–200, 210;
National HIV Prevention and Control Center in Beijing, 195; and
nation-state concept, 191, 212n3;
and needle exchange programs,
201; and NGOs intervention in HIV
crisis, 23, 191, 199, 207, 210, 211;
and the "other" and HIV disease,
200; and police force, 189, 192,
209; and policies for HIV disease,
23, 190, 191, 195, 201, 203, 204,
210, 253; and prevention of HIV
disease, 23, 190, 191, 199, 202,
203–6, 208, 209, 211; and prostitution industry, 199, 202, 208,
209, 210; and the Public Security
Bureau narrative, 203, 206–7; and
qigong fever, 191; and rates of new
HIV infections, 196; and recidivism
rates, 208; and risk groups for HIV
disease, 23, 190, 195, 196; and
risky behaviors of persons with
HIV, 23, 190, 196,210; and seroprevalence rate for HIV disease,
196; and sex tourism, 202; and
sexual transmission of HIV disease,
194–95, 200; and socialist civil
society, 191, 211, 212n3; and sovereignty, 23, 190, 191, 200; and
spread of HIV disease into Han
interior, 189; and state boundaries,
191–92; and state surveillance and
control over HIV crisis, 23, 189,
192, 193, 200; and statistics for
HIV disease, 196; and survey information about HIV, 205; and Tai-Lüe
kingdom, 194; and Tai peoples'
relationships with Han Chinese, 23,
194, 204; and video-tape of people
with HIV disease, 205; and *yangui*
(cigarette addicts), 208, 213n10. *See
also* borderlands; everyday AIDS
practices in China; illegal drug-use
in China; Jinghong, China; Sipsongpanna Prefecture, China
Chomsky, Noam, 133
Christianity: and church bombings during Suharto era, 96; and conflicts
between Muslims and Christians in
Indonesia, 83, 120; and feminine
Christ label for Jacobina Mentz
Maurer, 282, 295; and Iwa (ancestors, divine spirits), 145; and religious persecution in Germany,

Haiti (*continued*)
postcolonial reconstructions, 133,
134; and post-Duvalier/post-Aris-
tide society, 18; and poverty, 132,
133, 134; and power shift caused
by humanitarian intervention, 134;
and Préval, 134, 152; and prostitution industry, 148–49; and PTSD,
21, 138–39, 148, 153n9; and rape
survivors, 135; and routines of
rupture, 139; and *sanpwèl* (secret
society), 143; and the self, 144;
and *siyon/sillon* (open-walled Penta-
costal church), 140; and sociocentric "self/body" serving spirits,
144, 146, 153n12; and sociopolitical instability, 133, 152n2; and
spaces of death, 18, 21, 151; statistics, 132; and Trager Approach,
134–35, 138; and transitional
nations, 133; and unemployment,
132; and UN peacekeeping mission, 151; and *viktim* (victims of
organized violence), 134, 135,
139, 149, 152n5; and violence,
133, 136, 152n4; and women,
134, 141–42, 148–49, 153n10. *See
also* culture of insecurity (*ensekirite*);
Martissant, Haiti; Vodou in Haiti
Hamas, 263, 266
Hardt, Michael, 159, 179n6
Harris, J., 247
Harvard's Friday Morning Seminar on
Medical Anthropology and Cultural
Psychiatry, 4–5, 29n3
Harvey, David, 232n9
hauntology, 3, 15, 21
Hayami, Yoko, 401
healing practices, 330, 331, 332
health intervention: and depressing
speech, 364–66, 373; and India,
27, 360, 361–64, 366, 367; and
knowledge display, 364, 365; and
naming death, 359; and narratives
of infant death, 369, 371; and rural
villages in India, 27, 361–64, 366,
367; and sterilization of women in

India, 367; and suffering theory,
365–66; and veil of ignorance in
India, 366; and WHO as ministry
of health in Kosovo, 171. *See also*
humanitarian intervention
Heifetz-Yahav, Deborah, 266, 269, 270
Henan Province, China, 195–96
Herman, Judith, 139
Hersak, D., 254n9
Hertz, Barbara, 365, 366
Herzfeld, Michael, 7
Hillebrand, João Daniel, 280, 286, 288,
295
Hinduism, Balinese, 110
Hinton, P., 401
HIV (human immunodeficiency virus),
211–12n1. *See also* sexually trans-
mitted infections (STIs); *specific
countries*
Hollifield, Michael, 380
Hooper, E., 254n8
House of Glass (Pramoedya Ananta Toer),
102n11
Hovermyr, A., 401
Hsieh Shih-Chung, 193
Huang, Shirlena, 228, 230, 232n14,
233–34n26
Hug (artwork), 86
Hugo, Graeme, 219, 228
Human Development Report 2000, 132
human immunodeficiency virus (HIV),
211–12n1. *See also* sexually transmitted infections (STIs); *specific
countries*
humanitarian intervention: and Albania,
169, 181n16; aphorism about,
163; and the Balkans, 161–63; and
categories applied to territories,
170–71; and "complex emergencies," 158, 159, 170, 179n5,
182n22; and creation of emergencies, 170, 179n5; defined, 158;
and diplomacy, 167, 169, 175,
176, 177, 181n19; and distance
suffering, 172–73; and donor priorities, 171–72; and ethics, 166;
and ethnographic studies, 157; as

foreign-policy tool, 158, 159, 160; and geography of occupied spaces, 163, 164–66; and globalization, 161; and governmental institutions, 173, 174; and gray zone between humanitarian intervention, 22, 158, 160, 164, 166, 180n13, 261, 270–72; and green zone, 164; and Haiti, 133, 134, 136, 151; and inherent innocence, 166–67; and international law, 161, 179n8; and international marketplace, 167, 171; and intervention studies, 22, 157, 158–61; and Kosovo, 169, 181n16; and laboratories of democratization, 168; and legitimacy, 158–59, 166, 173, 175; and local contexts, 157, 158, 175–76, 177; and marketplace, 163–64, 166–68; and morality, 180–81n14; and natural catastrophes, 177; and neutrality, 160, 175; and Palestine/Israel borderland, 25, 261; participants in, 157, 158, 175; and permanent transition phenomenon, 180n10; and politics, 160, 166–67, 177; and power, 25, 134, 159, 164, 165, 175–77, 181n15, 182n26; and privatization, 167–68, 181n15; and privatized management, 167–68, 174–75, 181n15, 182n24; and professionalization of emergencies, 179n5; social effects of, 159–60, 167; and sovereignty, 159, 163, 179n6; and "state of exception," 159; and strongmen/new elite, 175–77, 182n26; theoretical examination of, 168–69; and "the responsibility to protect," 158; and transformations of lived experience, 177; and Westernization, 157, 160. See also globalization; health intervention; international community; intervention studies; military humanitarianism

human rights: and international law, 160, 399; and juridical-ethical universalism, 28, 160, 168; and military humanitarianism, 160, 180–81n14; and one-size-fits all principle, 180–81n14; and Palestine/Israel borderland, 261; and privatized management of humanitarianism, 168. See also human rights abuses

human rights abuses in Burma: and beliefs of refugees about Unocal, 412, 413–14; and globalization, 28, 402–4, 414–15; and intersubjectivities, 398–99; and Karen peoples, 397, 402; and legal investigations, 398–99; and mental health assessments, 26, 398–99; and subjectivity, 28–29; and Unocal Corporation, 28, 397, 402–4, 412, 413–14, 414–15. See also human rights

Human Rights as Politics and Idolatry (Ignatieff), 168

Human Rights Watch, 230, 233n17, 233–34n26, 234n27,28

Human Rights Watch and National Coalition for Haitian Refugees, 136, 152–53n8

Hunsche, Carlos, 280, 282, 287

Hurbon, Laënnec, 143

Hurting Landscape exhibit, 65, 94, 104n25,29

Hutter, Lucy Maffei, 303n5

Hyde, Sandra Teresa, 190, 194

Ibn al-Arabial-ᶜArabi, 354

Ibu Mega. See Megawati Sukarnoputri

IDF (Israel Defense Forces), 263, 266, 268–69, 270, 271, 273n4,6. See also Palestinian-Israeli joint patrols

IEC (information, education, and communications) materials in China, 197, 199

Igert, M., 335

Ignatieff, Michael, 168, 180–81n14, 270

pelago, 218, 219, 224, 225, 231; and Ruwantan Bumi, 1998 (Earth Exorcism, 1998), 68, 102–3n12; and secret student reading groups, 112; and self-identity experience, 68, 103n13; and Sukarno era, 68, 103nn13,16; and trafficking in women and children, 225. *See also* the Growth Triangle; Lombok, Indonesia; militias in Indonesia; post-New Order/post-Suharto period; separatist movements in Indonesia; Soleh (Indonesian leader); Suharto era; *specific artists; specific artworks*

Indonesian Democratic Party (PDI-P), 62, 100n1, 104n19, 111, 112, 114, 120–21, 123, 127n3

Indonesian political party (PPP), 127n3

Indonesia Sakit (Indonesian Disorders) (artwork), 20, 62, 63, 64, 79–82

inequality issues, 152n7, 220–21, 232n7

infant death in India: and causality, 369, 370, 371, 373; and fatalism, 363–64, 367; and grief of women, 27–28, 368–74; and hauntology, 368, 374, 375; and healing, 372, 373; and health intervention, 360; and human inaction, 375; and India, 27, 359–60; and intersubjectivities in India, 28, 360, 372–73; and knowledge display of rural women in India, 364; and melancholia, 374; and modernity, 363, 372–73; and narratives, 368–74; and normality, 359, 366, 370, 372, 374; and poverty, 360, 363; and split self experience of grieving women, 360, 365; and statistics India, 362–63; and structural violence, 372; and suffering, 360, 365–66, 368, 371–72; and tetanus, 363, 369, 370

information, education, and communications (IEC) materials in China, 197, 199

INGOs international nongovernmental organizations, 136

insecurity, culture of. *See* culture of insecurity (*ensekirite*)

intergovernmental organizations (IGOs), 19, 133

International Commission on the Balkans, 162

international community: and the Balkans, 162; and effects on local political practices, 163; and geography of occupied spaces, 164; and Haiti, 21, 133, 134, 135, 151; and Iraq, 170; and multilateral organizations, 177; and national/territorial parliaments, 163, 180n10; and political space, 160; and power of political civil societies, 164, 165, 175–77, 182n26; and power relations, 164, 181n15; presence of, 180n11; representatives of, 180n11; and "right of interference," 158, 169, 173, 175; and role of international hotels, 165–66; and standardized practices, 163. *See also* globalization; humanitarian intervention; military humanitarianism

international law, 160, 161, 179n8, 399

International Military Force (AFOR), 169, 179n3, 180n11, 181–82n20, 181n18n

International Organization for Migration (IOM), 157, 171, 182n21,23, 212–13n8

Internet, 112, 219, 220, 223, 226

intersubjectivities: and borderlands, 22–25, 192; and human rights abuses in Burma, 398–99, 414–15; and infant death in India, 28, 360, 372–73; and legal investigations of human rights abuses, 398; and reformation art/artists in Indonesia, 99; and Vietnamese refugees, 380–82, 385, 392. *See also* subjectivity

Kosovo (continued)
  national/territorial parliaments,
  163, 180n10; and Surroi, 176–77,
  182n26; and UNMIK, 171,
  179–80n9, 181n18; and violence
  under Milosevic, 162, 181–82n20;
  and war in Kosovo, 165, 169,
  179n8; and WHO as ministry of
  health, 171. See also the Balkans
Kouchner, Bernard, 173, 181n15
KRIS (T) IS (Raging Bull) (artwork), 82
krismon ([Asian] monetary crisis), 24,
  65, 102n12, 221, 224
Kristeva, Julia, 3, 27, 88, 365, 366, 373
Kulahirkan Untuk Tidak Menjadi Bebek (I Gave
  Birth [to You] Not to Be Ducks)
  (artwork), 88, 89
Kultur, German, 26, 284, 285–87,
  289–90, 296, 301
Kunming, China, 193, 201, 202, 203,
  210, 212n5

labor migrants in Asia: and Batam
  Island, 23–24, 224; and circuit of
  debt and servitude, 231; and cultural contexts, 221; and de facto
  divorce in Indonesia, 229, 233n23;
  and factories offshore employment
  of women, 223, 226; and family
  obligations felt by women, 226,
  227, 228; and flow in contemporary processes of globalization,
  223–24; and globalization, 228;
  and the Growth Triangle, 22,
  23–24; and Indonesia, 22, 23–24;
  and Islamic norms, 22, 23; and
  Jamal (janda Malaysia, "Malaysian
  widow"), 233n23; and labor
  recruiters (tai kong), 225; and
  maids, 221, 224, 232n14; and
  men, 224, 229; and migration
  (rantau) culture, 24, 227, 228–29,
  233n21; and moral economy of
  women, 227, 228, 231, 233n22;
  and narratives of eviction, 24; and
  prostitution industry, 194, 221,

223–24; and rantau (migration,
  space of migration), 227, 228; and
  shame (malu) culture, 24, 221, 227,
  228, 229, 231; and victimhood of
  women, 219, 229, 230, 232n2,
  233n25; and women in the
  Growth Triangle, 219, 221,
  223–24, 227, 228, 231, 233n22
Lacan, Jaques, 53, 54, 297, 298
Lacanian analysis, 3, 16, 17, 19, 336
Lacoue-Labarthe, P., 337
Lafontaine, Annie, 159
Laguerre, Michel S., 143, 146
Laïdi, Zaki, 179n5
Lambek, Michael, 380
Langewiesche, William, 164
language: and Arabic language in
  Morocco, 27, 330–31, 337–39,
  342, 344, 345, 347–48, 350, 351,
  356n9; and censuring/satirizing
  function of Irish poets, 314–15,
  326n3; and depressing speech
  about infant death, 364–66, 368,
  373; and experience-near language
  analysis, 5, 10, 28–29; and French
  language in Morocco, 27, 330–31,
  337–38, 342–43, 344, 346, 350,
  351, 356n9; and Israel, 261; and
  naming death, 359–60; and Palestinians, 261, 264; and psychological experience, 3. See also speech
Laos, 189, 192, 193, 194, 208
Lao Yan and the Security Drug Center
  narrative, 206–7
Larose, Serge, 143, 145
Lear, D., 254n5
Leaving the Yellow Sperm Community
  (artwork), 91, 93
Lebanon, 170, 267–68, 269
LeClerc-Madlala, S., 251
Lee, Ching Kwan, 212n3
Lee, S., 192
Legal Aid Institute, 112, 114
LEKRA—The Insitute for People's Cul-
  ture (Lembaga Kebudayaan
  Rakyat), 68, 102n11

military humanitarianism (*continued*)
261, 270–72; and Haiti, 136,
151; and human rights, 168,
180–81n14; and international law,
179n8; and international marketplace, 167; and Kosovo, 169–70,
181n17; and nation-state interests,
173; and permanent transition
phenomenon, 180n10; and "right
of interference," 158, 169, 173,
175; and tensions, 271; and "the
responsibility to protect," 158; and
transformations of lived experience, 177. *See also* globalization;
humanitarian intervention
militias in Indonesia: Amphibi militia,
116, 117–18, 119, 120, 128n10;
Bujak militia, 116, 117, 118; and
community vigilantism, 116,
125–26; and FUIB, 126–27n1; and
pamswakarsa (anticrime militia),
111, 115, 126–27n1, 127–28n8;
and power from Islamic scripture,
118; and Soleh, 111, 126–27n1;
types of, 126–27n1
Milosevic, Slobodan, 162, 181–82n20
Ministry of Health, Joint UN Programme on HIV/AIDS, and World
Health Organization, 195, 196
Mitchell, Timothy, 360
Mizrahim, 261, 267, 268
MLNV (*Movimiento de Liberación National
Vasco*; Basque Movement of National
Liberation), 53
Mollica, R. F., 410
Moradi, Robert, 379
moral economy, and female labor
migrants, 227, 228, 231, 233n22
moral militias. *See* militias
Morocco: and Arabic language, 27,
330–31, 337–39, 342, 344, 345,
347–48, 350, 351, 356n9; and
biopolitics, 333, 334, 335, 336,
355–56n6; and *chomeur* (unemployed person), 334, 355n5; and
cultural-linguistic translations,
330–31; and *dahir* (decree) of psy-

chiatry, 332, 333; and French language, 27, 330–31, 337–38,
342–43, 344, 346, 350, 351,
356n9; and healing practices, 330,
331, 332; and health care, 331,
355n4; and health rights, 331, 333;
and Hospital Arrazi, 330, 335; and
jinn stories, 27, 340, 341, 345, 347,
348, 351, 354; and "knottedness,"
27, 349–50; and modern culture vs.
cultural traditions, 329–30, 335–36;
and the Mother-Tradition in literature, 353; and narratives of patients
at mental hospital, 329, 333–34;
and psychiatry, 27, 330–32,
332–37, 335n2; and Salé's Hospital
Arrazi, 330, 335; and struggles for
place in the world, 339, 356n10;
and topography of the unlivable,
339–43; and truth commission,
355–56n6; and *twkkel* (magical oper-
ation/illness attack), 338, 339, 340,
353. *See also* literature in Morocco
mortality, infant. *See* infant death
Mother India (Mayo), 366
the Mother-Tradition in literature of
Morocco, 353
Le Moustique (newspaper), 255n13
Movimiento de Liberación National Vasco/Basque
Movement of National Liberation
(MLNV), 53
Mrázek, Rudolf, 228
Die Mucker (The Muckers) (Schupp), 298
Mucker cult: and alterity, 282, 291,
303n12; and articulation of theological ideas, 282; and civil war,
299–301; and daily life, 282, 293,
296; definition of label, 281; and
deviltries, 290, 303n11; and
enlightenment, 288–89; and free-
spirited label, 294–95; and German upper class attitudes, 26, 281,
282, 290; and herbal medicines,
281; history of, 281; and Jesuit
missionaries, 280, 289, 291, 293,
295, 296, 298; and Koseritz's anti-
Mucker cult campaign, 279,

281–82, 284, 294; as label for violence, 281, 302; and Maurer, João
Jorge, 281, 288–89, 295–96,
303n8; memory of, 280, 301–2;
and military intervention, 295–96,
299–300; and narratives about,
281–82, 284, 286, 291, 293–94,
298–301; as the "other," 26, 302;
and persecution against, 26, 279,
282, 298; and progress notions,
282, 301–2; and rationality
notions, 282, 293; and the Real
(local Real) concept, 284–85; and
redefinition of common sense,
282, 293–97; and social sciences,
293–94; and statistics on membership, 292–93; and the uncanny,
297–99. *See also* Maurer, Jacobina
Mentz

The Muckers (Die Mucker) (Schupp), 298
El Mundo, 52
Myanmar. *See* Burma
Myers, Fred, 101n6

Nahdlatul Wathan (NW), 117–18,
118n12
Naim, Mochtar, 227
naming death, 359–60, 366, 373,
374, 375
Nancy, J.-L., 337
Nandy, Ashis, 12, 13, 135, 367
nanm (animating force of body), 145
National Blood Bank (Congo), 246, 250
National HIV Prevention and Control
Center in Beijing, 195
nation-state: and biopolitics, 133; and
borderlands, 22; and China, 191,
212n3; definition of state, 191; and
family structure in Indonesia, 229;
and govermentality, 133; interests
vs. military humanitarianism, 173;
and rational order vs. postcolonial
disorders, 8, 30n8; and reformation art/artists in Indonesia, 20,
64, 69, 75, 78, 81, 99, 103n18;
subjectification of, 64, 78, 101n4;
and supranational disorders, 28;

and transformations of lived
experience, 378, 379. *See also* state
nation-states: and disordered states,
18, 19
NATO (North Atlantic Treaty Organization), 169, 179n8, 180n11,
181n17,18, 181–82n20, 182n27,
273–74n7
Negri, Antonio, 159, 179n6
neocolonialism. *See* globalization;
humanitarian intervention; international community; military
humanitarianism
nervousness, 19, 21, 137
New Asia concept, 222
*The New Face of the Mucker (A Nova Face dos
Muckers)* (Domingue), 299
New God Series (artwork), 87, 88, 93,
104n25
New Mexico Refugee Project, 385,
394n3
the New Order. *See* Suharto era
the *New York Times* (newspaper), 105n32
nganga ngombo (specialist in divination),
249
NGOs (nongovernmental organizations):
and development of political civil
societies, 173–74, 182n24; and
disordered states, 23; and govermentality, 133; and HIV prevention
work, 23, 191, 199, 207; and
humanitarian-military intervention,
19, 136, 151; and hybridization
with state governments, 191, 207;
and privatized management of
humanitarianism, 174–75,
182n24; and theory-minded
activism, 114, 123, 127n6; and use
of communication technologies in
Somalia, 273–74n7; and without
borders label, 22
Ničija Zemlja (No Man's Land) (film), 260,
272n1
Nietzsche, Friedrich, 284, 301
9/11 attacks, 94–95, 96, 393
Noé, Miguel, 288–89, 292, 299, 300,
301

Nogueira, Arlinda Rocha, 303n5
No Man's Land (*Nićija Zemlja*) (film), 260, 272n1
nongovernmental organizations (NGOs). *See* NGOs (nongovernmental organizations)
North Atlantic Treaty Organization (NATO), 169, 179n8, 180n11, 181n17,18, 181–82n20, 182n27, 273–74n7
North-South relations: and globalization, 262
North Vietnam, 378, 384, 386, 391, 393
Le Nouvellist (newspaper), 151
A Nova Face dos Muckers (The New Face of the Mucker) (Domingue), 299
NusuAmuk series exhibition (artwork), 20, 64, 84, 85, 87–93

OAS (Organization of American States), 136
Obbo, Christine, 242, 251
Oberacker, Carlos, 283, 285, 286, 287
Occupied Territories: and Gaza Community Mental Health Program, 265; and Gaza psychiatrist's narrative, 263–64; and Israeli reservists, 266, 273n4,6; and West Bank, 268, 269, 272–73n3,4. *See also* Palestine/Israel borderland
O'Connor, Tomás: biography of, 310, 316, 319; and bureaucratic structures, 311, 313, 322, 325; and colonial landscapes, 313; described, 310; and DPMA, 310; and drinking/drunkenness,311, 321; and gifts of sweets, 320–21; and labels, 320; and local frames of reference for understanding characterhood, 316–19, 320, 322, 325, 326n5; and medications, 320; and mental hospital, 310, 316, 318, 322, 323; and mental patient, 26; and postcolonial landscapes, 313; and poverty, 310–11, 319; psychology of, 310, 316, 319–20; and

resistance, 324; and respectability/unrespectability status, 318, 319, 325; and social experience, 321–22; and socio-political speeches, 321; and speech as production of self-identity, 312–13, 326n2; and wanderings, 311–12, 319, 320, 321–22, 324
Oei Hong Djien, 102n11
Ohmae, Kenichi, 219
Ó'hógáin, D., 321
Ong, Aihwa, 9, 222, 230
ontological security, 138, 151–52
Operation Allied Harbour, 169, 179n3, 181–82n20
Operation Go Away, 224, 227
Operation Restore Hope, 267, 271
Organization for Security and Co-operation in Europe (OSCE), 158, 177, 179n3, 180n11, 181n19
Organization of American States (OAS), 136
OSCE (Organization for Security and Co-operation in Europe), 158, 177, 179n3, 180n11, 181n19
Oslo Agreements, 263, 266, 267
Otegi, Mikel, 17, 51
the "other": and assemblages for construction of colonialism, 7–8; and Basque radical nationalists self vs. dominant the "other" experience, 54–55, 60; and ethnographic studies, 4; and German immigrants, 283, 298; and HIV disease in China, 200; and Mucker cult, 26, 302; and Palestine, 268; and postcolonial disorders, 25; and Reda (Moroccan mental patient), 353, 354–55; and subjectivity, 2; and Vietnamese refugees, 382, 383, 384, 385, 387, 388, 392, 393, 394; vs. national self, 54–55, 60. *See also* alterity; marginality
Outpatient Care Center, 245
outsiders: and borderlands in Asia, 230, 243; and globalization, 415; and Indonesia, 113; and Israeli out-

sider/insider power struggles,
267, 268–69; and maids as
moral outsiders, 230; and Palestinian outsider/insider power
struggles, 268–69; and Vietnamese
refugees, 392

PA (Palestinian Authority), 266, 273n6.
See also Palestine; Palestine/Israel
borderland; Palestinian-Israeli joint
patrols
Paci, Eugenio, 248
painting. See specific genres
El País, 52, 53
Pak Alex. See Luthfi, Alex
Pak Harto, 79. See also Suharto era
Palestine: and aggressive actions, 263;
and al-Aqsa Brigade, 266; and attitudes towards government, 264;
and community concept, 264; and
fear of attending school, 263, 265;
and Gaza Community Mental
Health Program, 265; and grieving
process, 264; and humanitarian
aid, 262; and Intifada, 263, 264,
269, 270; and Islamic jihad, 266;
and martyrs, 263, 264; and North-
South relations, 262; and the
"other," 268; and outsider/insider
power struggles, 268–69; and PA,
266, 273n6; and Palestine Security
Forces, 266; and paradigm shifts of
state-led modernization, 262; and
PLO, 261, 268; and postcolonialism, 264; and power of father-
hood, 263; and public apologies by
Israelis, 264; and radicalization of
women, 263; and revenge, 264;
and riot control in North-South
networks, 262; and state concept,
264; and trauma, 263; and violence, 263. See also Palestine/Israel
borderland; Palestinian-Israeli joint
patrols
Palestine/Israel borderland: and communications technologies, 271–72;
and disorders, 23, 272; and eco-

nomic dynamics, 265; and elementary forms of social life, 25; and el-
Sarraj, 263–64, 265, 266,
272–73n3; and emergency, 272;
and EU solutions, 264–65; and
family dynamics, 265; and Gaza
psychiatrist's narrative, 263–64;
and geopolitical space, 264; and
gray zone between military and
humanitarian intervention, 261,
270–72; and historical fault lines,
23; and humanitarian intervention,
25, 261; and IDF invasion of Jenin
narrative, 266, 273n4,6; and Israel,
22–25; and judgements of ethical
action, 25; and nonviolence, 265;
and Oslo Agreements, 263, 266,
267; and Palestine, 22; and political dynamics, 265; and psychiatrists, 23, 25; and psychoanalytic/
psychotherapeutic discourses,
263–65; and psychotherapy certificate program, 265, 272–73n3; and
the Real (local Real) concept, 272;
and right of return, 264; and situations of trauma, 25, 263; and
soldiers, 23, 25; and split self
experience, 266; and standing
state of emergency, 272; and subjectivity, 25; and Tamari, 264–65;
and third-party intervention,
272; and three-state solution,
265, 272n2; and violence, 263,
265. See also Palestine
Palestine Liberation Organization (PLO),
261, 268. See also Palestine; Pales-
tine/Israel borderland
Palestinian Authority (PA), 266, 273n6.
See also Palestinian-Israeli joint
patrols
Palestinian-Israeli joint patrols: and al-
Aqsa Intifada, 263, 270; described,
266, 268, 270; and dramaturgy or
theater, 267, 270; and emotionality, 269, 270; and empowerment
of Palestinians, 269; and game of
provocations and score keeping,

Pollack, Sheldon, 164
pornographic films, 121–22, 124
Porter, Doug, 190, 195
Porto, Aurélio, 286, 290
Porto Alegre, Brazil, 280, 282, 286, 296
Portugal, and history in Brazil, 280, 302n2
postcolonial disorders: and altered mental states, 25; and borders, 22; and cultural traditions vs. modern culture, 335–37; and ethnographic studies, 26; and ethnographic studies of anxiety, 4; found in contemporary social life, 2; and health care, 331; and mental illnesses, 25–26; and nation-state rational order, 8, 30n8; and the other, 25; and postcolonialism, 8; and postcolonial order/realities, 25; and psychiatry, 25; and repression, 331; and subjectivity, 2, 8, 11, 26; and supranational disorders, 28; and toleration, 7
postcolonialism: and classic scholarship, 12; defined, 6–7; and ethnographic studies, 4–7; and global hierarchies, 7; and global public health, 379, 386–87, 394, 414–15; and historical legacy of violence, 7–8; and history of Vietnam, 378, 382–84, 394–95n4, 394n2; and human rights, 379; and knowledge displays, 367; landscapes, 313; and landscapes, 313; and language, 9, 10, 13, 27, 350, 352; and memory, 380, 381; and naming death, 359; and the "other," 380; and political conditions, 6, 8; and political violence, 8; and self-identity, 381; and split self experience, 12–13, 367; and subjectivity, 2, 5–7, 8–9; and terrorism, 8; and trauma, 380; and traumatic memory, 381; and truth commission in Morocco, 355–56n6
postcommunist Balkan territories. See the Balkans

post-New Order/post-Suharto period: and accountability of Suharto family, 83; and community vigilantism, 113; and democratization of violence, 111; and East Timor, 83, 115, 127–28n8, 128n10; and fantasies of state, 112, 113, 121–22, 123, 124, 127n4; and moral militarism, 116; and Muslim anticrime militias, 111; and oknum-oknum gelap (dark conspirators), 113, 119, 127n4; and political madness, 18, 21–22; and political reforms, 113; and presidential elections, 62, 83; and reformation art/artists, 20, 66–68, 100; and reform era (reformasi) in Indonesia, 62, 63, 64, 65, 66, 67, 84; and "run amok" (mengamuk) experience, 20, 29n2, 84; and security issues, 84, 104n21; and theory-minded activists, 114, 123, 127n6; and violence, 83, 87. See also Lombok, Indonesia; reformation art/artists
poststructuralist writings, 3, 9, 29n1
post-Suharto period. See post-New Order/post-Suharto period
post-traumatic stress disorder (PTSD): and Burmese refugees, 410, 411; and culture of insecurity (ensekirite) in Haiti, 21, 138–39; and diagnosis across cultures, 28; and Haiti, 21, 138–39, 148, 153n9; Haitian Creole version of Clinician Administered PTSD Scale (CAPS), 153n9
Povinelli, Elizabeth, 303n12
power: and biopower in borderlands, 22; and character's fear/authority powers, 318; and distortion of state power representations in artwork, 69; and empowerment of Palestinians through joint patrols, 269; of fathers in Palestine, 263; and humanitarian intervention, 25, 134, 159, 164, 165, 175–77, 181n15, 182n26; and Islamic calligraphy, 101n3, 118; and marginality, 309–10, 318; and

power (continued)
  outsider/insider power struggles,
  267, 268–69; and place in shaping
  subjects/subjectivity, 9; and political
  civil societies, 164, 165, 175–77,
  182n24,26; and resistance, 109;
  and shifts through globalization,
  181n15; and subjectivity, 9
PPP (Indonesian political party), 127n3
Prakash, Gyan, 333
Pramoedya Ananta Toer, 102n11
PRD (Democratic People's Party),
  102n11
preman (roughhouse youth), 114, 127n6
Prendergast, John, 160
Préval, René, 134, 152
prostitution industry: and anticrime
  campaigns (yanda yundong), 189,
  209; and Asia, 231; and Batam
  Island, 219–20, 223, 230; and
  Batam/Riau entertainment Web
  site, 219, 220, 223, 226; and borderlands, 194, 202; and Cambodia,
  220; and China, 194, 199, 202,
  208, 209, 210; and circuit of debt
  and servitude by prostitutes, 231;
  and condoms, 199, 201, 202; and
  everyday AIDS practices in China,
  199, 210;and family obligations
  felt by prostitutes, 227; and female
  labor migrants in Asia, 194, 221,
  223–24; and flow in contemporary
  processes of globalization, 205,
  223–24; and forced HIV tests,
  205–6, 210; and the Growth Triangle, 221, 223–24; and Haiti,
  148–49; and Han beliefs about
  sexual promiscuity of Tai peoples,
  194; and Han Chinese female
  migrants, 194; and HIV prevention
  education, 205; and illegal drug-
  use in China, 199, 202, 208, 209,
  210; and Indonesia, 220, 233n25;
  and maids' transition to prostitution, 221, 224–28, 230; and
  Malaysia, 219; and mass media in
  Asia, 219, 220, 232n3, 232n5; and

political economy in Asia, 226; and
  Putri narrative, 227; and Singapore,
  220, 229, 231; statistics, 226; and
  structural violence, 220, 230,
  233n25; and Thailand, 205, 219;
  and trafficking in women and children, 212–13n8, 408; and victimhood of women, 230, 233n25; and
  Web site pages, 219.
Proudhon, 163
La psychanalyse à l'épreuve de l'Islam
  (Benslama), 336
The Psychiatric Services, 322, 323
psychiatry: and APA, 410; and auditory
  hallucination/voices, 343–44,
  345–46; and biological components of trauma, 28; and borderland conflicts, 265; and chomeur
  (unemployed person), 334,
  355n5; and dahir (decree) in
  Morocco, 332, 333; and diagnostic
  criteria, 28; and DSM-IV, 345, 410;
  and espace originaire (primal space),
  356n7; and ethnographic studies
  of colonialism, 26; and Gaza psychiatrist's narrative, 263–64; Harvard's Friday Morning Seminar on
  Medical Anthropology and Cultural
  Psychiatry, 4–5, 29n3; and healing
  practices, 330, 331, 332; and insti-
  tution/deinstitution of the subject,
  355n3; and international guidelines for medical legal investigation
  of human rights abuses, 398–99;
  and intersubjectivities in legal
  investigations of human rights
  abuses, 398, 414–15; and kanarrab
  b-la littérature (I escape, save myself
  with literature), 343–44, 352; and
  l-ʾaquda nefsyia (knot of the soul)
  diagnosis, 27, 349–50; and manual
  therapies, 134–35; and marginality,
  414–15; and Morocco, 27,
  330–32, 332–37, 335n2; and
  Palestine/Israel borderland, 23, 25,
  263–64; and postcolonial disorders, 25; The Psychiatric Services,

epidemic, 239, 246, 248, 253. *See also* language

Sperb, Angela T., 291

Spiegelman, Art, 260

spirit theft/recovery (*ketemuq/nebusang*), 117, 118, 128n9, 128–29n11

Spivak, Gayatri C., 180-81n14, 324

split self experience: and ETA, 60; of grieving women over infant death, 360, 365; and India, 12–13, 360, 365, 366–67, 368, 373; and Palestine/Israel borderland, 266; and Reda (Moroccan mental patient), 339

squatter settlement/shantytown (*bidonvil*), 134, 135, 149

le *Stade Cervantes*: and Reda, 344, 346–47, 350, 351, 352, 353, 354; and symbolic geography, 353–54

Stadler, J., 251

the Stage. *See* le *Stade Cervantes*

State Law and Order Restoration Council (SLORC), 402

state of emergency, 16, 31n23, 272

states of exception, 16, 31n25

Stavrakakis, Yannis, 3

STDs. *See* HIV (human immunodeficiency virus); sexually transmitted infections (STIs)

stealing. *See* theft

Steedly, Mary, 64

Steinmetz, George, 283

Stern, T., 401

Stiglitz, Joseph E., 161

STIs (sexually transmitted infections), 194, 212n5

Stoler, Ann, 30n20

Stomp (rock band), 66

Straits Times (newspaper), 219, 232n3, 234n27

Strecker, Robert, 254n6

strike-hard anticrime campaigns (*yanda yundong*) in China, 189, 209

structural violence: and culture of insecurity (*ensekirite*) in Haiti, 136, 152n7; and globalization, 231; and infant death in India, 372; and

meaningful structures, 54; and prostitution industry, 220, 230, 233n25; and social systems, 137, 152n7; and structural inequalities, 152n7. *See also* violence

Subandi, 83

subjectivity: and borderlands, 23, 25; and colonialism, 2, 15–16; defined, 1; and disordered states, 29; and economic resources, 2; and ethnographic studies, 2–4, 9, 13–14, 29n2, 64, 261, 380; and human rights abuses in Burma, 28–29; and language, 3, 9–10, 28–29, 29n2, 264; and marginality, 23, 313–14; and the "other," 2; and postcolonial disorders, 2, 8, 11, 26; and postcolonialism, 2, 5–7, 8–9; and power, 9; and psychiatry, 28, 265; and psychological experience, 2, 3, 333, 337, 355n3, 356n7; and returns to subjectivity, 261, 262–66, 273n6; and state as social subject, 69; and states of emergency, 16, 31n23; and subjectification of nation-state, 64, 78, 101n4; and traumatic experiences, 16, 265–66; and unspeakable/unspoken concepts, 11, 14–15; and Vietnamese refugees, 28, 378. *See also* intersubjectivities; political subjectivities

Sublime Tunnel (artwork), 98

Südhaus, Fritz, 285

Sudiamo, Tarko, 102n11

suffering: and Burmese refugees, 397, 404–5, 406–7, 412–13; defined, 10; distance suffering, 172–73; and distance suffering in humanitarian intervention, 172–73; and documentation by psychiatrists, 397–98; experience-near language of, 5, 10, 28–29; and infant death in India, 360, 365–66, 368, 371–72; and suffering theory in health intervention, 365–66; and Vietnamese refugees, 378, 379, 382, 383–84, 386–87, 388–89, 391, 393

United States (U.S.): and autonomy-control narrative, 247; and colonialism, 18, 393; and *Doe v. Unocal*, 403–4, 415; and mental health issues of ethnic group, 5–6; and military humanitarianism in Haiti, 136; and postcolonialism of peoples, 5–6; and self-identity, 393; and September 11, 2001 attacks, 94–95, 96, 393; and Somalia Operation Restore Hope, 267, 271; as source for HIV/AIDS HIV/AIDS epidemic beliefs in Africa, 243; and U.S. Geological Survey in Palestine, 272n2; and xenophobia, 393

University of California, San Francisco, 255n42

UNMIK (United Nations Mission in Kosovo), 171, 179–80n9, 181n18

Unocal Corporation: and beliefs of Burmese refugees about communication about human rights abuses, 412, 413–14; and Burmese military, 397, 402–3, 404, 406, 412, 413; and *Doe v. Unocal*, 403–4, 415; and human rights abuses by transnational corporation, 28, 402–4, 414–15; and human rights legal case, 397; and SLORC, 402; and Unocal Myanmar Offshore Company, 402; and Yadana Pipeline Project, 28, 402–4

UN Office of the High Commissioner for Human Rights (UNHCHR), 399, 400

unspeakable/unspoken concepts, 11, 14–15, 16–17

U.S. Geological Survey, 272n2

USAID, 233n25

The Use and Abuse of History (Nietzsche), 284

Uttar Pradesh (U.P.), India, 359, 361, 362–63

Valley of the Squinting Windows I (MacNamara), 309, 314–15, 318, 326n4

van der Kolk, Bessel A., 139

Van Gennup, Arnold, 192

Vansina, J., 254n9

Varnedoe, Kirk, 101–2n6

Vasquez, Paula, 161

veil (*purdah*) of ignorance in India, 366

veils of fantasy, 3, 15

victimhood: and culture of insecurity (*ensekirite*) in Haiti, 135, 136, 142, 150, 152n6; and female labor migrants, 219, 229, 230, 232n2, 233n25; and maids portrayed by Indonesian mass media, 219, 229, 232n2; and sexual relationships with persons with HIV/AIDS in Uganda, 250; trauma of, 170–72; and victim as sociopolitical category of activism, 152n5; and *viktim* (victims of organized violence) in Haiti, 134, 135, 139, 149, 152n5; and women in prostitution industry, 230, 233n25

Viet Minh (Viet Cong), 378, 384, 386, 391, 393

Vietnam: history of, 378, 382–84, 388, 390–91, 394–95n4, 394n2. *See also* Vietnamese refugees

Vietnamese refugees: and alterity, 28, 379, 380–81, 385, 387, 388, 392, 393; and body-self, 392, 393–94; and case studies, 385–92; and history of Vietnam, 378, 382–84, 388, 390–91, 394–95n4, 394n2; and intersubjectivities, 380–82, 385, 392; and memory, 385, 391, 392–93; and migration, 384–85; and Mr. H. case study, 386–90; and Mr. T. case study, 390–92; and national identity, 382, 383; and New Mexico Refugee Project, 385, 394n3; and the "other," 382, 383, 384, 385, 387, 388, 392, 393, 394; and outsiders, 392; and paternally complex relationships, 393; and public health care, 386–87; and self-identity, 381, 384, 385, 389–90, 391–92; and subjectivity, 28, 378; and suffering, 378, 379,

visions, 67, 79, 80–81, 82; *Yang Kuat Tidak Lagi Perkasa* (Those Once Strong Are No Longer Powerful) (artwork), 81. *See also* reformation art/artists in Indonesia

Yunjinghung, China. *See* Jinghong, China

Yunnan Centers for Disease Control and Prevention, 196

Yunnan Province: and AIDS epidemic (1996–2000), 190; and epidemiology of HIV on borderlands, 195–96; and everyday AIDS practices, 190, 205–6; and harm reduction projects in China, 207, 213n9; and importance of family unit, 205, 206; and political subjectivities regarding everyday AIDS practices, 190, 205–6; and video-tape of people with HIV disease, 205

Yunnan Provincial Department of Health, 203

Zaire: and HIV/AIDS epidemic, 248

Zambian Copperbelt, 229

zenglendo (armed civilian gangs), 137–38, 152–53n8

Zero Hora (newspaper), 280, 281

Zhang Konglai, 195

Zhang Li, 191, 212n3

Zhang Xiobo, 196

Zhang Zizhuo, 201

Zheng Xiwan, 195

Zhou Yan, 201

Žižek, Slavoj, 3, 15

Zolo, Danilo, 163, 168, 180–81n14

zonbi (metaphysical double) in Haitian Vodou, 145–46, 149–50, 151, 153n13

Text:	10/13 Joanna
Display:	Joanna, Syntax
Compositor:	BookComp, Inc.
Indexer:	J. Naomi Linzer
Printer and Binder:	Sheridan Books, Inc.